Nursing Consultation

A Framework for Working with Communities

Susan L. Norwood

Professor and Chairperson
Department of Nursing
Gonzaga University
Spokane, Washington

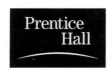
Prentice
Hall

Upper Saddle River, New Jersey 07458

Library of Congress Cataloging-in-Publication Data
Norwood, Susan Leslie.
Nursing consultation : a framework for working with
communities / Susan L. Norwood. — 2nd ed.
p. ; cm.
Rev. ed. of: Nurses as consultants / Susan L. Norwood.
c 1998.
Includes index.
ISBN 0-13-061798-9
1. Nursing consultants.   I. Norwood, Susan Leslie.
Nurses as consultants.   II. Title.
[DNLM: 1. Nurses.   2. Consultants.   WY 90 N895na
2003]
RT86.4 .N67 2003
610.73'06'9—dc21   2002017067

Notice: Care has been taken to confirm the accuracy of information presented in this book. The authors, editors, and the publishers, however, cannot accept any responsibility for errors or omissions or for consequences from application of the information in this book and make no warranty, express or implied, with respect to its contents.

The authors and publisher have exerted every effort to ensure that drug selections and dosages set forth in this text are in accord with current recommendations and practice at time of publication. However, in view of ongoing research, changes in government regulations, and the constant flow of information relating to drug therapy and drug reactions, the reader is urged to check the package inserts of all drugs for any change in indications of dosage and for added warnings and precautions. This is particularly important when the recommended agent is a new and/or infrequently employed drug.

Publisher: *Julie Levin Alexander*
Executive Editor: *Barbara Krawiec*
Executive Assistant: *Regina Bruno*
Editorial Assistant: *Sheba Jalaluddin*
Director of Manufacturing and Production:
  Bruce Johnson
Managing Production Editor: *Patrick Walsh*
Production Management: *Rainbow Graphics*
Production Editor: *Linda Begley*

Production Liaison: *Mary Treacy*
Manufacturing Buyer: *Pat Brown*
Creative Director: *Cheryl Asherman*
Senior Design Coordinator: *Maria Guglielmo Walsh*
Marketing Manager: *Nicole Benson*
Product Information Manager: *Rachele Strober*
Printing and Binding: *RRD Harrisonburg*
Cover Printer: *Phoenix Color*

Pearson Education LTD.
Pearson Education Australia PTY, Limited
Pearson Education Singapore, Pte. Ltd
Pearson Education North Asia Ltd
Pearson Education Canada, Ltd.
Pearson Educación de Mexico, S.A. de C.V.
Pearson Education–Japan
Pearson Education Malaysia, Pte. Ltd
Pearson Education, Upper Saddle River, NJ

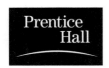

10 9 8 7 6 5 4 3 2
ISBN 0-13-061798-9

Contents

Preface

Providing consultation services is an increasingly important nursing role. Indeed, nurse leaders recognize that the formal title of "nurse consultant" is not needed to provide consultation; the consultation role is, rather, an integral part of being a nurse in today's health care environment. Thus, the theory behind and principles of nursing consultation are a critical part of contemporary nursing education.

Nursing Consultation: A Framework for Working with Communities (previously published as *The Nursing Consultation Process: Essential Concepts and Principles*) presents nursing consultation as a five-phase process for working with individuals or groups to help them resolve actual or potential problems related to the health status of clients or to health care delivery. The content is appropriate for senior-level leadership and community health courses in baccalaureate nursing and RN to BSN programs, as well as for nurses who are pursuing graduate degrees and preparing themselves to assume advanced roles in nursing (e.g., as clinicians, educators, or managers/administrators).

While the first edition of this text promoted nursing consultation as a dimension of contemporary, everyday nursing practice in all settings, many of the examples in the text focused on nurses providing consultation in organizational settings. This may have inadvertently reinforced nursing consultation as only a career option, rather than as something nurses do on a daily basis. Since the first edition of this text was published, a community perspective in health care has become increasingly apparent—and important. This perspective presents new needs and opportunities for nurses to take on the consultant role and was the impetus behind the changes that have been incorporated into the revised edition of this text.

The revised edition of this text retains the basic structure that shaped the first edition: its organization (foundational concepts, contextual issues, the consultation process, and professional issues), its pedagogy (an integration of theory-based and application-oriented approaches), and special features (a chapter overview and guiding questions, boxed features of consultation strategies and scenarios, documentation guidelines, examples of consultation contracts, and end-of-chapter learning activities). At the same time, the revised edition is enhanced by several new features:

- A new title reflecting the text's emphasis on providing consultation to communities
- Three new chapters: Chapter 2—"Communities, Nurses, and Consultation"; Chapter 12—"Team Building in Nursing Consultation"; and Chapter 18—"Working with Consultants"
- Community-oriented examples of nursing consultation
- Key search engine terms at the beginning of each chapter
- Updated references
- A new, more reader-friendly design and layout

A frustration encountered while updating and revising this text was the paucity of new references about consultation processes in general, and about nursing consultation in particular.

So, while nursing leaders advocate consultation competencies and a community perspective (with its inherent need for nurse consultants), the nursing profession has lagged behind in terms of reporting consultation strategies, success stories, and lessons learned from less-than-successful consultation engagements. This situation challenges readers of this text to share their consultation experiences so that their experiences become learning tools for colleagues and communities. As did the first edition of this text, this edition of *Nursing Consultation: A Framework for Working with Communities* provides nurses with both the theoretical background and practical strategies that are needed to successfully respond to the exciting and challenging opportunities for nurses to provide consultation in today's health care environment.

Acknowledgments

Revising an existing text presents its own special challenges, and—as is the case with any challenging project—it is made easier when there is a cast of supporters, assistants, and just plain friends in the background. To this end, I would like to extend my gratitude to the following persons:

Thanks, first, to the students in the MSN program of the Department of Nursing at Gonzaga University, whose enthusiastic response to the first edition of this text motivated me to take on this revision. Thanks also to my colleagues in the Department of Nursing and the School of Professional Studies. Our discussions of trends in nursing, health care, and nursing education helped me to clarify my own thoughts about nursing and the value of using the nursing consultation process as a framework for practice. A special thank you is owed to Marnie Broughton—not only the best assistant I could ask for, but also a good friend. Marnie's energy and sense of humor keeps me from taking myself too seriously.

I would also like to acknowledge and thank the staff at Prentice Hall Health: Maura Connor, who helped get this project under way; and Barbara Krawiec, Michael Sirinides, and the production staff, who picked it up at its midpoint and saw it through to completion. Thank you, too, to the anonymous reviewers who endorsed the project and helped me refine my ideas.

The final group I would like to acknowledge is my family, who put up with my compulsiveness to meet and beat deadlines as I tackled this project. A special thanks to my brother Geoff, whose superb computer fix-it skills saved the day when I was in the middle of final revisions and getting scary messages on my computer screen!

Reviewers

Randy M. Caine, EdD, RN, CS, CCRN, ANP-C
Professor of Nursing and Director of Nurse
    Practitioner Programs
California State University
Los Angeles, CA

Margaret P. Leider
Marquette University College of Nursing
Milwaukee, WI

Carol Green-Hernandez, PhD, ANP/FNP-C
Associate Professor and Director, Primary Care
    Nurse Practitioner Program
The University of Vermont
Burlington, VT

Renee Hoeksel, PhD, RN, CCRN
Associate Professor of Nursing
Coordinator Nursing Programs
Washington State University College of Nursing
Vancouver, WA

Carol M. Brown, PhD, MS, ARNP
Associate Clinical Professor
Washington State University College of Nursing
Vancouver, WA

Ruby S. Morrison, DSN, RN
Capstone College of Nursing
The University of Alabama
Tuscaloosa, AL

INTRODUCTION
TO NURSING CONSULTATION

SECTION 1

The Nature of Nursing Consultation

Few nurses regarded themselves, or were regarded by others, as experts in the field with credentials worthy of consultation until after the 1950s. (Robinson, 1982)

 KEY CONCEPTS:

consultation, consultee, client, client system

 KEY TERMS FOR YOUR SEARCH ENGINE:

nurses and consultation

INTRODUCTION

The word "consultant" often brings to mind the picture of an expensive outside expert who has been brought in to fix an organization-wide problem. Many nurses have been on the "receiving end" of consultation, often in connection with team-building efforts, and work redesign or downsizing experiences at their place of employment. However, whether they recognize it or not, most nurses have also been on the "doing end" of consultation.

Consultation is fundamentally a process of working with individuals or groups to help them solve work-related problems. More specifically, nurse consultants address work-related problems that concern the health status of individuals or groups or health care

delivery processes. Nursing consultation, then, means *working with individuals or groups to help them resolve actual or potential problems related to the health status of clients or to health care delivery.*

Consultation skills have been recognized as a core competency for advanced practice nurses (i.e., clinical nurse specialists, nurse practitioners, nurse-anesthetists, and certified nurse-midwives) as well as for nurses assuming advanced nursing roles as educators and administrators (American Nurses Association (ANA), 1995; Fenton & Brykcynski, 1989). However, as health care delivery increasingly moves into community settings and the environmental determinants of health are recognized, baccalaureate-prepared nurses are finding themselves taking on the role of nurse consultant. Indeed, when the American Association of Colleges of Nursing's *Essentials of Baccalaureate Education* (1998) states that "Nurses focus not only on individual health care, but also manage, monitor, and manipulate the environment to foster health," it is referring to consultation activities.

When nurses practice consultation, their ultimate goal is to enhance the well-being of patients or health care consumers. Yet in most cases, nurses learn consultation skills through trial and error, a method that is both inefficient and potentially harmful to a client's well-being. Consultation can be harmful to a client, for example, if an assessment is incomplete or a recommended intervention doesn't address the real problem issue or if a consultant fosters dependency rather than self-reliance. Rather than continue to rely on trial and error, nurses who expect to provide consultation services need to base their actions on theory. A theory-based approach to consultation helps promote successful outcomes in the widest variety of problem situations.

This book presents the theoretical concepts and pragmatic processes that are the foundation of effective nursing consultation. By implementing these concepts and processes, nurses can enhance their consultation skills and, ultimately, improve the well-being of patients. While many of the references cited throughout the text may at first glance appear dated, they represent classic consultation content and are still very relevant.

This first chapter begins with a general description of consultation and the consultation relationship. It describes nursing consultation and compares it with consultation as practiced by professionals in other disciplines. Nursing consultation is then compared with the nursing process and other nursing activities. In the final section of this chapter, variables in nursing consultation are discussed.

As you read this chapter, consider the following questions:

- What types of experiences have you had with consultants? Were they positive or negative experiences? What do you think explains these different experiences?
- How have you practiced nursing consultation? What was that experience like?
- How do you envision yourself incorporating consultation into your practice of nursing?
- What skills and assets do you have that should facilitate your practice of nursing consultation? What gaps in knowledge and skill can you identify?

BASIC CONSULTATION CONCEPTS

One way to begin to understand the nature of nursing consultation is to examine how consultation is described by other professions in which consulting has evolved into a highly developed practice and a more recognizable role.

Defining Consultation

The word "consultation" is often used ambiguously. The common element of virtually all definitions of consultation, however, is prob-

lem solving. The two definitions that follow, while drawn from disciplines or perspectives other than nursing, illustrate both the problem-solving focus of consultation and the characteristics of consultation relationships.

One expert team of organization development consultants (specialists concerned with helping organizations function more effectively) defines consultation as a two-way process of problem solving: "a process of seeking, giving, and receiving help. Consultation is aimed at aiding a person, group, organization, or larger system in mobilizing internal and external resources to deal with problem confrontations and change efforts" (Lippitt & Lippitt, 1986).

Human resource professionals, individuals who work in administrative or direct service roles within such settings as school systems and community social service agencies, have their own definition of consultation. According to one well-respected human services theorist, consultation occurs when a professional "assists a consultee with a work-related (or caretaking-related) problem with a client system, with the goal of helping both the consultee and the client system in some specified way" (Dougherty, 1995).

Both of these definitions reveal that consultation is a process that is intended to solve a problem and, by doing so, bring about change. The two definitions also reveal that the focus of consultation is helping individuals or groups learn to solve their own problem(s), rather than solving problems for them. Finally, these definitions indicate that consultation involves a consultant who is the professional guiding the process, the consultee or individual (or group) who is receiving the help, and other parties who hold a stake in both the consultation process and its outcomes. These ideas are explored further in the following sections.

The Characteristics of Consultation Relationships

The characteristics of consultation relationships can be grouped into three categories: the parties involved in the consultation process, the "phenomena of interest" in consultation, and the roles and responsibilities of consultants.

The Parties Involved in Consultation

Consultation typically involves three parties: a consultant, a consultee, and a client. The consultant is the helper. More precisely, the consultant provides the leadership for the problem-solving efforts. The consultee is the person or group that is working directly with the consultant to learn problem-solving skills. In some cases, the consultee is the person who has asked for help on behalf of a client. In other cases, a "contact person" who is not directly involved in the problem-solving activities may have requested the consultation. For example, the administrator of a community health agency might ask a consultant to work with selected personnel (the consultees). The client is the individual, group, organization, or community that is the intended beneficiary or target of the consultation. In other words, the client is the party on whose behalf help has been sought. It is important to understand that clients are not usually active participants in the consultation process. Thus, consultation is a tripartite (three-party) relationship that involves cooperative efforts between a consultant and consultee in order to enhance a client's well-being.

Consultation takes place within an environment called the "client system." The client system includes the physical setting in which the consultation is taking place, as well as anyone who, in addition to the consultant, consultee, and client, may have some stake in the consultation process and its outcomes. It is important to note that these *consultation stakeholders* are neither involved in the consultation process nor a target of its results. The relationships among the parties in a consultation relationship are illustrated in Figure 1-1.

The Phenomena of Interest in Consultation

A profession's "phenomena of interest" are the range of problems that give it purpose and define its scope of practice. Consultation has as its phenomena of interest work-related problems, or problems in which role implementation interferes with optimum functioning and achievement of client goals. Because

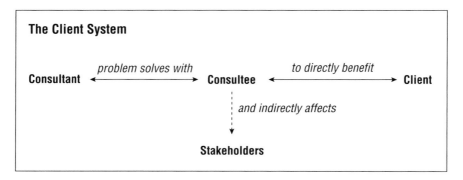

Figure 1-1   The Consultation Relationship.
During the consultation process, the consultant and consultee collaborate to solve problems that are affecting a client's well-being. The client is the intended beneficiary of the interactions between the consultant and consultee. Stakeholders are other individuals who are indirectly affected by the consultation process and its outcomes. Together, these parties comprise the client system.

consultants help consultees resolve work-related (as opposed to personal) problems that affect client well-being, they deal with the issues that are causing a problem rather than consultees' personal or emotional reactions to the problem situation, unless consultees' reactions to a situation are the source of the problem.

The Roles and Responsibilities of Consultants

Consultants work with consultees to help them incorporate behavioral, cognitive, attitudinal, or organizational/structural changes that will result in problem resolution. While helping consultees make these changes, consultants are also striving to empower consultees and increase their self-sufficiency. In fact, a professional goal and responsibility of a consultant is to become progressively unnecessary (Lippitt & Lippitt, 1986). Consultants accomplish this goal through a "skills transference" process that helps consultees learn to make better use of their own personal and professional resources. Hence, consultants have remedial as well as preventive responsibilities toward their consultees: They want to help consultees resolve their present problem

as well as learn to respond more effectively to similar problems in the future (Zins, 1993).

Consultants not only offer education and clarify situations, but they diagnose a presenting problem's likely cause and suggest problem-solving strategies (Barron, 1989). Consultees, however, are always free to accept or reject a consultant's opinions and advice. In a sense, then, a consultant is only an "option-giver." In other words, consultants "do not, indeed cannot tell managers [or other consultees] what to do, nor do they actually effect change, unless of course they are specifically employed to supervise a process of transition" (Windle & Boyd, 1989).

Consultants are responsible for projecting the likely effects and side effects of their recommendations. For example, a consultant who recommends downsizing as a solution to an organization's financial problems has the responsibility to not only predict the effects of downsizing on the organization's budget. The consultant must also predict the effects on worker productivity and morale, quality of service, and the organization's public image. Consultants bear only limited responsibility for change in a client's status or problem resolution because change is ultimately contingent on a consultee's implementation of a consultant's recommendations. Consultants do, however, bear responsibility for the quality of the options they present to a consultee and for informing the consultee about the limitations of any proposed problem solution.

NURSING CONSULTATION

Consultation is not a new role for nurses. Florence Nightingale, for example, acted as a consultant during the Crimean War when she worked with British Army officials developing strategies to stem the post-battlefield mortality rate. Following the war, she consulted with nurses throughout the world on issues regarding nursing education, hospital organization, and patient care. Lillian Wald is another nurse who practiced consultation when she provided advice to schools and other public health agencies. For many years after Miss Nightingale and Miss Wald, consultation among nurses was so informal and taken for granted that it failed to receive notable publication. It was not until the 1950s, when more nurses were visible in academic settings and earning graduate degrees, that accounts of nursing consultation began to appear in the professional literature (Robinson, 1982). These initial accounts described nursing consultation as a service provided primarily by nurse-educators and nurse-administrators. By the late 1960s, however, accounts of clinical consultation were becoming more common. The majority of the accounts at this time focused on the then-evolving clinical specialty role of psychiatric consultation–liaison nurse.

Today, consultation is formally recognized as an important component of nursing practice. Patricia Benner (1984) implied that skill in consultation is a competency of expert nurses within the practice domain of "Organizational and Work-Role Competencies." Fenton (1985) identified consultation as a specific practice domain for clinical nurse specialists

by citing examples of how clinical nurse specialists provide "expertise and guidance, both formally and informally, to other health care providers." In addition, Brykcynski (1989) related how nurse practitioners provide "consultation to physicians and other staff on patient management." Thus, at every level of professional nursing practice, consultation skills are now a role expectation and core competency. These skills are especially important for nurses who wish to assume leadership roles in resolving current nursing and health care problems.

Nursing consultation, like other forms of professional consultation, involves a tripartite relationship (consultant + consultee + client). Nurse consultants work with consultees to help them resolve problems that affect a client's well-being. Nursing consultation is unique, however, in that health care consumers are always the ultimate beneficiaries (or victims) of the consultation process. For example, even if the client in a nursing consultation relationship is an organization (as in a work redesign effort), it is the patients who ultimately benefit (or suffer) from the consultation process and its outcomes. In a nursing consultation relationship, patients may be either the intended beneficiary—that is, the client—or, as illustrated in the previous example, an unintended beneficiary or stakeholder.

Consultees with whom nurse consultants work include staff nurses, families, nursing faculty, community members, and other health care providers. A nurse consultant's clients include patients, family members, work units, organizations, students, and communities. Stakeholders in the nursing consultation process may include, in addition to health care consumers, other health care providers. For example, work redesign efforts, as mentioned above, affect patients, but may also affect other providers and support personnel in a health care delivery setting. Client systems within which nursing consultation occurs include nursing units, hospitals, community-based health care agencies, private medical practices, academic institutions, and communities. The relationships between the parties involved in nursing consultation are illustrated in Figure 1-2. Examples of client systems, problem situations, consultees, and clients encountered in nursing consultation are described in Box 1-1.

In summary, nursing consultation has as its phenomena of interest problems related to the health status of clients or to health care delivery processes. The ultimate goal of nursing consultation is enhanced well-being for individual health care consumers or communities. Thus, nursing consultation and its phenomena of interest are an extension of nursing's concern: "the diagnosis and treatment of human responses to actual or potential health problems" (ANA, 1980).

Nursing Consultation Compared to Consultation in Other Professions

A nurse consultant's roles and responsibilities are similar to those of consultants in other professions in that nurse consultants work with consultees to develop problem-solving options (Alvarez, 1992). In addition, like consultants in other professions, nurse consultants seek to improve their consultees' problem-solving skills so that they are better able to respond to similar problems in the future. Advanced practice nurses who are functioning as consultants assume even more specialized roles. Consultants who are clinical nurse specialists, for example, may act as expert advisors, role models, and advocates. Working in these consultant roles, clinical nurse specialists (1) provide expert guidance and advice

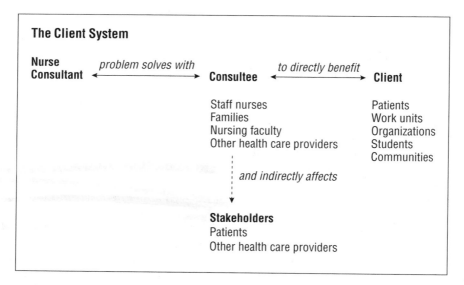

Figure 1-2   The Nursing Consultation Relationship.
Like consultation that is practiced by other professionals, nursing consultation involves a tripartite relationship that occurs within the context of a client system. Nursing consultation, however, is unique in that patients are always affected—either intentionally and directly or unintentionally and indirectly—by the nursing consultation process and its outcomes. The client systems in which nursing consultation may occur include hospital units, organizations, academic institutions, private health care practices, community-based health care agencies, and communities.

BOX 1-1   NURSING CONSULTATION: CLIENT SYSTEMS, PROBLEM SITUATIONS, CONSULTEES, AND CLIENTS

Following are examples of the types of problem situations in which a nurse consultant might be involved. Who would be possible stakeholders in each of these examples?

Client System	Problem Situation	Consultee	Client
Nursing unit	Complex patient with unfamiliar treatment plan	Staff nurses	Patient
Hospital	Poor results on patient satisfaction survey	Nurse managers	Hospital Patient(?)
Nursing unit	Family needs help preparing for home care needs of ill family member	Family members	Patient
Academic institution	Need to revise curriculum	Faculty	Students
Community	Meningitis outbreak	Health care providers	Community members
Private medical practice	Declining patient volume	Office staff	Medical practice

about patient problems both formally and informally, (2) interpret the nursing role for nursing staff in specific patient situations by identifying patient needs not apparent to less expert nurses, and (3) serve as patient advocates by broadening the staff's understanding of the experience of the patient and family, and helping staff to change their responses to the patient (Fenton, 1985). Nurse practitioners function as consultants when they provide advice to physicians and other health care providers on patient management (Brykcynski, 1989).

As is the case with other forms of professional consultation, the consultee in a nursing consultation relationship is free to accept or reject the nurse consultant's recommendations and opinions. The consultee, then, bears the ultimate responsibility for whether or not a problem is resolved and patient well-being is enhanced. Even in situations in which the client is a patient and the consultee a staff nurse, the direct responsibility for enhancing the patient's well-being rests with the consultee. The only exception to this is when a consultee's lack of skill presents a serious threat to patient well-being. In this situation, the nurse consultant has the ethical responsibility to assume direct caregiving activities on a temporary basis until the consultee or another staff nurse is able to do so.

Like other professional consultants, a nurse consultant is responsible for the effects of an intervention on a client (Barron, 1989). The nurse consultant has the additional responsibility, however, of considering the effects of a recommended intervention on patient or group of health care consumers even when they are not the client. For example, work redesign may resolve a hospital's (the client's) financial problems, but its effects on patient care must also be projected and articulated by the nurse consultant.

Nursing Consultation Compared to the Nursing Process

Nursing consultation and the nursing process share similar phenomena of interest and both work toward similar goals. Nursing consultation differs significantly from the nursing process, however, because it involves an indirect rather than a direct intervention. Indirect interventions such as nursing consultation are "performed away from the patient but on behalf of a patient or group of patients" and are "aimed at management of

the care environment and interdisciplinary collaboration" (ANA, 1995). In the nursing process, nurses usually interact directly with health care consumers to enhance their well-being rather than on their behalf through an intermediary (such as a consultee). The nursing process is a dyadic helping relationship that contrasts with the tripartite relationship of nursing consultation (see Figure 1-3).

Nurses involved in the nursing process often assume similar roles to those engaged in the nursing consultation process. In the nursing process, however, nurses enact these roles (teacher, coach, advisor, etc.) directly with patients rather than through an intermediary (a consultee). In the nursing process, the patient is both the intended and ultimate beneficiary of nursing interventions as well as a participant in them. Recall that in nursing consultation, health care consumers are, again, the ultimate beneficiaries of the con-

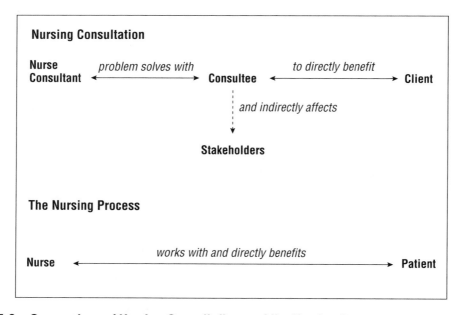

Figure 1-3   Comparison of Nursing Consultation and the Nursing Process.
Despite their differences, both nursing consultation and the nursing process work toward the same goal: promoting a patient's well-being.

sultation process even when they are not the intended beneficiaries and a participant in the consultation interventions.

As a final point of comparison, in the nursing process it is the nurse who is directly responsible for patient outcomes. In nursing consultation, however, the consultee bears this responsibility. The nurse consultant only maintains responsibility for the quality of options that are proposed for responding to a problem. Chapters 9 through 14 clarify further the differences between the nursing process and the nursing consultation process.

Nursing Consultation Compared to Other Nursing Activities

Nurses engage in a variety of activities (such as medication administration, teaching, and counseling) that are intended to promote patient well-being. Some of the activities—such as teaching—may be used as an intervention in nursing consultation. Aspects of other common nursing activities (such as collaboration and managing) are incorporated into the nursing consultation relationship. Other nursing interventions or activities (e.g., counseling) may be confused with consultation, however, and actually contradict characteristics of a consulting relationship. The following section discusses differences between nursing consultation and other nursing activities.

Consultation Compared to Counseling

Nursing consultation is often confused with counseling because both activities involve giving advice. Counseling is a direct service to an individual or group that is provided for the purpose of stimulating self-awareness, helping to solve problems and make decisions, and promoting emotional and personal growth (Collins, 1989). The phenomena of concern in counseling are personal issues. In contrast, consultation is an indirect service to clients that focuses on work-related issues, or

issues in consultee role implementation that interfere with the client's health. Although a consultee may derive personal benefits (e.g., learning problem-solving skills) from a nurse consultant's assistance, the goal of consultation is enhanced client (not consultee) well-being. Consider the following difference between counseling and consulting: A nurse counselor might work with nurses who are struggling with their feelings about working with AIDS patients; a nurse consultant might work with the setting in which these nurses work to establish a support group for the nurses.

Consultation Compared to Teaching

Nurse consultants teach, but nursing consultation is different from teaching. When teaching is used in the nursing process, it is a direct patient care intervention—for instance, a nurse teaching an individual who is newly diagnosed with diabetes how to adapt his or her diet. Nurse consultants frequently use teaching as an intervention when working with consultees as well, though in the nursing consultation process, teaching is an indirect patient care intervention. For example, a nurse consultant might develop teaching sessions to help staff (the consultees) in a diabetes clinic learn new teaching strategies they can use when working with patients (the clients) in regard to dietary management.

The teaching role in nursing also differs from teaching during consultation, specifically in terms of the nature of the relationship between those involved. Formal teaching is an unequal relationship to the extent that it incorporates evaluation and the giving or withholding of rewards (e.g., grades for students or hospital discharge for a diabetic patient). Because a nurse consultant works with consultees as peers, the evaluation that occurs during the nursing consultation process is intended to promote professional growth and problem solving rather than form the basis for reward or punishment.

Consultation Compared to Managing and Supervising

Nurse consultants incorporate supervisory and managerial activities into the consultation process when they direct problem-solving activities. For example, a nurse consultant might manage the logistics of a needed skills-training session. The practice of these activities in nursing consultation is different, however, from enacting a formal supervisory relationship. Whereas nurse supervisors are administratively responsible and accountable for their supervisees, nurse consultants and their consultees interact as peers. Finally, supervisory relationships tend to be ongoing, whereas consultation relationships are only temporary and are terminated once the consultee has learned problem-solving skills.

Consultation Compared to Change Agency

Change agents engage in deliberate processes to precipitate and accomplish change (Hansen, 1995). Because a successful consultation relationship accomplishes changes in behaviors, attitudes, or beliefs, consultants are often considered to be change agents. Change agency differs from nursing consultation, however, because it involves unilateral identification by the change agent of both the opportunity for change and the desired change outcomes. The need for change in nursing consultation is identified by the consultee. The nurse consultant's task is to provide options about how the desired change can be brought about. It is the consultee who establishes the goals and implements the change strategies.

Consultation Compared to Co-Management

Co-management entails two or more professionals, each with a distinct area of expertise, working together to manage different aspects of a client's care (Barron & White, 2000). A familiar co-management situation in patient care is an oncologist and surgeon working together. An example of co-management with a community client would be an epidemiologist and public health nurse working together during a hepatitis outbreak. Co-management tends to be a direct care activity in which the "co-managers" share responsibility for the outcome of the relationship. In contrast, nursing consultation is an indirect care activity, and the outcome is the responsibility of the consultee.

Consultation Compared to Referral

Nurse consultants may use referral as a nursing consultation intervention, but the nursing consultation relationship itself is different from accepting a referral. The goal of referral is to enhance patient care by relinquishing care, or aspects of it, to another professional who is perceived to have the needed expertise (Barron & White, 2000). The relinquishment of care may be either temporary or permanent, and the professional who is accepting the referral assumes the responsibility for the outcome of the care he or she provides. Nursing consultation, in contrast, is always a temporary relationship, and the consultee, rather than the nurse consultant, is responsible for the outcome.

Consultation Compared to Collaboration

Collaboration is a partnership established for the purpose of accomplishing a commonly held goal (Kyle, 1995). Although nursing consultation involves a collaborative relationship (i.e., one that is based on authenticity and constructive problem solving) between a nurse consultant and consultee (Barron & White, 2000), it differs from collaboration per se because the goal of a consultation relationship is specified by the consultee. Collaboration also differs from nursing consultation because it presumes joint involvement in the "action phase" of the relationship as well as joint responsibility for the outcome of the relationship. In consultation, however, both the

BOX 1-2   NURSING CONSULTATION COMPARED TO OTHER NURSING ACTIVITIES

Nursing consultation is often confused with the following activities in which nurses engage. As you study these different helping activities, consider the following questions:

- How is the activity different from nursing consultation?
- Who is responsible for the outcomes of the activity?
- Is the relationship to the client direct or indirect?
- How might a nurse consultant incorporate aspects of this activity in the nursing consultation role?

Activity	Focus	Goals
Nursing consultation	Work-related problems	Enhance client and patient well-being
Counseling	Interpersonal problems	Promote emotional and personal growth
Teaching	Knowledge and skill deficits	Impart new knowledge and skills
Managing/Supervising	Resources (personnel, time, money)	Effective use of resources
Change agency	Change	Precipitate and accomplish change
Co-management	Share care responsibilities	Enhance patient well-being
Referral	Relinquish care responsibilities	Enhance patient well-being
Collaboration	Partnership	Accomplishment of mutual goals through joint action

"action" (implementation of recommended problem-solving activities) and the outcome of the relationship are the responsibility of the consultee.

Box 1-2 summarizes the differences between nursing consultation and other nursing activities.

VARIABLES IN NURSING CONSULTATION

While nursing consultation is always a tripartite relationship within the context of a client system, the nature of a nurse consultant's relationship to the client or client system may vary. Important variables in a nurse consultant's relationship to a client or client system are insider versus outsider status and intra- and interprofessional interactions, that is, whether the interaction is with nurse consultees or with consultees who have other professional backgrounds.

Insider/Outsider Status

An internal consultant ("insider") is a member of a client system who is asked to assume a temporary and additional role as a problem solver within the system. An external consultant, on the other hand, is an outsider who establishes a temporary relationship with some members of a client system (the consultees) for the express purpose of helping them resolve a problem. Clinical nurse specialists practice internal consultation when they work with nursing staff to address problems related to the care of specific patients. These same clinical nurse specialists would be practicing external consultation if they worked with nurses in a home health care agency to address patient care problems.

Both internal and external nursing consultation relationships have advantages and disadvantages. An internal nurse consultant has the advantage of being preacquainted with the client system and the issues underlying the consultation problem; this often facilitates the development of rapport with the consultees. Furthermore, because an internal nurse consultant has a vested interest in successful consultation outcomes, there may be less resistance to developing an effective problem-solving relationship. Finally, because of an internal consultant's familiarity with the client system, the consultation process may take less time and therefore be less costly to the system.

The disadvantages of practicing internal nursing consultation relate to the consultees' preconceptions, the consultant's inability to exit the client system, and the issue of fees. First, a nurse working as an internal consultant may be perceived as having less ability, credibility, and authority than an external consultant. Nursing staff tend to relate to internal nurse consultants in their "known role" (e.g., as their supervisor) and often have difficulty accepting them in a role that involves a different set of tasks and responsibilities. Additionally, because internal consultants cannot completely exit the client system once the consultation relationship has ended, consultees may tend to rely too much on the nurse consultant's expertise and problem solving. This may lead to resentment and burnout on the part of the nurse consultant as well as dependency on the part of the consultee.

The issue of reimbursement for consultation services can also create dilemmas for nurses practicing internal consultation. Internal nurse consultants are rarely paid a fee that is commensurate with what would typically be negotiated by an external consultant. Furthermore, nurses who are asked to take on internal consulting projects are too often expected to do so in addition to meeting their other responsibilities. The issue of reimbursement in internal nursing consultation is discussed further in Chapter 17.

Nurses practicing external consultation enjoy certain advantages made possible by their unique role. Because they are outsiders to the client system, external consultants are more readily perceived as having expertise and credibility by consultees. External consultants tend to be less constrained by a client system's politics and internal rules so they "can ask the unaskable and suggest the unsuggestable" (Furlow, 1995). Because external consultants can leave the client system at the conclusion of the consultation relationship, they generally have an easier time than do internal consultants recommending unpopular problem solutions, such as eliminating staff positions.

External consultants, however, also face distinct disadvantages. A nurse who is an external consultant will need to spend time learning how to effectively interact within a client system. Being less acquainted with the client system, external consultants run the risk of unknowingly violating a system's rules and cultural norms; this can slow down or temporarily derail consultation efforts. To gain a sense of the impact of these disadvantages, recall some of the "adjustment challenges" you may have experienced the last time you entered a new setting, during a job change perhaps, or when starting school or moving to a new neighborhood.

Intra- and Interprofessional Interactions

Nurses practice intraprofessional consultation when their consultees are other nurses. In interprofessional consultation relationships, nurse consultants work with consultees who are from other professions. Interprofessional consultation offers the opportunity to generate a wider range of possible problem solutions because professionals from other disciplines bring different perspectives to a consultation situation. The challenge of interprofessional consultation is learning the philosophy, language, standards, and methodology of another profession.

CHAPTER SUMMARY

Nursing consultation is fundamentally a problem-solving process. Consultation is not a new role for nurses but rather something that nurses have always done and a nursing activity that has long been taken for granted. Consultation is well recognized as an integral part of advanced practice nursing and advanced nursing roles. Consultation skills are also being increasingly used by baccalaureate-prepared nurses as health care moves into communities and health promotion activities become aimed at addressing environmental variables in health. In short, in today's health care environment, consultation is an integral part of the role of a nurse, and the formal title "nurse consultant" is not needed to function in this capacity. Consultation theory and skills, thus, are an essential part of contemporary nursing education.

Consultation has been recognized as a domain of nursing practice with its own specific competencies. While nursing consultation shares features of consultation as practiced by other professions and incorporates selected activities of the nursing process, the collective attributes of nursing consultation distinguish it as a unique activity. Nurses who practice any form of consultation will become more effective nurse consultants by studying the concepts and processes that provide the basis for successful consultation.

APPLYING CHAPTER CONTENT

1. Explore the nursing (periodical) literature for 1980 and the present. What examples can you find of nursing consultation? How are the examples for these two points in time different? What do you think accounts for these differences?
2. Examine how nursing consultation is practiced in your own work setting. What situations can you identify in your work setting that could benefit from nursing consultation?
3. What situations can you identify in your community that could benefit from nursing consultation?

References

Alvarez, C. (1992). Let's talk about clinical consultation. *Clinical Nurse Specialist, 6*(2), 117.

American Association of Colleges of Nursing. (1998). *The essentials of baccalaureate education for professional nursing practice.* Washington, DC: Author.

American Nurses Association. (1980). *Nursing: A social policy statement.* Kansas City, MO: Author.

American Nurses Association. (1995). *Nursing's social policy statement.* Kansas City, MO: Author.

Barron, A. (1989). The CNS as consultant. In A. Hamric & J. Spross (Eds.), *The clinical nurse specialist in theory and practice* (2nd ed.) (pp. 125–146). Philadelphia: Saunders.

Barron, A., & White, P. (2000). Consultation. In A. Hamric, J. Spross, & C. Hanson (Eds.), *Advanced nursing practice: An integrative approach* (2nd ed.) (pp. 217–244). Philadelphia: Saunders.

Benner, P. (1984). *From novice to expert: Excellence and power in clinical nursing practice.* Menlo Park, CA: Addison-Wesley.

Brykcynski, K. (1989). An interpretive study describing the clinical judgment of nurse practitioners. *Scholarly Inquiry for Nursing Practice, 3*(2), 75–103.

Collins, B. (1989). Do you need an external consultant? A model for decision-making. *Clinical Nurse Specialist, 3*(2), 90–96.

Dougherty, A. (1995). *Consultation: Practice and perspectives in school and community settings* (2nd ed.). Pacific Grove, CA: Brooks-Cole.

Fenton, M. (1985). Identifying competencies of clinical nurse specialists. *Journal of Nursing Administration, 15*(12), 31–37.

Fenton, M., & Brykcynski, K. (1989). Qualitative distinctions and similarities in the practice of clinical nurse specialists and nurse practitioners. *Journal of Professional Nursing, 9*(6), 313–326.

Furlow, L. (1995). So what good are consultants anyway? *Journal of Nursing Administration, 25*(7/8), 13, 15.

Hansen, H. (1995). The advanced practice nurse as a change agent. In M. Snyder & M. Mirr (Eds.), *Advanced practice nursing: A guide to professional development* (pp. 197–213). New York: Springer.

Kyle, M. (1995). Collaboration. In M. Snyder & M. Mirr (Eds.), *Advanced practice nursing: A guide to professional development* (pp. 169–182). New York: Springer.

Lippitt, G., & Lippitt, R. (1986). *The consulting process in action* (2nd ed.). San Diego: University Associates.

Robinson, L. (1982). Psychiatric liaison nursing: A review of the literature, 1962–1982. *General Hospital Psychiatry, 4*(2), 139–146.

Windle, G., & Boyd, R. (1989). Working with management consultants: Collaboration to a common end. *Senior Nurse, 9*(10), 6–8.

Zins, J. (1993). Enhancing consultee problem-solving skills in consultative interactions. *Journal of Counseling and Development, 72,* 185–190.

Communities, Nurses, and Consultation

In many ways, the nursing profession is the most qualified to respond to current changes in the health system. (Institute for the Future, 2000)

 KEY CONCEPTS:

community, community based, community focused, partnership

 KEY TERMS FOR YOUR SEARCH ENGINE:

nurses and community based and consultation

INTRODUCTION

Over the last 20 to 30 years, there has been a growing realization that our nation's current systems do a good job of addressing illness care needs and a fair job of addressing health care needs, but, to a large extent, do not address health issues per se. This realization is slowly but surely leading to a change in perspective—namely, the recognition that health issues are better addressed by communities than by centralized and hierarchical institutions. This change in perspective calls for a change in nursing roles and creates new needs and new opportunities for nurses. In many ways, this "new" community perspective is an invita-tion to the nursing profession to return to its roots.

Moving from institutions into communities, and focusing on health rather than only illness care or health care, means, however, that as nurses we need to look at the frameworks we are using to deliver nursing services. To this end, the premise of this text is that the nursing consultation process is a "good fit" as a framework for providing nursing services in, to, and with communities.

This chapter begins by briefly reviewing the key economic, social, and scientific forces that have brought about a refocus on the concept of community as an integral part of health and the health care delivery system. Next, "community" is defined, ways in which the concept of community applies to health care are explored, and nursing implications of a community perspective in health care are considered. The chapter ends by presenting the nursing consultation process as a framework for nursing practice in the evolving health care system. As you read this chapter, think about the following questions:

- What examples can you think of in your own city or region that indicate a community perspective in health care?
- How are nurses utilized in these examples? Or, how could they be utilized?
- What facilitators and barriers to the adoption of a community perspective in health care exist both nationally and in your own city or region?

THE EVOLUTION OF A COMMUNITY PERSPECTIVE

The current community perspective is the result of a constellation of economic, social, and scientific forces that has evolved over the past 50 years. The seeds for this perspective can be traced to the 1950s and the postwar expansion of hospitals and related facilities. This expansion was funded primarily with federal dollars. At the same time, third-party health insurance rapidly developed as a reimbursement mechanism. The widespread availability of health insurance as an employment benefit resulted in increased access to and utilization of health care services for millions of Americans.

The 1960s saw the rise of federal policy and legislation (e.g., Medicaid and Medicare) aimed at increasing access to health care services for those without third-party insurance and/or with inadequate personal financial resources. Federal funding and scientific advances also gave rise to new technologies for illness diagnosis and treatment, life support, and life extension. These technologies resulted in further increases in health care costs as consumers gained access to them and demanded their utilization.

Concern about rapidly increasing government expenditures for health care began to appear in the 1970s. These concerns were expressed as increasing governmental regulation and mandated community-based planning as strategies to limit hospital-related expenses and duplication of services. At the same time, consumerism in the form of expecting quality and positive outcomes for dollars spent began to appear.

Concerns about health care expenditures (personal and governmental) and the outcomes associated with those expenditures became a dominant theme in the 1980s and 1990s. The aging population and the costs of treating chronic disease came to be recognized as a significant factor in increasing health care costs. Technology increased health care costs in a couple of ways—by facilitating the development of more expensive treatment options and by fueling consumer demands (via information technology and the widespread use of personal computers and the Internet) for the latest (and often most expensive) treatments. Managed care and cost-containment pressures pushed health care delivery into noninstitutional settings such as urgent care centers and outpatient surgery centers.

It was also during the 1980s and 1990s that we came to realize that spending more money on institutionally-based health care did not necessarily result in improved health statistics. In spite of spending more per capita on health care, the United States continued to lag behind many other developed nations on such

BOX 2-1   THE EVOLUTION OF A COMMUNITY PERSPECTIVE: KEY ECONOMIC, SOCIAL, AND SCIENTIFIC FORCES

Economic Forces

- Increasing personal and governmental expenditures on health care, without a corresponding improvement in key health statistics
- Cost-containment pressures result in an increasing amount of care that is delivered in community-based settings

Social Forces

- The aging population and cost of treating chronic diseases
- Consumer demands for quality and positive outcomes for dollars spent
- Increasing poverty and inequities in access to even basic health care begin to tug at the collective social conscience and are recognized as contributing to increased health care expenditures in the long term

Scientific Forces

- Costly technological advances in illness diagnosis and treatment, life support, and life extension
- Information technology increases consumer demand for application of the latest technology
- Scientists verify that many chronic diseases are a result of personal behaviors and/or environmental factors

key health indicators as infant mortality rate, perinatal mortality rate, and life expectancy at birth (Helvie, 1998). Researchers also realized that, taken together, access to basic health care, environmental factors, and health behaviors determined 90 percent of an individual's health (Institute for the Future, 2000). Indeed, personal habits such as smoking, alcohol use, poor diet, inadequate exercise, seat belt use, and sexual practices were identified as being responsible for the major diseases, killers, and health care costs of the 1980s and 1990s (Anderson & McFarlane, 1988, 2000).

Finally, the 1990s also saw increasing concern about the millions of Americans who lack access to even basic health care and who

live in unsafe and unhealthy environments. These trends and concerns continue today and call for changes in how and where we deliver health care. These trends and concerns clearly support a community perspective.

Key forces that have led to the community perspective of health care are summarized in Box 2-1.

THE CONCEPT OF COMMUNITY

While it is clear that the health problems of the twenty-first century will require broad-based health promotion efforts and that a community perspective makes good sense, what is less clear is what this really means. This section presents definitions of "community" and discusses the various ways in which the concept of community can be linked to health care delivery.

Defining Community

"Community" can mean different things, depending on the perspective of its participants. Anderson and McFarlane (2000) define a community as "complex webs of people shaped by relationships, interdependence, mutual interests, and patterns of interaction." While a community encompasses people in a particular time and place, it is the quality of relationships more than sharing a piece of geography that defines a community (Sullivan, 1998). Members of a community share a history, a language, and a sense of purpose and responsibility. Thus, a community involves a place but is really a network of persons having common interests. In a very real sense, then, community is a "state of mind" (Tagilareni & Sherman, 1999). According to these defining characteristics, a hospital, a unit within a hospital, a neighborhood, a school, a

support group, or a community agency could all be considered communities. Box 2-2 summarizes characteristics of communities.

Communities and Health Care

Adopting a community perspective of health care is complicated by labels such as "community-based," "community-focused," "public health," and "population-focused." Each of these labels means something different for nursing roles and nursing interventions, and each viewpoint brings important contributions to health care. In this section, these various labels are redescribed as four different relationships between communities and health care: community-based, community as context, community as client, and community as partner.

Community-Based Health Care

Community-based health care refers to providing care for individuals, families, or groups wherever they are located. Community-based, however, means more than just deinstitutionalized health care services. It also means incorporating community values, needs, culture, and concerns into health care delivery

BOX 2-2   CHARACTERISTICS OF COMMUNITIES

Communities are complex and interdependent webs of people who share

- Space and time
- A history
- A language
- Interests
- A sense of purpose
- A sense of responsibility
- Patterns of interaction and communication

(Alexander, 2001). For example, community-based women's health care services might need to include translator and child care services if they were located in a multilingual, low-income neighborhood.

Community as Context

When the community is used as the context of care, not only is care community-based, but the community's impact on individual health status, health-seeking behaviors, and the ability to participate in health promotion and disease management activities is considered. In other words, this viewpoint acknowledges the strong relationship between a person's daily environment and individual or family health. This means that information about community variables is gathered during the health history or assessment process and community variables (assets and barriers) are addressed during the care planning process. Health care delivered through the viewpoint of community as context has a holistic orientation. A basic premise of this text is that considering community as context is foundational to successful health care and nursing consultation services.

Community as Client

When a community is the client in a health care relationship, the community itself, as an aggregate entity, is the target beneficiary of health care activities. In other words, of concern is the well-being of the community as a whole, and services are delivered to the community rather than to individual community members. Sometimes care that has a community client is differentiated as "community-focused" (focus = total regional community) or "aggregate-focused"

(focus = high-risk subgroup of a regional population) (Helvie, 1998).

Delivering health services to community clients is an efficient way of addressing issues that foster disease. What is more, it is a more efficient use of nursing and economic resources than is providing care to individuals whose health is compromised by environmental conditions (Koerner, 2001). Consider, as an example, the difference in nursing and economic resources needed to (a) treat individuals with asthma who suffer exacerbations when local grass growers burn their fields, and (b) work with local health and governmental agencies to develop guidelines for "safe burning days" and an air-quality warning system. Another example of care for a community client is working with employers (community client = worksite) to develop health promotion activities that will reduce the company's health insurance premiums and health care expenditures.

The labels of "public health nursing" and "community health nursing" are consistent with the viewpoint of community as client. Public health nursing has as its mission fulfilling society's interest in ensuring that the conditions in which people live are healthy (Alexander, 2001). The focus of community health nursing is improving the health of populations by promoting healthy lifestyles, preventing disease and injury, and protecting the health of communities (Alexander, 2001; Helvie, 1998). Figure 2-1 depicts the nursing consultation relationship (as described in Chapter 1) with a community client. The consultee in this type of relationship is often an interdisciplinary team.

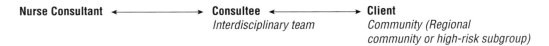

Figure 2-1   The Nursing Consultation Relationship with a Community Client.
The consultee in this type of relationship is often an interdisciplinary team.

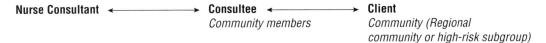

Figure 2-2   The Nursing Consultation Relationship When the Community Is a Partner.
In this relationship, the consultee is members of the community. The client is the community as an entity.

Community as Partner

When the community is a partner in a health relationship, representatives of the community work with health care providers to address health concerns of the community. In other words, community members would be the consultees in a nursing consultation relationship. This type of relationship is depicted in Figure 2-2.

Working with a community as a partner brings a powerful social resource to problem-solving efforts and helps to ensure a viewpoint of community as context. Partnerships also provide access to larger and more diverse social, economic, and political environments in a community. This access can elicit problem-solving resources and assist in identifying potential barriers to problem solving that will need to be addressed. A basic premise of the nursing consultation process is that community members should always be included as consultees whenever a community is the client or a key stakeholder in the consultation relationship.

IMPLICATIONS OF A COMMUNITY PERSPECTIVE FOR NURSES

Through cooperation and co-creation, a synergy will be formed that can transform the total well-being of society. Alone nursing cannot do it. Without nursing it cannot be done. (Koerner, 2001)

Experts predict a 44 percent increase in the number of full-time equivalent registered nurses needed in community-based health settings between now and 2010 (Institute for the Future, 2000). Some authorities (e.g.,

Helvie, 1998) differentiate generalist or baccalaureate-level community nursing practice as working with individuals and families in community settings and specialist or master's-level nursing practice as focusing on the community as client and engaging in activities such as community development, community empowerment, and policy formation. The reality is, however, that as a community perspective takes hold in health care, supply issues within nursing may cause this distinction of roles to become merely academic. In short, a community perspective brings with it new opportunities for nurses at all levels of practice. It also calls for an expanded set of competencies.

Nursing Roles and Opportunities

Historically, the community has been where nurses have engaged most imaginatively. Key roles that nurses assume when a health care system has a community perspective are those of educator, collaborator, change agent, and leader (Helvie, 1998). Recall from Chapter 1 that these roles are distinct from but incorporated in the more global role of nurse consultant. Nurses in the twenty-first century will also be advocates, catalysts, and monitors. They will be "enablers" in the sense of helping individuals and communities to increase control over and improve their own health (Anderson & McFarlane, 2000).

With a community perspective in health care, nurses will form partnerships with community leaders, entrepreneurs, businesses, other health care providers, government and community agencies, and health care consumers as they engage in efforts to restructure the health care system. Nurses will also have opportunities to engage in program planning to address the biological, environmental, lifestyle, and health care delivery determinants of health (Alexander, 2001). Nurses will find themselves increasingly needed and valued as translators of community issues into language that can be understood by makers of social policy (Koerner, 2001). A community perspective in health care will need nurses who act as spokespeople for health care consumers and as the social conscience for the health care system. Nurses can, for example, call to attention policy issues that are counterproductive to community well-being—such as paying for amputations that result from complications of diabetes but not paying for diabetes screening or education.

Competencies for a Community Perspective

Basic competencies for nursing consultation are discussed in Chapter 5 of this text. This section highlights additional competencies that relate specifically to a community perspective in health care.

The core competency for nurses working in a health care system that is driven by a community perspective will be community-focused skills (Balik, 1998). Specifically, nurses must be able to work with community groups to recognize and tap power existing within the community. Nurses need to be able to integrate diverse ideas, people (and their values, backgrounds, and skills), and resources in both developing and implementing problem solutions from a community's vantage point (Anderson & McFarlane, 2000).

A community perspective of health care calls for nurses to expand their holistic assessment skills and simultaneously consider and address the multiple human and structural determinants of health and health behaviors

(Institute for the Future, 2000). Nurses will find themselves charged with improving access to care for those with unmet needs. As nurses develop skills in forming partnerships and developing policy, they will also need to ensure that problem solutions balance individual, professional, system, and societal needs (O'Neil & The Pew Health Professions Commission, 1998).

Nurses working in a health care system that has a community perspective will also need empowerment skills. Empowerment can take place only when nurses interact with communities in a nonjudgmental manner, truly allow communities to make their own informed decisions, and ensure that the decisions made have the possibility of being both implemented and effective (Anderson & McFarlane, 2000).

A final competency needed for working in a community perspective is a community mindset. This mindset entails more than recognizing the impact of a community on individual health. It is a mindset that acknowledges and values communities as resources in and of themselves, and recognizes the impact of community health on societal health. Box 2-3 summarizes nursing roles and competencies that are needed with a community perspective in health care.

CONSULTATION AS A FRAMEWORK FOR NURSING PRACTICE IN A HEALTH CARE SYSTEM WITH A COMMUNITY PERSPECTIVE

In Chapter 1, nursing consultation was defined as the process of "working with individuals or groups to help them resolve actual or potential problems related to the health status of clients or to health care delivery." Nursing consultation describes what nurses do when working in a health care system that has a community perspective.

BOX 2-3   NURSING ROLES AND COMPETENCIES FOR A COMMUNITY PERSPECTIVE

Nursing Roles

- Consultant
- Educator
- Collaborator
- Partner
- Change agent
- Leader
- Advocate
- Catalyst
- Monitor
- Enabler
- Program planner
- Translator of community issues

Needed Competencies

- Partnership skills
- Ability to recognize and tap into community power
- Ability to integrate diverse ideas, people, and resources into problem solutions
- Holistic assessment skills
- Empowerment skills
- A community mindset

With a community perspective of health, health professionals are partners rather than authorities. With their history of strong support for health promotion and client advocacy, nurses will be at the forefront of this evolution (Hollinger-Smith, 2001). This emphasis on partnership is consistent with the peer relationship between consultee and consultant that characterizes the nursing consultation process. Likewise, the concept of community empowerment is consistent with the notion of "skills transference" as a goal of nursing consultation. Finally, because community partnerships means working with and through intermediaries (i.e., community rep-

resentatives) to improve the well-being of a community client, a community perspective, like nursing consultation, entails and values indirect nursing activities.

The nursing consultation process is a logical framework for providing nursing services to communities for additional reasons. First, the consultation process facilitates the creation of networks focused on offering and receiving advice and information that can improve the health status of populations. Consultation also offers nurses the opportunity to positively influence health and health care beyond a direct patient care encounter (Barron & White, 2000). This makes a consultative approach an efficient use of nursing and other resources. Finally, as consultants, nurses reweave the traditional nursing roles of community health nurse, public health nurse and educator, and individual and family care provider and work with individuals and families as community members to show them how to share responsibility for healthier lifestyles and the health of their community (Koerner, 2001). For many nurses, the consultation process and the autonomy and types of relationships it involves may increase job satisfaction.

CHAPTER SUMMARY

A range of economic, social, and scientific forces have converged to give rise to a new and evolving community perspective in health and health care. For nurses, this new perspective means new practice settings, as well as more autonomy and closer relationships with individuals and families in the context of their home, family life, and community. Partnerships with other health care providers and relationships with community leaders and policy makers will be inherent in all levels of nursing practice in the twenty-first century. With its emphasis on collaboration and empowerment, the nursing consultation process is a logical framework for nursing practice from this new perspective.

APPLYING CHAPTER CONTENT

Visit a local community-based agency that focuses on a health issue. What partnerships or relationships exist between this agency and (a) other health care providers and (b) community members? If these relationships are present, what impact do they have on the agency's services and their effectiveness? If these relationships do not exist, what opportunities are there for relationships and how would these improve the agency's services?

References

Alexander, J. (2001). Community health service. In N. Chaska (Ed.), *The nursing profession: Tomorrow and beyond* (pp. 537–546). Philadelphia: Saunders.

Anderson, T., & McFarlane, J. (1988). *Community as client: Application of the nursing process.* Philadelphia: Lippincott.

Anderson, T., & McFarlane, J. (2000). *Community as partner: Theory and practice in nursing* (3rd ed.). Philadelphia: Lippincott.

Balik, R. (1998). The impact of managed care and integrated delivery systems on registered nurse education and practice. In E. O'Neill & J. Coffman (Eds.), *Strategies for the future of nursing* (pp. 41–63). San Francisco: Jossey-Bass.

Barron, A., & White, P. (2000). Consultation. In A. Hamric, J. Spross, & C. Hanson (Eds.), *Advanced nursing practice: An integrative approach* (2nd ed.) (pp. 217–244). Philadelphia: Saunders.

Helvie, C. (1998). *Advanced practice nursing in the community.* Thousand Oaks, CA: Sage Publications.

Hollinger-Smith, L. (2001). Building and sustaining community partnerships. In N. Chaska (Ed.), *The nursing profession: Tomorrow and beyond* (pp. 547–559). Philadelphia: Saunders.

Institute for the Future. (2000). *Health and health care 2010: The forecast, the challenge.* San Francisco: Jossey-Bass.

Koerner, J. (2001). Nightingale II: Nursing in the new millennium. In N. Chaska (Ed.), *The nursing profession: Tomorrow and beyond* (pp. 17–28). Philadelphia: Saunders.

O'Neil, E., & The Pew Health Professions Commission. (1998). *Recreating health professional practice for a new century.* San Francisco: Pew Health Professions Commission, Pew Charitable Trust.

Sullivan, T. (1998). *Collaboration: A health care imperative.* New York: McGraw-Hill.

Tagliareni, M., & Sherman, S. (1999). When community becomes more than a place. In M. Tagliareni & B. Marckx (Eds.), *Teaching in the community: Preparing nurses for the 21st century* (pp. 35–50). Sudbury, MA: Jones & Bartlett Publishers.

Overview of the Nursing Consultation Process

The consultation process is the "science" of consultation. . . . As with a person learning a new skill, the initial task is to learn the basics. The next transition is to move from the "science" or technique of the consultation process to the "art" of the process. (Ulschak & SnowAntle, 1990)

 KEY CONCEPTS:

entry, assessment, formative evaluation, summative evaluation, ownership

---

 KEY TERMS FOR YOUR SEARCH ENGINE:

consultation and process

INTRODUCTION

When nurses rely on the steps of the nursing process to guide their interactions with patients, they increase the likelihood that nurse–patient interactions will both meet a patient's needs and enhance a patient's well-being. In the same way, nurse consultants who follow the five steps or phases of the nursing consultation process increase the likelihood of a successful consultation outcome.

In Chapter 1, nursing consultation was described as a collaborative interaction between a nurse consultant and a consultee that occurs on behalf of a client and takes place within an environment called the client

system. The nursing consultation process is, more specifically, a systematic and scientific approach to problem solving that a nurse consultant carries out with a consultee or group of consultees for the purpose of enhancing client well-being. The process involves five sequential and ongoing phases that provide a framework for nursing consultation relationships.

This chapter introduces the phases of the nursing consultation process and discusses the tasks or activities that characterize each phase. (Chapters 9 through 14 explore these phases in greater detail.) The chapter concludes by considering some of the potential problems encountered in implementing the nursing consultation process. As you read this chapter, consider the following questions:

- How is the nursing consultation process different from the nursing process?
- What specific tasks or activities seem to occur on a more or less continual basis throughout the nursing consultation process?
- Will completing the activities of the nursing consultation process always ensure a successful consultation outcome? Why or why not?

THE NURSING CONSULTATION PROCESS: AN OVERVIEW

The nursing consultation process consists of five interrelated phases (see Figure 3-1):

1. Gaining entry
2. Problem identification
3. Action planning
4. Evaluation
5. Disengagement

Each phase in the nursing consultation process has its own purpose, tasks, concerns, and potential problems. The essential tasks of each phase must be completed in order

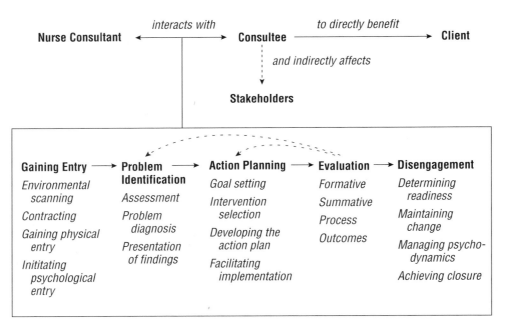

Figure 3-1   The Nursing Consultation Process.
The nursing consultation process represents the interaction between a nurse consultant and consultee. The process consists of five phases, each of which has its own tasks. Note that there is a certain amount of back-and-forth movement or recylcing between these phases. Recycling should occur when new information is uncovered or a proposed problem solution is either unacceptable to the consultee or unsuccessful. Recycling allows refinement of the action plan and increases the likelihood that the consultation will be successful.

to achieve a successful consultation out- come. Omitting a phase or failing to com- plete the tasks associated with a specific phase may cause a nurse consultant to miss gathering essential information, overlook intervention opportunities, or rush the con- sultee to proceed prematurely with problem solving.

Each phase of the nursing consultation process is essential to the success of the con- sultation relationship, yet the associated tasks and activities of each phase need to be imple- mented with a flexibility that allows for the unique characteristics of each problem-solving situation. Some activities of the nursing con- sultation process, while they begin or are most important during a specific phase, occur to some degree throughout all phases of the process. A nurse consultant, for example, engages in a continual process of assessing, diagnosing, intervening, evaluating, and working to develop a trusting relationship with the consultee and other members of the client system.

Sometimes the phases of the nursing con- sultation process overlap, leading to a back- and-forth movement or recycling between phases. For instance, a nurse consultant may find that as a consultation relationship pro- gresses, new information about a problem sit- uation makes it necessary to repeat earlier activities and phases of the process. Repeating phases of the nursing consultation process as needed increases the likelihood that the con- sultation problem will be resolved.

The nursing consultation process provides a necessary guide for achieving a successful consultation outcome. The manner in which a nurse consultant completes the tasks of the process, however, is just as important as per- forming the tasks themselves. The human processes and technical skills a nurse needs to bring to a consultation relationship are dis- cussed in Chapter 5; competencies for work- ing with community consultees and clients were discussed in Chapter 2.

Gaining Entry

The gaining entry phase of the nursing consul- tation process centers around relationship building and defining. The specific tasks that need to be accomplished during this phase are:

- Environmental scanning
- Contracting
- Gaining physical entry into the client sys- tem
- Initiating psychological entry

These tasks or activities get under way at the time of initial contact between the consul- tee (or contact person) and the nurse con- sultant. Different ways in which initial contact might occur are described in Chapters 4 and 9.

Environmental Scanning

Environmental scanning is the informal assessment or "scouting" process that a nurse consultant begins at the time of initial contact with a consultee. During this process, a nurse consultant gathers information and forms impressions in order to determine whether there is a fit between the needs, skills, inter- ests, and personality ("chemistry") of the nurse consultant and those of the consultee and problem setting.

Because environmental scanning occurs before a nurse consultant and consultee have agreed to a contract, the nurse consultant is usually limited to gathering data through indirect observation and informal interviews. Publicly available information about a client system—such as mission statements and news reports—can also help a nurse consultant form impressions about the system's needs, values, and personality.

The nurse consultant uses the information gathered during environmental scanning to decide whether to continue a consultation relationship. The goal of scanning activities here is to learn about the need for, rather than to sell, consultation services. In fact, if a nurse consultant determines that involvement in a problem situation would not be mutually beneficial, the consultant is obligated to help the consultee see that their needs would be better met by someone else. Box 3-1 highlights the questions a nurse consultant may have during the environmental scanning process.

Contracting

If environmental scanning results in a mutual decision by the nurse consultant and consultee to enter into a problem-solving relationship, the second task of the gaining entry phase—contracting—gets under way. Contracting is the process of identifying "mutual wants" (Dougherty, 1995), the result of which is a formal agreement or "contract" between the consultant and consultee. A contract sets forth the purpose and goals of the nursing consultation relationship and delineates tasks, relationships, responsibilities, expectations, accountability, and the anticipated timeline for the consultation project. The contract should state the nurse consultant's expectations for evaluation of the consultation process and spell out how the nurse consultant's and consultee's personal and professional needs will be met throughout the process. Examples of nursing consultation contracts are included in Chapter 17.

Gaining Physical Entry

The third task associated with gaining entry in the nursing consultation process is gaining physical entry into the client system. This task usually begins when the consultee or contact person formally introduces the nurse consultant to members of the client system. An important part of gaining physical entry (especially in systems-wide consultation situations) is sanctioning of the consultation relationship and activities by a community leader or someone in an administrative-level position. Clearly articulated support at the community or administrative level can largely determine the speed at which change occurs. In a smaller-scale consultation scenario such as a clinical nurse specialist providing consultation to one or two staff nurses about a patient care issue, the consultee/staff nurse (who likely initiated the consultation relationship) might facilitate physical entry by introducing the clinical nurse specialist to other nurses on the unit and, perhaps, the patient's physician.

On the nurse consultant's part, physical entry into the problem setting can be accomplished by establishing the parameters of availability (such as work space and work hours) as well as by meeting or mingling with members of the client system on their own turf. For example, a clinical nurse specialist consulting with staff on a particular hospital unit may gain physical entry by working each of the unit's shifts in order to spend time with nurses. Additional activities that can be used to gain physical entry are discussed in Chapter 9.

Initiating Psychological Entry

The final task associated with gaining entry—initiating psychological entry—is an activity that continues throughout the entire nursing consultation process. Put simply, psychological entry involves "engaging the consultee" (Ross, 1993). The nurse consultant accomplishes this task by engaging in actions that are intended to establish the nurse consultant's credibility and promote a sense of trust on the part of the consultee.

An important aspect of psychological entry is clarifying the consultant's roles and correcting distorted expectations. For example, clinical nurse specialists who provide consultation to staff nurses about problematic patient situations may need to correct the expectation that they, rather than the nursing staff, will be providing direct care to the patient. Consultation involves working with staff so they can learn to provide more effective care on their own; it means "doing with" rather than "doing for." The outcome of psychological entry is decreased resistance to problem-

BOX 3-1   QUESTIONS FOR ENVIRONMENTAL SCANNING

The purpose of environmental scanning is to determine the fit between the needs, skills, interests, and personality of the nurse consultant and the consultee and client system. The following are typical questions a nurse consultant tries to answer during environmental scanning:

Questions About the Problem Situation

- What problem "symptoms" are bothering the consultee?
- How long have the symptoms been present?
- What attempts have been made to resolve the problem?
- What prompted the consultation request? That is, why does this problem seem particularly bothersome now?

Questions About the Consultation Outcome

- What is the desired (stated) outcome for the consultation?
- Does the consultee seem to have any hidden agendas?

Questions About the Client System

- Who does the client system consist of?
- Who will I be working with?
- What is the nature of the relationship between the person requesting the consultation and (a) the consultee, (b) the client, and (c) the consultation fee payer?
- Are the appropriate people involved in preliminary discussions about this problem and the need for consultation?
- What is the level of administrative support for solving this problem?
- What is the level of motivation and readiness to change within the client system?
- Is the client (or contact person) leveling with me?
- Are the values of the client system compatible with my own? What about other compatibility issues such as work and communication styles?

Questions About the Consultant's Skills and Interests

- Is there something I can do to help resolve this problem? Do I have the skills to resolve the problem?
- Can I achieve a favorable outcome within the time frame the consultee is requesting?
- Are there political considerations I need to think about in terms of continuing (or not continuing) involvement in this situation?
- Am I interested in working on this project?

solving activities and the establishment of a relationship of mutual respect and cooperation between a nurse consultant and a consultee. Box 3-2 illustrates how the gaining entry phase of the nursing consultation process might take place in a community consultation scenario.

Problem Identification

The goal of the problem identification phase is to determine the cause of the "symptoms" or presenting problem. The tasks associated with the problem identification phase are:

BOX 3-2   GAINING ENTRY IN A COMMUNITY CONSULTATION SCENARIO: THE MERGER, PART 1

Under pressure to avoid costly duplication of services, two competing emergency response services, both of which are staffed largely by volunteers, decide to undergo a merger. As a result of the proposed merger, some current members of the two services may lose their position; others will be forced to assume new roles and learn new ways of doing things. Faced with increased staff and community anxiety and low morale among staff, and realizing that a successful merger is dependent on staff and community acceptance and commitment to the changes in service operation, a well-respected nurse in the community is asked by several community members to help accomplish the merger. The specific consultation request is "Help us make this work."

Following this consultation request, the nurse consultant immediately begins *environmental scanning.* Informal conversations and a review of recent emergency calls reveal that competition between the two services has not always been friendly, that both services have been losing money, and that the two services tend to respond to different types of emergencies. The nurse consultant arranges for a meeting with the contact person, who is the supervisor of the older of the two services but is considered "neutral." Getting answers to the following questions is particularly important:

- Who will I be working with? What do they know about the merger and its implications?
- What do you really want me to do? For example, will I be expected to make any specific personnel decisions?
- What is the timeline for the merger?

Following this meeting, the nurse consultant decides the situation is a "good fit." Another meeting is scheduled for the purpose of *developing a contract.* The nurse consultant agrees to work with the client system at least until the merger is finalized, with need for continued services to be established at that time.

Physical entry gets under way when the contact person introduces the nurse consultant to the staff of each of the merging services. The nurse consultant gains further physical entry by spending time with the staff of the two services (on all shifts)—including going on some actual emergency calls. This latter activity also helps establish the nurse consultant's credibility and therefore initiates *psychological entry.* Psychological entry is further facilitated when the nurse consultant shares personal experiences of working as a volunteer with an emergency service in another rural community.

- Assessment
- Problem diagnosis
- Presentation of findings

Assessment

Assessment activities actually begin while the nurse consultant is initiating psychological entry into a client system. Because assessment and information gathering conveys interest in the client system, these activities can facilitate psychological entry. To conduct an assessment of a client system, a nurse consultant systematically collects data from multiple sources using a variety of methods. This assessment is more intensive than that conducted during the gaining entry phase (environmental scanning) because now the nurse consultant and consultee have established a contract. The contract both legitimizes the nurse consultant's data-gathering activities and facilitates access to confidential information such as financial records or results of patient satisfaction surveys.

Information obtained during the assessment phase provides a foundation on which to design strategies for resolving the consultation problem. Examples of the issues a nurse consultant explores during assessment are presented in Box 3-3. Frameworks for conducting an assessment are described in Chapter 10.

BOX 3-3   ISSUES TO EXPLORE DURING ASSESSMENT

The purpose of the assessment activities that take place during the problem identification phase is to identify the cause of the problem and factors that can affect the problem-solving process. Issues to explore during assessment include:

Issues Related to the Consultation Problem

- What is the consultee experiencing as a result of the problem?
- What is the client experiencing as a result of the problem?
- Who are the stakeholders affected by this problem? How are they affected?
- How do consultee attitudes, beliefs, and behaviors affect this problem?
- What features of the problem setting might contribute to this problem?
- What factors in the external environment might contribute to this problem?

Issues Related to Planning Problem Solutions

- What supports and blocks are there to the problem-solving process? Do these come from within the client system or are they external to the client system? What is the relative strength of each?
- What assets does the consultee bring to the problem-solving process?
- What will be gained and lost by solving this problem?
- How will solving this problem affect the consultee? The client system? The stakeholders? Who stands to win or lose by solving this problem?

Sources: Barron, A., & White, P. (2000). Consultation. In A. Hamric, J. Spross, & C. Hanson (Eds.), *Advanced nursing practice: An integrative approach* (2nd ed.) (pp. 217–243). Philadelphia: Saunders; and Price, J., & Reiss-Brennan, B. (1989). Consulting telesis: A systems approach. *Nursing Management, 20*(11), 80A–80F.

Assessment activities assume primary importance during the problem identification phase, but occur to some extent throughout the entire nursing consultation process. The nurse consultant uses the information gained through ongoing assessment to confirm that problem-solving activities are proceeding in the right direction.

Problem Diagnosis

Problem diagnosis is the process of attaching meaning to assessment findings and drawing conclusions about the cause of a nursing consultation problem. During this process, the nurse consultant must determine the scope of a problem—that is, how much of the client system is affected, what factors in the client system contribute to the problem, and what resources exist within the client system for solving the problem.

Nursing consultation outcomes will only be successful if problem diagnosis results in an accurate and acceptable problem definition (Kurpius, Fuqua, & Rozecki, 1993). Part of diagnosing a problem, then, is creating "ownership" of the problem, or getting consultees to accept a problem's cause and agree to assume their share of responsibility for its solution. This is facilitated by involving the consultee in assessment and diagnosis activities.

Presentation of Findings

Presenting assessment findings and problem diagnosis to consultees and other key members of the client system is important because it creates awareness of the problem and its causes, as well as motivates those in the client system to give support and input regarding problem-solving strategies. The challenge of presenting assessment findings is in packaging them effectively for different audiences. Findings need to be translated into familiar language, and the problem and its likely causes should be confirmed with the audience.

A nurse consultant should make an effort to reframe diagnostic conclusions and present them as opportunities for change and improvement rather than as problems (Cohen & Murri, 1995). Take, for example, the case of a group of home health care nurses who are unable to meet established productivity goals (i.e., number of patients seen per day). Rather than presenting the problem as the result of inefficiency on the part of staff nurses, a nurse consultant may reframe the problem as a need to explore factors within the agency which, if changed, might facilitate meeting productivity goals. Note how reframing the problem "depersonalizes" the problem's cause and creates a situation that challenges the nursing staff to find more effective ways of delivering care rather than blames them for the problem.

Box 3-4 illustrates how the problem identification phase might unfold in a community consultation situation.

Action Planning

During the action planning phase of the nursing consultation process, the nurse consultant and consultee identify specific goals for the nursing consultation relationship, select interventions for achieving those goals, and develop an action plan for implementing the interventions. Also during this phase, the nurse consultant facilitates activities such as team building and puts into place supports that will facilitate implementation of the action plan.

Goal Setting

Goal setting involves articulating the desired consultation outcome, or formulating a goal statement. In a situation where a clinical nurse specialist is providing consultation to nursing staff about a patient care issue, the goal statement would describe exactly how patient outcomes are expected to improve as a result of the nursing consultation: increased

BOX 3-4   PROBLEM IDENTIFICATION IN A COMMUNITY CONSULTATION SCENARIO: THE MERGER, PART 2

The nurse consultant working with the merging emergency services begins the assessment activities of the problem identification phase at the same time efforts are being made to establish psychological entry. Conversations and separate meetings with, first, members of the two services and, second, the community provide the nurse consultant with the opportunity to gather information about the feelings and concerns about the merger. Additional information is gained from the supervisors of the two services about exactly how the merger is likely to affect services to the community (number of positions that will be lost, training that will be needed, etc.).

Assessment reveals a high level of administrative support for the merger but a low level of support among personnel; the community has mixed feelings. Everyone does, however, express commitment and motivation to "give it a good try for the sake of the community." The two services themselves are willing to commit adequate time and resources to facilitate the merger process.

Based on these assessment findings, the nurse consultant identifies anxiety and fear as the major problems threatening a successful merger. A lack of information about what exactly the merger will involve on a day-to-day personal level is identified as a major cause of the problem.

The assessment findings and problem diagnosis are presented separately to the supervisors and staff of each service, and to the community itself in an open meeting. All parties concur with the diagnosis. "Ownership" of the problem is indicated by their agreement to address the issues that are contributing to the problem.

---

satisfaction with care, fewer complications, lower cost of care, and so forth.

Meaningful goals are based on what is both feasible and desirable as a consultation outcome. Thus, when goals are being established, needs of the client, consultee, and stakeholders need to be considered; resources and constraints imposed by the client system also need to be kept in mind as goals are formulated. It might be desirable, for example, that a nursing consultation relationship results in home health care nurses seeing more patients each day. This goal, however, might not be feasible if the problem setting lacks the financial resources to hire more assistive personnel or purchase a computer software program that will map out the most efficient sequencing of a

nurse's visits for the day, or implement any other possible problem-solving strategy.

Selecting Interventions

Most nursing consultation goals can be achieved through more than one intervention. Intervention selection begins by brainstorming about all of the strategies or interventions that could be used to achieve a goal. Once potential interventions are identified, each is evaluated in terms of its "fit" with the needs and resources of the client system. Strategies for increasing productivity among home health nurses might include hiring more staff, paying nurses on the basis of number of visits made, not accepting patients who will need time-consuming and poorly reimbursed visits, or seeking grant funding. In order to determine which of the interventions would work best in the client system, the nurse consultant and the consultee need to consider such factors as financial resources, number of staff and their capabilities, and desired timeline for goal achievement.

Developing the Action Plan

The best predictor of success for a consultation relationship is an accurate problem definition that is owned by or acceptable to the consultee. The next best predictor is selection of the correct set of interventions that also are acceptable to the consultee (Kurpius et al., 1993). Collaborative development of a detailed action plan is one way of creating ownership of goals and interventions. Even though a nurse consultant is not responsible for implementing the recommended interventions, it is necessary to help a consultee explore ways of doing so. An action plan provides this direction.

The nursing consultation action plan should identify the specific steps involved in carrying out a recommended intervention as well as the resources needed to implement each step. The nurse consultant should also check resources needed against those of the consultee (knowledge, skill) and the problem setting (time, money, equipment) to make sure that proposed interventions are feasible. The nurse consultant also needs to explore any consultee objections to the action plan and determine whether they reflect valid objections or represent resistance to change (Mendoza, 1993). The final action plan should be practical, workable, and mutually agreed upon. Characteristics of effective action plans are summarized in Box 3-5.

Facilitating Implementation of the Action Plan

Even though a consultee is free to accept or reject a nurse consultant's recommendations, and implementation of the action plan is not the nurse consultant's responsibility, part of the action planning phase involves putting supports in place to facilitate implementation of the action plan. Two sets of strategies that are frequently used by nurse consultants to facilitate implementation of the action plan are team building and transition management. The goal of team building is to create cohesiveness and effective working relationships among a group of consultees. Transition management strategies focus on helping consultees anticipate and cope with the ways in which an action plan will affect them on a personal level. Transition management strategies are discussed in Chapters 8 and 11; team-

---

BOX 3-5   CREATING AN EFFECTIVE ACTION PLAN

Action plans are most likely to be effective when they are characterized by:

- Collaborative development
- Clear specification of the sequence in which interventions need to occur
- Identification of resources needed for each intervention
- Verification of the availability of needed resources
- Acknowledgment and exploration of consultee objections to the plan

building strategies are discussed in Chapter 12. Box 3-6 describes how the problem identification phase might occur in a community consultation scenario.

Evaluation

Evaluation activities in the nursing consultation process have a multidimensional focus. Evaluation activities should be reflected in the action plan. Areas to be evaluated, evaluation criteria, relevant information sources, and the timing of evaluation activities should all be detailed. Chapter 13 provides a more detailed discussion of developing an evaluation plan.

Evaluation should focus on more than just the outcomes of the nursing consultation process; it should also consider consultee reactions to how the process was carried out. Information obtained from the evaluation of consultation outcomes—summative evaluation—can indicate success or can point to the need for additional interventions (in the case of an unresolved or newly developed problem, for instance).

Even though evaluation activities are most important during the fourth phase of the nursing consultation process, evaluation occurs during the other phases of the process as well. Evaluation of the nursing consultation process as it is unfolding—formative evaluation—provides a nurse consultant with the opportunity to make midcourse corrections, thereby increasing the likelihood that the consultation will be successful. As an example, evaluation of the problem identification phase might reveal a lack of consultee acceptance of the nurse consultant's conclusions about a problem's cause. Based on this information, the nurse consultant can gather additional data and reformulate the problem diagnosis in order to increase its acceptability before proceeding to the action planning phase. Evaluation activities that might take place in a community consultation scenario are presented in Box 3-7.

BOX 3-6   ACTION PLANNING IN A COMMUNITY CONSULTATION SCENARIO: THE MERGER, PART 3

After the supervisors and staff of the merging emergency response services agree that communication issues are the cause of the anxiety among the staff and community and threaten the success of the merger, they work with the nurse consultant to establish goals, select interventions, and develop an action plan. One of the goals they establish is increased communication between the two services and the community.

After brainstorming ideas for interventions and considering the needs and resources of the two services and the community, it is agreed that a biweekly newsletter and weekly joint staff meetings will be initiated as strategies for increasing communication. The action plan details responsibilities for contributing to and producing the newsletters as well as for arranging and facilitating the meetings.

Collaborative development of the action plan serves as a team-building strategy. To help with transition management, the nurse consultant agrees to be a participant in the first four staff meetings and to contribute columns to the newsletter about dealing with change.

BOX 3-7 EVALUATION IN A COMMUNITY CONSULTATION SCENARIO: THE MERGER, PART 4

The nurse consultant, along with the staff and supervisors of the merging emergency response services, decides to gather two different types of evaluation data. First, an evaluation of the perceived effectiveness of both the nurse consultant and the consultation process itself will be obtained. This information will be collected by means of anonymous surveys distributed to the participants once the nurse consultant has left the client system. Since the administrators of the services believe that meaningful indicators of the consultation's success would be reasonable response times, volume, and community satisfaction with the merged services, plans are made for these data to be collected six months after the completion of the merger.

Disengagement

The final phase in the nursing consultation process—disengagement—is a series of strategically planned activities designed to increase the likelihood that problems resolved as a result of the nursing consultation process remain resolved after the nurse consultant leaves the client system. The four specific tasks of the disengagement phase are:

1. Determining readiness to disengage
2. Maintaining change
3. Managing the psychodynamics of disengagement
4. Achieving closure

The disengagement phase often begins with summative evaluation activities.

Determining Readiness to Disengage

The activities of the disengagement phase should not get under way until both the nurse consultant and consultee agree that it is appropriate to terminate the nursing consultation relationship. In most situations, the criteria for beginning the disengagement phase include evaluation findings that indicate a consultee's ability to proceed with the action plan. In other cases, disengagement needs to begin when it becomes clear that a successful outcome to the consultation is unlikely. Additional indicators of readiness to disengage are considered in Chapter 14.

Maintaining Change

A nurse consultant's second task in the disengagement phase is developing change maintenance strategies. These strategies should support the consultee in maintaining changes that have occurred as a result of the consultation process. This is referred to as putting "continuity supports" into place (Lippitt & Lippitt, 1986).

Reducing contact with a consultee while still being available for troubleshooting and follow-up is one strategy that can be used to encourage a consultee to assume ongoing responsibility for problem solving. Another strategy for maintaining change is to work with consultees on developing a regular schedule of self-evaluation that will monitor whether goals established during the action plan continue to be met, and whether desired changes in behavior continue.

Managing the Psychodynamics of Disengagement

Disengagement activities may cause consultees to feel abandoned and inadequate. Often, as disengagement gets under way, consultee dependency and conflict seem to increase. Anticipating and managing these psychodynamics, or emotional reactions to disengagement, helps prevent a consultee from becoming overwhelmed and consequently regressing to old patterns of behavior. Providing evidence to consultees about their readiness to disengage as well as reframing disengagement as a vote of confidence are two ways in which a nurse consultant might address the psychodynamics of disengagement.

Achieving Closure

A nurse consultant's final task in the disengagement phase (and in the nursing consultation process) is to achieve closure. The purpose of closure activities is to leave both the nurse consultant and the consultee with a sense of satisfaction about what they have accomplished. In community consultation situations, closure is often achieved when the nurse consultant submits a final report to the contact person or consultee group. A variety of symbolic rituals such as celebrations can also be used to signify closure. Clinical nurse specialists providing consultation to staff nurses might achieve closure by simply thanking the consultee for the consultation opportunity and offering to be of service in the future. Further examples of closure activities are provided in Chapter 14. Box 3-8 illustrates how disengagement might take place in a community consultation scenario.

BOX 3-8   DISENGAGEMENT IN A COMMUNITY CONSULTATION SCENARIO: THE MERGER, PART 5

The nurse consultant's disengagement from the merger scenario begins by decreasing contact with the client system. More specifically, the nurse consultant limits contact with the client system to attendance at staff meetings. During this "weaning period," the nurse consultant remains available for troubleshooting as needed.

Disengagement also involves developing continuity supports within the client system to help maintain the outcomes of the consultation relationship. One type of continuity support that often is developed by nurse consultants is training one of the consultees to act as an internal consultant. In support of this strategy, the supervisor of the merged services creates a position for a volunteer coordinator/community liaison.

The nurse consultant anticipates increased anxiety and morale problems as disengagement (and the merger) becomes a reality. To address this possible emotional response to disengagement, the nurse consultant writes a series of articles on coping with change for use in the staff's newsletter.

To celebrate the completion of the merger, the emergency response service plans an open house at its new facility and has a contest to design a new logo. These activities help bring closure to the consultation relationship. As another closure strategy, the nurse consultant writes a "closing memo" to both the supervisor and staff of the merged service. This memo summarizes the initial problem, the consultation activities that were carried out, the nurse consultant's impression of the current status of the initial problem, and suggestions for future actions. The nurse consultant considers the "case closed" when a return letter of thanks and acknowledgment and the final portion of the consultation fee are received.

POTENTIAL PROBLEMS IN IMPLEMENTING THE NURSING CONSULTATION PROCESS

Problems that a nurse consultant might encounter while implementing the nursing consultation process can originate either with the consultee and client system or with the nurse consultant.

Problems that Originate with the Consultee or Client System

Several consultee characteristics can cause problems during the nursing consultation process. These may include denial about the need for change, a lack of a sense of shared responsibility for problem solving, or not being ready to enter into a change effort. When nurse consultants interact with a group of consultees, they may discover that not everyone in the group is ready to become involved in problem solving at the same time. Another common setting-based or consultee-based problem is misunderstanding about the identity of the client (e.g., the patient or the organization) or about which outcomes (patient well-being or cost containment) ought to drive goal setting. Finally, a consultee might put pressure on the nurse consultant to skip steps in the consultation process (assessment and evaluation activities are the usual targets) in order to save time and money. The risks of rushing the consultation process—solving the wrong problem, developing an unworkable action plan, and causing disorder and frustration—need to be pointed out to consultees when this pressure occurs.

Problems that Originate with the Nurse Consultant

Other problems that can complicate the nursing consultation process originate with the nurse consultant. Sometimes nurse consultants mistakenly assume that the problem presented by the consultee or contact person is

---

BOX 3-9   POTENTIAL PROBLEMS IN IMPLEMENTING THE NURSING CONSULTATION PROCESS

Problems that Originate with the Consultee or Client System

- Consultee lacks self-awareness or denies the need for change
- Consultee lacks a sense of shared responsibility for problem solving
- Consultee is not ready to enter into a change effort
- Different levels of readiness to problem solve among members of a consultee group
- Misunderstanding about who the client is in the situation
- Misunderstanding or conflict about goals
- Pressure to rush through the consultation process

Problems that Originate with the Nurse Consultant

- Failure to validate the nature of a consultation problem
- Relying on the same interventions for all problem situations
- Assuming problem-solving responsibilities that belong to the consultee

the real problem. Failing to gather assessment data to validate the nature of a problem can lead to irrelevant, unworkable, and possibly harmful interventions. A related problem is trying to use the same package of interventions to solve all problems in all client systems. Finally, nurse consultants may take on the consultee's responsibilities in the problem-solving process. A nurse consultant may, for example, implement a recommended intervention rather than give the consultee this responsibility. Should this occur, future problems that arise in the client system may be blamed on the nurse consultant because the client system has not been given the opportunity to develop its own problem-solving skills. Box 3-9 summarizes problems that can interfere with effective implementation of the nursing consultation process.

Most of the problems that can derail the nursing consultation process can be avoided or overcome by completing (and being willing to repeat) the necessary phases and tasks of the process, being clear about the purpose of each phase, and attending to issues that arise throughout the process. Continual monitoring of both progress in problem solving and consultee reactions to the consultation relationship can help a nurse consultant identify these problems before they threaten to derail the entire consultation process.

CHAPTER SUMMARY

The nursing consultation process is the systematic approach to problem solving that is enacted with consultees in order to enhance client well-being. While the activities of the nursing consultation process occur in a progressive or forward-moving sequence, there is some degree of back-and-forth movement between phases. In fact, some activities occur continually throughout the entire process. Following the phases of the nursing

consultation process and completing its tasks offers the nurse consultant the best chance that a consultation relationship will be successful. Implementing the tasks of the process with a flexibility that acknowledges the uniqueness of each consultation problem and client system helps to ensure that problem solutions will be relevant, feasible, and long lasting.

APPLYING CHAPTER CONTENT

1. Analyze two nursing consultation efforts in which you have been involved, one of which you would label *successful* and the other *unsuccessful*. Which components of the consultation process were present and which were absent in each of these situations? How do you think this contributed to their success or failure? What could have been done differently in the unsuccessful situation?

2. Describe how the nursing consultation process might need to be adjusted for internal versus external nursing consultation situations. Why do you think these adjustments might need to occur?

3. How would you implement the evaluation and disengagement phases of the nursing consultation process if the action plan was rejected by the consultee?

References

Cohen, W., & Murri, M. (1995). Managing the change process. *Journal of AHIMA, 66*(6), 40–41.

Dougherty, A. (1995). *Consultation: Practice and perspectives in school and community settings* (2nd ed.). Pacific Grove, CA: Brooks-Cole.

Kurpius, D., Fuqua, D., & Rozecki, T. (1993). The consulting process: A multidimensional approach. *Journal of Counseling and Development, 71,* 601–606.

Lippitt, G., & Lippitt, R. (1986). *The consulting process in action* (2nd ed.). San Diego: University Associates.

Mendoza, D. (1993). A review of Gerald Caplan's theory and practice of mental health consultation. *Journal of Counseling and Development, 71,* 629–635.

Ross, G. (1993). Peter Block's Flawless Consulting and Homunculus Theory: Within each person is a perfect consultant. *Journal of Counseling and Development, 71,* 639–641.

Ulschak, F., & SnowAntle, S. (1990). *Consultation skills for health care professionals.* San Francisco: Jossey-Bass.

Interaction Patterns
for Nursing Consultation

The time to be aware of the choice among models is at that moment in a relationship when one party says to another: "Can you give me some help?" or "I don't know what to do with this problem I've got," or, simply, "What should I do?" (Schein, 1988)

 KEY CONCEPTS:

interaction pattern, content variables, process variables, process consultation

 KEY TERMS FOR YOUR SEARCH ENGINE:

process consultation, consultation and styles

INTRODUCTION

Just as nurses interact with patients in different ways to provide nursing care (e.g., through team nursing and primary care nursing), nurse consultants interact with consultees in different ways to solve problems. Different nursing care delivery patterns describe the specific tasks and roles (e.g., team leader versus direct care provider) a nurse must carry out in a patient care relationship. Similarly, a nursing consultation interaction pattern describes the roles and interactions of a nurse consultant and consultee in a problem-solving relationship. In nursing consultation, "interaction pattern" refers to the approach to problem solving that a nurse consultant uses in a specific

situation. An interaction pattern can be thought of as a "model of delivery" for consultation services or a "style" of carrying out the nursing consultation process.

An interaction pattern provides guidelines that help a nurse consultant determine how to approach a specific problem situation. This is valuable because the way in which a nurse consultant provides help when a particular interaction pattern is used has a powerful influence on almost every aspect of the nursing consultation process. If the interaction pattern being used fits poorly with a consultee's beliefs, values, real and perceived needs, skills, and preferences, the nursing consultation relationship will likely fail.

Because a single interaction pattern will not work in all problem situations, nurse consultants need a working knowledge of a variety of interaction patterns. Nurse consultants who are familiar with and able to selectively apply different interaction patterns are more likely to be helpful to their consultees because they are better able to individualize the nursing consultation process.

This chapter describes the three interaction patterns that predominate in nursing consultation: providing a solution, prescribing a solution, and facilitating a solution. While these interaction patterns are derived from classic models of organizational consultation, they are equally useful in nursing consultation situations. This chapter also describes the role and task implications of each interaction pattern for the consultee and nurse consultant, as well as each pattern's advantages and disadvantages. The final section of the chapter discusses factors to consider when selecting an interaction pattern and combining interaction patterns. As you read this chapter, think about the following questions:

- What are the distinguishing features of the different interaction patterns?
- How do the nursing consultation skills needed vary with each pattern?
- How would you choose which pattern to use?
- What challenges would you face implementing each of these interaction patterns as an internal and external nurse consultant?
- Which interaction pattern seems most "comfortable" to you? How might this affect your practice of nursing consultation?

PROVIDING A SOLUTION: THE PURCHASE OF EXPERTISE INTERACTION PATTERN

"Purchase of expertise" describes an approach to organizational consultation in which a consultant provides specific services that have been requested by a consultee (Schein, 1988). The interaction pattern represented by this consultation model is likewise applicable to selected nursing consultation situations.

The Interaction Framework

In a typical purchase of expertise scenario, a consultee identifies a specific need and contracts with a consultant for the provision of specific services. The consultee in this scenario identifies the problem, its cause, and the desired solution. However, despite wanting the problem solved and knowing how the problem should be solved, the consultee may lack the time, skill, or interest needed to solve the problem alone and thus hires a consultant. The following scenarios are examples of nurse consultants applying a purchase of expertise interaction pattern:

- A nurse-educator is asked to develop a survey and collect and analyze data for a small community hospital. The hospital wants to learn about the general health status of the community so that it can develop programs the community needs.
- A psychiatric nurse practitioner is asked by a rehabilitation facility to develop protocols for diagnosing and managing depression in the facility's patients.
- A school board is alarmed about the increase in pregnancies among the district's high school students. They ask a nurse to develop a class on assertiveness and safe sex.
- A nurse manager is asked to develop staffing patterns for a Saturday walk-in clinic for children.

The common thread in these scenarios is that the consultee has identified both the problem and the desired solution. Each scenario is characterized by a request for nursing consultation that is something like, "I have this problem that I can't solve on my own. Fix it for me and bring me the bill." Note that part of this interaction pattern is the expectation that the nurse consultant will provide the specified problem solution. As discussed in Chapter 3, providing the problem solution or implementing the intervention is not typically a part of the nursing consultation process. Note also that the purchase of expertise interaction pattern is "content-oriented." That is, it focuses on the "what variables" in the problem situation—what the problem is and what needs to be done to resolve it.

Task Implications

The purchase of expertise interaction pattern implies tasks that both the consultee and nurse consultant must complete in order to obtain a satisfactory nursing consultation outcome. The consultee's tasks center around purchasing the "right" expertise for the problem solution. The nurse consultant's tasks focus on verifying the appropriateness of the purchased services and providing the problem solution.

The Consultee's Tasks

The purchase of expertise interaction pattern is unlikely to be effective unless the consultee successfully carries out four important tasks. First, the consultee is responsible for correctly identifying the problem. Moreover, the consultee needs to accurately identify what is causing the problem and what needs to be done to resolve it (Rockwood, 1993). If the consultee identifies the wrong problem and the wrong solution, the consultation process is unlikely to produce satisfactory results.

Consider the first scenario in the preceding examples. A nurse-educator is asked to provide research expertise to a hospital. The implied problem is that the hospital needs (or wants) to offer community education programs but doesn't know where to start. The consultee's assessment is that more information is needed about the health status of the community in order to develop these programs. The consultee also believes that a survey is the best way of gathering this information. The implied cause of not knowing where to start is a lack of knowledge. However, if the real problem is not a lack of knowledge about the community's needs but rather a lack of knowledge about how to put together and offer community programs, the consultation process is heading in the wrong direction and will likely be unsuccessful.

The consultee's second task in the purchase of expertise interaction pattern is to correctly assess the consultant's ability to solve the problem. In the previous example, if the nurse-educator who has been hired to conduct the desired survey lacks data analysis skills, the problem-solving effort will have an unsatisfactory outcome (even though the consultee has correctly diagnosed the problem).

Third, the consultee must accurately communicate to the nurse consultant the nature of the perceived problem and its desired solution. Again, using the previous scenario, if the consultee fails to clarify the exact population to survey or that the nurse consultant is expected to analyze as well as collect the data, the consultee's needs will go unmet and the problem will remain unresolved.

Finally, the purchase of expertise interaction pattern is unlikely to result in a satisfactory outcome unless the consultee provides the time and resources that will be needed to implement the proposed solution and accepts any temporary side effects, such as decreased productivity, of working to solve the problem. The consultee also needs to plan for possible long-term effects of the proposed consultation services. Consultees often overlook resources such as time, money, equipment, and personnel needed to solve a problem. In our working example, the resources required to conduct the desired survey might include postage costs, staff time (to administer the surveys), and a computer with data analysis capabilities. The possible long-term effects of this project on the client system might include hiring an additional staff person or remodeling a facility to accommodate the community education programs. In the purchase of expertise interaction pattern, it is the consultee's responsibility to identify any constraints that might affect the nurse consultant's ability to offer the desired service.

The Nurse Consultant's Tasks

At first glance, it appears that the consultee bears all of the responsibility for a successful outcome when the purchase of expertise interaction pattern is used to guide the nursing consultation process. The nurse consultant's task is often interpreted as simply providing the contracted service. However, the nurse consultant must do more than just perform the requested service if the desired consultation outcome is to be achieved (Kurpius & Fuqua, 1993).

The nurse consultant's tasks in the purchase of expertise interaction pattern can be described as verification and validation activities. The nurse consultant's first task is to verify that the consultant has correctly identified a problem's cause and is proposing a solution that will resolve the problem. In our working example, the nurse consultant would be responsible for verifying that what the hospital really needs in order to start offering education programs is more information about the community's health status. The nurse consultant would also verify that the proposed solution—gathering information through a survey—is in fact the best solution.

Second, in a purchase of expertise interaction pattern, the nurse consultant needs to verify that she or he is the right consultant for the problem situation. As discussed in Chapter 3, if a nurse consultant realizes that there is a lack of fit between his or her skills and those needed for a consultation project, the nurse consultant is responsible for helping the consultee see the need for a different consultant. Consultant skills in instrument design and data analysis would be imperative for a successful outcome in the example scenario. A nurse consultant lacking these essential skills would be responsible for referring the consultee to someone who could better meet their needs.

The nurse consultant's third task in a purchase of expertise interaction pattern is to verify that the consultee is communicating everything that needs to be communicated. The nurse consultant must actively listen and ask questions so that a consultee's problems, desires, needs, resources, and constraints are accurately understood. Again, using our working example, the nurse consultant would be responsible for verifying exactly what services the consultee wants—the exact population to survey, the nature of data analysis desired, and so forth.

The nurse consultant's final task in a purchase of expertise interaction pattern is to verify that the consultee has thought through the possible consequences of carrying out the proposed problem solution. This responsibility is a part of effective action planning (discussed in Chapters 3 and 11). In our working example, the nurse consultant would verify that the consultee has the resources needed to complete the consultation process. In addition, the nurse consultant would help the consultee think about possible long-term consequences of the consultation project. For example, what if the survey suggests a need for education about workplace hazards present in the community's major industry—could this need really be addressed or would community politics force the issue "under the table" and leave survey respondents frustrated because their needs are not addressed?

Box 4-1 summarizes the tasks that the consultee and nurse consultant need to complete if the purchase of expertise interaction pattern is to result in a satisfactory consultation outcome.

Advantages and Disadvantages

A purchase of expertise interaction pattern is attractive to consultees because it allows them to temporarily turn a problem situation over to the consultant. In situations in which the proposed intervention would have negative effects, such as job losses, a purchase of expertise interaction pattern allows the consultee to maintain an appearance of detachment from the problem solution, while the consultant takes the "heat" for any adverse side effects of the consultation. A purchase of expertise interaction pattern can also be attractive to consultants in that the consultation relationship tends to focus on a very specific problem and tends to be relatively short term in nature. The nurse consultant can perform the contracted service and leave the client system without the added burden of needing to develop a long-term working relationship with the consultee.

The disadvantages of a purchase of expertise interaction pattern relate to the consultant's limited role in initially defining the problem and identifying possible solutions. The nurse consultant can be put in the difficult position of discovering that the wrong problem is being addressed or that the desired intervention is unsuitable. How should a nurse consultant respond, for example, if it becomes apparent the problem solution proposed by the consultee will only resolve the problem on a temporary basis or may actually be an avoidance tactic? A consultee's request for team building, for instance, will not likely

---

BOX 4-1   TASK IMPLICATIONS OF THE PURCHASE OF EXPERTISE INTERACTION PATTERN

In order for the purchase of expertise interaction pattern to result in a satisfactory nursing consultation outcome, the following tasks must be completed:

Consultee Tasks	Nurse Consultant Tasks
• Correctly identify the problem.	• Verify the consultee's diagnosis of the problem and appropriateness of problem solution.
• Choose the right consultant.	• Verify one's own abilities to help with problem solving.
• Communicate clearly and accurately with the consultant.	• Verify what the consultee is communicating; listen, question, and clarify.
• Identify and accept the possible costs and side effects of solving the problem.	• Verify that the consultee has thought through the consequences of proceeding with problem solving.
	• Develop the action plan.
	• Implement the problem solution.

BOX 4-2   THE PURCHASE OF EXPERTISE INTERACTION PATTERN: ADVANTAGES AND DISADVANTAGES

Advantages

- Consultee can turn the problem situation over to the nurse consultant.
- Consultee can appear detached from a problem solution that may have adverse side effects.
- Nurse consultant can avoid the burden of needing to establish a long-term problem-solving relationship.

Disadvantages

- Nurse consultant may discover consultee is trying to solve the wrong problem.
- Nurse consultant may discover consultee's desired problem solution will not solve the problem.
- Consultee may not learn problem-solving skills for future use.

resolve (on a long-term basis) morale problems within a work unit if those problems are occurring as a result of the management style being practiced. In a situation such as this, the nurse consultant is faced with the choice of either exiting the consultation relationship or changing the interaction pattern in order to solve the problem in a different way. Another disadvantage of the purchase of expertise interaction pattern is that the consultee, in turning over the problem-solving task to the nurse consultant, does not learn problem-solving skills for future use.

Box 4-2 summarizes the advantages and disadvantages of the purchase of expertise interaction pattern.

Indications for Use

As suggested in the preceding discussion, a purchase of expertise interaction pattern, when misused, can become a means of avoiding a persistent problem and applying only a "band-aid" solution. This is more likely to happen when the consultation problem involves complex human relations issues, such as burnout and low morale, rather than technical issues. Because of this, a purchase of expertise interaction pattern is most appropriate when a consultee's problem is straightforward and the requested expertise is for help with problems of a technical nature.

PRESCRIBING A SOLUTION: THE "DOCTOR–PATIENT" INTERACTION

Nurse consultants can also address consultation problems by interacting with consultees in a prescriptive interaction pattern. The prescriptive interaction pattern describes a content-oriented consultation model in which the consultant diagnoses and prescribes what is needed to solve a problem. This consultative approach is commonly referred to as the "doctor–patient" interaction pattern (Schein, 1988). This label, while likely offensive to some people, is derived from the roles and tasks typically assumed by the consultant and consultee when this interaction pattern is used.

The Interaction Framework

The prescriptive (or "doctor–patient") interaction pattern gets its name from the way in which the typical consultation scenario unfolds: The consultee senses something is wrong (experiences a symptom) and seeks help for both a diagnosis and prescription. A typical consultation request would be something like, "Something is wrong. Tell me what it is and what to do about it." The consultee wants to learn about the problem and its cause, as well as what to do about it. This contrasts with a purchase of expertise interaction pattern in which the consultee has identified both the problem and the desired solution before seeking consultation.

Task Implications

In a doctor–patient interaction pattern, the consultee's tasks are analogous to behaviors associated with being a "good patient." The nurse consultant's task, in turn, is to be a "good doctor."

The Consultee's Tasks

In order to achieve a satisfactory outcome using a doctor–patient interaction pattern, the consultee must successfully complete five tasks (Dougherty, 1995; Rockwood, 1993). First, the consultee must correctly identify where in the client system the problem exists. To understand the importance of identifying the problem sources in a nursing consultation scenario, consider the example symptom of "increased absences because of diarrheal illness (subsequently diagnosed as hepatitis A) among the children in a certain school district." The consultee needs to help the consultant by isolating the part of the client system in which this problem is arising. For example, is this "symptom" occurring among

all of the students or among only those in a certain school or from a certain neighborhood or other subgroup? The location of the "symptom" helps the nurse consultant determine where to focus assessment activities.

The consultee's next two tasks are founded on a relationship of trust with the consultant. First, the consultee must be willing to provide the information that the nurse consultant needs to accurately diagnose the cause of the problem. To continue with the preceding scenario, the consultee would need to provide the nurse consultant with information about who has been ill. Second, the consultee must accept the consultant's diagnosis of the problem's cause; in the example, the hepatitis might be traced to poor handwashing practices among the food service personnel in a specific school.

Once the consultee has accepted the nurse consultant's diagnosis, the fourth task is to accept and comply with the consultant's problem solution or "prescription." In our working example, if the nurse consultant recommends hepatitis A vaccinations for all school personnel, "complying with the prescription" would mean ensuring that all personnel follow through with obtaining an immunization.

The consultee's final task in a doctor–patient interaction pattern is to want to remain healthy after the nurse consultant leaves the client system. That is, the consultee must be willing to engage in activities aimed at preventing similar problems in the future. In our working example, successfully completing this task would mean that the consultee demonstrates problem prevention behaviors such as requiring hepatitis A vaccinations for all new employees and, perhaps, arranging annual handwashing workshops for all students and school personnel.

The Nurse Consultant's Tasks

The nurse consultant must complete four tasks in the prescriptive (i.e., doctor–patient) interaction pattern if the nursing consultation relationship is to result in a satisfactory outcome. These tasks entail direct involvement in both problem diagnosis and intervention selection. Note that this is in contrast to the purchase of expertise interaction pattern, where the nurse consultant's tasks center around verifying the appropriateness of a problem diagnosis and problem solution generated by the consultee and implementing the desired intervention.

The nurse consultant's first task in a prescriptive interaction pattern is to gather enough assessment data to arrive at a problem diagnosis. This requires establishing a relationship of trust with the consultee. It also means gathering information from multiple sources using a variety of data collection strategies. In the working example—increased absences because of diarrheal illness—data sources might include students, their parents, and food service personnel; data collection strategies might include interviews, observation, and questionnaires.

The nurse consultant's second task in the doctor–patient interaction pattern is to correctly interpret the assessment data and make an accurate and acceptable diagnosis. As discussed in Chapter 3, nursing consultation outcomes will be successful only if a consultee "buys into" a problem's cause. Thus, a nurse consultant needs to carefully consider how the wording and presentation of a problem's cause will affect its acceptability. Think, for example, of the possible differences in consultee reactions to attributing the hepatitis A outbreak to "careless handwashing practices" rather than "ineffective handwashing." A diagnosis of "ineffective handwashing" suggests that a lack of knowledge might be contributing to the problem. In contrast, a diagnosis of "careless handwashing" suggests that the food service workers know what they are supposed to be doing but just aren't doing it. This diagnosis might be interpreted as implying laziness as the cause of the hepatitis out-

break, a connotation that could cause defensiveness among the personnel.

The third task that a nurse consultant must complete in this interaction pattern is to prescribe interventions that will be acceptable to the consultee and other members of the client system. The client system, of course, must have the abilities and resources needed to comply with the treatment plan. To continue with our working scenario, prescribing hepatitis A vaccinations for all school personnel might not make sense if the immunizations will not be covered by the employees' insurance and the district lacks the financial resources to pay for the vaccine. Of course, the nurse consultant could switch to a purchase of expertise interaction pattern and contract with the consultee to write a grant to obtain funding for the vaccine.

The nurse consultant's final task in the doctor–patient interaction pattern is to provide the consultee with enough support and direction to actually carry out the recommended intervention. The nurse consultant in our example would want to determine availability of the vaccine and, perhaps, arrange for an on-site immunization program.

Box 4-3 summarizes the tasks that the consultee and nurse consultant must complete if a doctor–patient interaction pattern is to be effective in resolving a nursing consultation problem.

Advantages and Disadvantages

The primary advantage of the prescriptive interaction pattern is that it enables problems to be resolved in a relatively short period of time. This is because the interaction pattern is consistent with "doing for" rather than "doing with" the consultee. In other words, the consultee is expected to contribute information but is not generally involved in the decision-making aspects of the nursing consultation process. Problem solutions are pre-

---

BOX 4-3   TASK IMPLICATIONS OF THE DOCTOR–PATIENT (OR PRESCRIPTIVE) INTERACTION PATTERN

The following tasks must be completed if the doctor–patient interaction pattern is to result in a satisfactory nursing consultation outcome:

Consultee Tasks	Nurse Consultant Tasks
• Correctly identify the source of the problem.	• Gather enough information to arrive at a diagnosis.
• Provide the nurse consultant with adequate and accurate information.	• Correctly interpret data; formulate an accurate and acceptable diagnosis.
• Accept the consultant's diagnosis of the problem.	• Develop acceptable problem-solving interventions.
• Comply with the recommended problem solution.	• Provide consultee with adequate support and direction to implement the intervention.
• Be willing to engage in problem-prevention activities.	

---

scribed for, rather than developed with, the consultee.

The chief disadvantage of this interaction pattern is that it can foster consultee dependency. This problem is likely to occur because the nurse consultant fixes the problem for a consultee rather than involves the consultee in the problem-solving process.

Box 4-4 summarizes the advantages and disadvantages of the doctor–patient interaction pattern.

Indications for Use

A prescriptive interaction pattern is most useful in two types of problem situations. First,

---

BOX 4-4   THE DOCTOR–PATIENT (OR PRESCRIPTIVE) INTERACTION PATTERN: ADVANTAGES AND DISADVANTAGES

Advantages

• Problems can be solved relatively quickly
• Enables an exhausted consultee to turn a problem over to someone else

Disadvantages

• Can foster consultee dependency
• Little opportunity for consultee to learn long-term problem-solving skills

because this interaction pattern enables problems to be resolved quickly, it is useful in crisis situations in which a timely problem resolution is of utmost importance. It is also useful in situations in which consultees are at their wits' ends and have exhausted their skills and energy trying to resolve a problem on their own; the model is useful in these scenarios because the doctor–patient interaction pattern allows a consultee to turn problem-solving responsibilities over to the consultant.

The doctor–patient interaction pattern could be utilized in the following problem situations:

• Increased incidence of job-related injuries among hospital workers
• Increased "no-show" rate at a community clinic
• Declining enrollment in a nursing program

In each of these scenarios, the nurse consultant has been presented with a troublesome "symptom" that needs to be diagnosed and "treated" with a prescription that will resolve the problem in a relatively short period of time.

FACILITATING A SOLUTION: THE PROCESS CONSULTATION INTERACTION PATTERN

"Process consultation" is a consultation approach that is concerned with long-term organization development and effectiveness (Schein, 1988). Process consultation emphasizes the process rather than the content variables in a problem situation (the "how" variables as opposed to the "what" variables). A nurse consultant using the process consultation interaction pattern is most interested in discovering how problems are related to group dynamics and communication patterns that exist within a client system (Rockwood, 1993).

The Interaction Framework

When a process consultation interaction pattern is used to guide the nursing consultation process, the nurse consultant and consultee function as "co-problem solvers" or partners. The chief difference between the process consultation interaction pattern and the two content-oriented consultation patterns that have been discussed so far in this chapter is that the nurse consultant and consultee work together to identify a problem's causes and develop satisfactory problem-solving strategies. In this interaction pattern, the nurse consultant assumes the role of facilitator in the nursing consultation relationship.

A consultee request of "I need help fixing this problem" (rather than "fix this problem for me") indicates that a process consultation interaction pattern might be the best way to approach the nursing consultation process. In a typical process consultation scenario, the consultee senses something is wrong but does not know what is wrong, why it is wrong, or what to do about it. The consultee also expresses desire to be involved in the problem-solving process. A clinic manager might, for example, initiate a process consultation interaction pattern with a request such as, "We've noticed lower patient satisfaction ratings lately and aren't sure why. We'd like someone to help us figure out what is going on and what to do about it."

Task Implications

In a process consultation interaction pattern, the nurse consultant's primary responsibility is to facilitate development of a consultee's problem-solving abilities. The consultee's responsibility, in turn, is to be a "good student."

The Consultee's Tasks

A process consultation interaction pattern will only be effective to the extent that the consultee accomplishes three tasks. First, the consultee must be willing to take responsibility for or "own" the consultation problem. When consultees own their problems, resistance and resentment to changes resulting from problem-solving efforts are likely to decrease. In the preceding example regarding concern about lower patient satisfaction ratings, the consultee must accept the possibility that staff behaviors might be contributing to the problem.

The consultee's second task in the process consultation interaction pattern is to want to learn how to solve the problem. This means the consultee must have an open mind about what the actual problem solution might be. In the working example, the clinic manager (i.e., the consultee) must be willing to consider problem solutions ranging from changes in personnel to staff education needs.

Finally, when the process consultation interaction pattern is used, the consultee must be willing to be an active participant in the problem-solving process. Consultees are expected to be involved in gathering assessment information, formulating the problem diagnosis, generating possible solutions, developing the action plan, and evaluating the nursing consultation process; in this interaction pattern, consultees "learn by doing" and are partners in the entire nursing consultation process. The clinic manager in our example would need to be personally involved in every phase of the nursing consultation process.

The Nurse Consultant's Tasks

The nurse consultant needs to accomplish two tasks in order to achieve a successful consultation outcome using the process consultation interaction pattern. The first task is cognitive in nature—the nurse consultant must genuinely believe that consultees are the experts in terms of knowing their own strengths, weaknesses, needs, abilities, and preferences. In a process consultation interaction pattern, the nurse consultant deliberately "taps into" the consultee's expertise and incorporates the consultee's insights, opinions, and preferences into the problem diagnosis and action plan. Note how this contrasts with the purchase of expertise interaction pattern where the consultee brings insights and preferences to the consultation relationship at the outset, and the nurse consultant has the task of verifying their accuracy and appropriateness.

The nurse consultant's second task in a process consultation interaction pattern is to actively involve the consultee in each step of the nursing consultation process. This is done by assuming the roles of teacher, guide, role model, mentor, and facilitator.

Box 4-5 summarizes the tasks that the nurse consultant and consultee need to complete when using a process consultation interaction pattern.

Advantages and Disadvantages

The primary advantage of using a process consultation (rather than a content-oriented) approach to the nursing consultation process is that problems are more likely to be resolved on a long-term basis. This interaction pattern leaves the consultee with problem-solving skills that can be used at the first sign of problem recurrence.

The main disadvantage of this interaction pattern is that it often takes longer to implement than do content-oriented interaction patterns. This is because of the teaching and learning that characterizes this interaction pattern. The problem-solving process may be further prolonged if the consultee initiated the process having only limited preexisting problem-solving skills. It is important to consider that needing more time to complete the problem-solving process can have negative financial implications for the client system.

BOX 4-5   TASK IMPLICATIONS OF THE PROCESS CONSULTATION INTERACTION PATTERN

If a process consultation interaction pattern is to be effective, the following tasks must be accomplished:

Consultee Tasks	Nurse Consultant Tasks
• Be willing to "own" the consultation problem. • Have a desire to learn problem-solving skills. • Actively participate in problem-solving activities.	• Believe that consultees are the experts in terms of knowing their own strengths, weaknesses, abilities, and preferences. • Actively involve consultee in problem-solving activities.

Box 4-6 summarizes the advantages and disadvantages of the process consultation interaction pattern.

Indications for Use

Because a process consultation interaction pattern facilitates the development of a consultee's problem-solving skills, it is particularly appropriate to use when the consultation problem is one that is likely to recur. This interaction pattern is also effective when the presenting problem is related to nontechnical issues such as the attitudes, beliefs, and culture of a client system that could be difficult for an external nurse consultant to diagnose alone, without consultee insight. On the other hand, because it often takes longer to implement, this interaction pattern is less appropriate as an approach in urgent situations. A process consultation interaction pattern would be appropriate to consider in the following problem situations:

BOX 4-6   THE PROCESS CONSULTATION INTERACTION PATTERN: ADVANTAGES AND DISADVANTAGES

Advantages

• Consultee learns problem-solving skills
• Increased likelihood of problems remaining resolved

Disadvantages

• Can take longer to carry out problem-solving process

- A diabetes educator is asked by the family of a teen client to help them learn strategies for facilitating compliance with dietary restrictions and glucose testing.
- A nurse-educator is asked by the staff development department of a local hospital to help them develop a peer evaluation process.
- A public health nurse is asked to develop an immunization tracking system for a network of day care providers.

These problem situations are all nonurgent in nature and involve nontechnical issues such as culture, knowledge, beliefs, and attitudes. Because each of these problems is likely to recur in one form or another, the consultee would derive long-term benefits from new skills learned through participating in the nursing consultation process.

MATCHING THE INTERACTION PATTERN TO THE CONSULTEE

The preceding sections of this chapter have linked the different interaction patterns to the nature of the consultation problem and the nature of a consultee's request for help. Another set of factors that can be used to determine which interaction pattern is most likely to be effective in a given problem situation is a consultee's willingness and ability to change. Taking into account these consultee characteristics reflects applying the classic principles of situational leadership (Hersey & Blanchard, 1982) to the selection of problem-solving strategies and a nursing consultation interaction pattern.

A consultee's ability to change is reflected by the amount of direction required during the problem-solving process. Some consultees may need to be told what to do as well as when and how to do it, or may need direction in setting goals and defining roles. A consultee's willingness to change is indicated by the

amount of support and encouragement needed to carry out problem-solving activities (Haffer, 1986).

Consultees are described as having a low willingness and ability to change when they are unsure, insecure, incompetent, unwilling, unmotivated, and unable to solve their own problems (due to exhaustion, time constraints, lack of skills, etc.). These consultees need "telling"—specific directions plus generous amounts of cajoling and encouragement—if they are to resolve their problems (Haffer, 1986). This style of interaction with consultees is most consistent with prescribing a solution, or using the doctor–patient interaction pattern.

Providing a solution or using a purchase of expertise interaction pattern is a good fit when consultees are willing to change but are unable to do so on their own because they lack time, self-confidence, or skill. These consultees will benefit from "selling"—being provided with knowledge and a demonstration of problem-solving skills (Haffer, 1986). These consultant behaviors are consistent with the purchase of expertise interaction pattern.

Other consultees will have preexisting problem-solving skills as well as some degree of motivation and willingness to engage in change efforts. These consultees will respond to an interaction pattern that is supportive, nondirective, and participatory in nature (Haffer, 1986). The interaction pattern that would best fit this nursing consultation situation is the process consultation interaction pattern.

Box 4-7 summarizes the factors to consider when selecting an interaction pattern for a nursing consultation relationship.

COMBINING INTERACTION PATTERNS

Many consultants are beginning to question whether the interaction patterns used in consultation are as mutually exclusive as they have

BOX 4-7 CHOOSING AN INTERVENTION PATTERN FOR A NURSING CONSULTATION RELATIONSHIP

Characteristics of the consultation problem and client system that a nurse consultant can use to guide the selection of an interaction pattern include the nature of the request for help, the nature of the problem, time and timing issues, and a consultee's willingness and ability to change.

Characteristic	Purchase of Expertise Interaction Pattern	Prescriptive Interaction Pattern	Process Consultation Interaction Pattern
Consulation request	"Solve this problem for me."	"Tell me what my problem is and how to fix it."	"I don't know what I need but I need help."
Nature of problem	Technical and straight-forward	Technical and straight-forward	Centered around human relations issues
Time and timing	Consultee is in a hurry	Crisis situation Consultee is at wits' end or is exhausted	Nonurgent problem
Willingness and ability to change	Willing to change but unable to do so alone	Low willingness and ability to change	Motivated to change and has some problem-solving skills

traditionally been presented (Dougherty, 1995; Rockwood, 1993). Because technical and human relations issues are often interrelated, the nursing consultation process may need to simultaneously address both types of issues in order to be most effective. If a combination of interaction patterns is used to guide the nursing consultation process in a given problem situation, the question the nurse consultant needs to ask becomes, "When should I use which model?" rather than, "What model should I use?"

One approach to combining nursing consultation interaction patterns is to start out with a process consultation approach (Rockwood, 1993). The advantage of this strategy is that the consultee's involvement in the activi-ties of the problem identification phase helps the nurse consultant learn the culture of the problem setting. Consultee involvement increases the likelihood that problem solutions that end up being prescribed will be feasible and acceptable to the consultee.

In other situations, a nurse consultant might want to begin the nursing consultation process using the purchase of expertise or doctor–patient interaction pattern and then change to a process approach once the initial crisis aspects of the problem have been resolved. A consultee often has more energy to devote to learning problem-solving skills and is more willing and able to learn once the most troublesome symptoms of a problem have been resolved.

CHAPTER SUMMARY

Nursing consultation interaction patterns reflect different ways of interacting with consultees to help them solve problems. For nurse consultants, an interaction pattern provides a guide for approaching the nursing consultation process in a way that will be most effective in a given situation. The interaction patterns that have been presented in this chapter differ in terms of their emphasis on the content ("what") or process ("how") issues of a problem situation. They also differ in terms of "working for" versus "working with" a consultee to solve problems.

A nurse consultant's selection of an interaction pattern should be based on the perceived needs and abilities of a consultee, including the consultee's willingness and ability to be involved in problem-solving activities. Problem situations in which nurse consultants are likely to be involved are often complex and rarely limited to only content or process issues. Therefore, nurse consultants need a working knowledge of a variety of interaction patterns, as well as the ability to apply these interaction patterns, if they are to be truly effective as problem solvers.

APPLYING CHAPTER CONTENT

1. Think of a consultation situation in which you have been involved. Identify the interaction pattern that was used. Was it a good fit for the situation? Why or why not? Speculate on how this same consultation experience might have been different if another interaction pattern had been used.

2. Refer to the merger scenario presented in Chapter 2 of this text. Which interaction would you use in this scenario? Explain your choice.

References

Dougherty, A. (1995). *Consultation: Practice and perspectives in school and community settings* (2nd ed.). Pacific Grove, CA: Brooks-Cole.

Haffer, A. (1986). Facilitating change: Choosing the appropriate strategy. *Journal of Nursing Administration, 16*(4), 18–22.

Hersey, P., & Blanchard, K. (1982). *Management of organizational behavior: Utilizing human resources* (4th ed.). Englewood Cliffs, NJ: Prentice Hall.

Kurpius, D., & Fuqua, D. (1993). Fundamental issues in defining consultation. *Journal of Counseling and Development, 71*, 598–600.

Rockwood, G. (1993). Edgar Schein's process versus content consultation models. *Journal of Counseling and Development, 71*, 636–638.

Schein, E. (1988). *Process consultation, volume I: Its role in organization development* (2nd ed.). Reading, MA: Addison-Wesley.

Nurse Consultant Roles and Skills

Things rarely, if ever, go in textbook fashion. Equal attention should be paid to both what you are doing and how you are doing those things. (Dougherty, 1995)

 KEY CONCEPTS:

task-oriented role, process-oriented role, universal role, competency, professionalism

 KEY TERMS FOR YOUR SEARCH ENGINE:

nursing and professionalism, consultation and professionalism, consultation and skills

INTRODUCTION

Nurse consultants find themselves taking on multiple roles when they work with consultees. The tasks associated with each phase of the nursing consultation process should readily suggest what some of these roles might be. As you may suspect, each role that a nurse consultant needs to assume is characterized by a set of competencies that reflect a skills base, a knowledge base, and a set of personal attributes. Consultation roles are supported by a set of competencies which, taken together, help to facilitate a successful outcome for the nursing consultation process (see Figure 5-1).

This chapter explores some of the roles and competencies involved in nursing consultation. The chapter begins with a description of the roles most commonly assumed by nurse consultants. It goes on to discuss the factors related to role choice as well as the skills, knowledge, and personal attributes needed to be an effective nurse consultant. The final section of this chapter considers strategies for developing the needed competencies for effective nursing consultation. (Recall that competencies related to working with communities were described in Chapter 2.) As you read this chapter, consider the following questions:

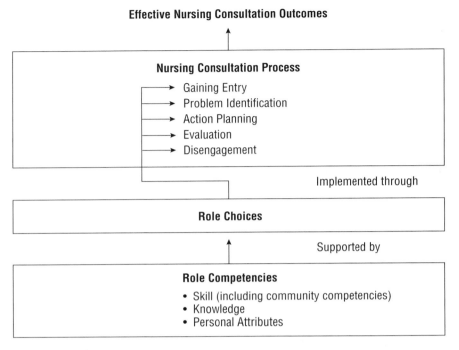

Figure 5-1   Components of Effective Nursing Consultation.
Effective nursing consultation relies on carefully selecting the roles needed to implement each phase of the nursing consultation process. Role competencies are the foundation of a nurse consultant's role choice. The nurse consultant may need to adopt a new role for each phase of the nursing consultation process.

- Which roles described in this chapter are most likely to be used in each phase of the nursing consultation process?
- How might these roles and their associated competencies differ for internal and external nursing consultation situations? How might they differ for community and individual client consulting situations?

- Which nurse consultant roles are most compatible or incompatible with your personal skills and attributes?
- How are the roles and competencies required for a nurse consultant similar to and different from traditionally recognized nursing roles and skills?

NURSING CONSULTATION ROLES

The roles that nurse consultants adopt most frequently in the course of the nursing consultation process can be clustered into three categories: task-oriented roles, process-oriented roles, and "universal" roles. Task-oriented roles are traditionally associated with technical expertise and tend to be directive in nature. Process-oriented nursing consultation roles are comparatively nondirective and more facilitative in nature. Universal roles tend to occur throughout the nursing consultation process and are often superimposed on other roles. It is rare that any nursing consultation role is enacted in isolation. It is more common, rather, for a nurse consultant to enact several roles throughout the course of the nursing consultation process, albeit in varying degrees. Box 5-1 describes the three types of nursing consultation roles in greater detail.

Task-Oriented Consultation Roles

Task-oriented nursing consultation roles tend to have a technical focus. These roles require specialized knowledge and skills and reflect the "technical work," or tasks, that must be accomplished to satisfactorily complete the phases of the nursing consultation process. (Note how the task-oriented roles in Box 5-1 "match" the tasks of the nursing consultation process identified in Chapter 3.)

Task-oriented roles are generally used when a consultee needs direction with problem-solving activities due to either the urgent nature of the problem or to the consultee's limited problem-solving abilities. Task-oriented roles are particularly apparent when a content-oriented interaction pattern (i.e., purchase of expertise or doctor–patient/prescriptive) is used to guide the nursing consultation process. Although many task-oriented roles exist, six are most commonly enacted in the nursing consultation process.

Fact Finding

One of the most frequently enacted nursing consultation roles is that of fact finder (McDougall, 1987; Monicken, 1995). Fact-finding activities predominate during the problem identification phase of the nursing consultation process. However, fact finding

BOX 5-1   TYPES OF NURSING CONSULTATION ROLES

Task-Oriented Roles

- Fact finding
- Diagnosing
- Advocacy
- Directing solution implementation
- Educating
- Coordinating resources

Process-Oriented Roles

- Joint problem solving
- Process counseling

Universal Roles

- Providing expertise
- Presenting information
- Role modeling
- Providing leadership

takes place during other phases of the nursing consultation process as well, because nurse consultants must constantly gather information to confirm that the consultation relationship is progressing satisfactorily. As a fact finder, the nurse consultant must know how, when, and from whom to obtain the data needed to clarify problems and identify meaningful goals and workable interventions. The following scenario illustrates a nurse consultant using the fact-finding role:

> A school nurse is asked to determine why there is an unusually high rate of absenteeism in one 4th grade class. The nurse interviews with the teacher, as well as students and their parents, and spends time observing classroom as well as after school and recess activities.

Diagnosing

The nursing consultation role of diagnostician is closely linked to the role of fact finder. Diagnosing entails analyzing, synthesizing, and attaching meaning to data in order to draw conclusions about the cause of a consultation problem. The role of diagnostician is also used when the nurse consultant is drawing conclusions about the feasibility and effectiveness of a potential problem-solving intervention. The preceding example can be extended to illustrate the following diagnostician role:

> The school nurse reviews the data gathered from multiple sources and draws conclusions about likely explanations for the high rate of absenteeism. She or he concludes that the absences are not related to illness.

Advocacy

When engaged in advocacy, a nurse consultant tries to persuade a consultee to take a specific course of action. Advocacy is based on a desire to protect the interests of those who are unable (because they lack skill, knowledge, or energy) to protect their own interests (Dougherty, 1995). Advocacy takes different forms depending on the particular interaction pattern being used to guide the nursing consultation process. When a content-oriented interaction pattern (i.e., purchase of expertise or doctor–patient/prescriptive) is being used, advocacy focuses on encouraging a consultee to take a specific course of action. This is known as "solution advocacy." This type of advocacy is appropriate because the nurse consultant is bringing objectivity and a broader perspective to a problem situation that is characterized by a sense of urgency and consultee frustration. In a process consultation interaction pattern, the focus of advocacy is encouraging the consultee to be an active participant in the problem-solving process. With this type of advocacy, known as "process advocacy," the consultee can benefit from learning problem-solving skills that can be applied to future problem situations. Following are examples of these two variations of advocacy:

- *Solution advocacy.* A nurse consultant is asked to improve patient flow in a family planning clinic. The clinic is losing money because of staff overtime and the fact that long waits often cause patients to leave without being seen. The clinic has already attempted to resolve flow problems through physical renovation of the facility. The nurse consultant persuades the clinic to revise both its appointment scheduling process and the tasks assigned to the clinical support staff.
- *Process advocacy.* A nurse consultant is asked to work with the staff of a family planning clinic to solve concurrent problems of prolonged waiting times for patients, "slow" times for the nurse practitioners, and consistent staff overtime. The nurse consultant persuades the clinic administrator to allow clinic staff to be involved in data gathering activities and brainstorming about possible problem solutions.

Directing Solution Implementation

When a nurse consultant is directing solution implementation, she or he delegates specific problem-solving tasks to the consultee. The role of director varies according to which nursing consultation interaction pattern is being applied. For instance, if a purchase of expertise interaction pattern is being used, the nurse consultant may direct the consultee to assist with specific components of the intervention. (Recall that in this interaction pattern, the nurse consultant is hired to implement a specific problem solution.) In contrast, with both the prescriptive and process consultation interaction patterns, directing solution implementation means providing the consultee with specific directions about how to implement the action plan. (Remember also that in a prescriptive interaction pattern, delegation decisions are made unilaterally by the nurse consultant; in a process consultation interaction pattern, the nurse consultant and consultee work together to decide how to delegate each task.) In these two interaction patterns, the nurse consultant directs solution implementation through the development of a comprehensive action plan. The following scenarios illustrate the nurse consultant directing solution implementation:

- A nurse practitioner accepts a contract to develop protocols for a telephone triage service. The nurse practitioner directs the consultee to gather protocols from other health care practices in the area.
- A telephone triage service is concerned about the high rate of hospitalizations among its callers. A nurse consultant develops an action plan for reviewing the calls made and the advice given over the past 12 months. The plan includes different assignments for various members of the client system.
- A telephone triage service is concerned about its low physician satisfaction ratings. The nurse consultant and consultee work

together to develop an action plan for ascertaining physicians' specific complaints and the types of calls that they refer to the service. Together the nurse consultant and consultee decide which members of the client system are best suited for surveying the various physicians from whom they hope to obtain information.

Educating

Nurse consultants assume the role of educator when they create learning experiences for a consultee. Typically, these learning experiences are directed at helping a consultee change their level of knowledge, understanding, or functioning. A nurse consultant's ultimate goals in providing education are to improve a client's well-being and develop a consultee's ability to respond to a problem situation that is likely to recur.

Like other nurse consultant roles, the role of educator changes its focus when different consultation interaction patterns are being used. In a purchase of expertise interaction pattern, a consultee may contract with a nurse consultant to provide a specific education service. In a prescriptive interaction pattern, a nurse consultant might teach a consultee how to follow through with the prescribed action plan. Because the focus of the process consultation interaction pattern is to help a consultee develop problem-solving abilities, here the nurse consultant may informally enact the role of educator throughout the nursing consultation process. The following examples illustrate different ways in which a nurse consultant may enact the role of educator:

- A nurse manager is hired by a home health care agency to teach assistive personnel about accepting delegated tasks.
- A nurse consultant develops an action plan that includes instructions (education) about how to assess the abilities of unli-

censed assistive personnel to carry out certain delegated tasks.

- A nurse consultant helps a consultee apply state rules and regulations to the development of a policy about delegating tasks to unlicensed assistive personnel.

Coordinating Resources

When assuming the role of resource coordinator, the nurse consultant finds resources that a consultee needs in order to be able to implement a problem solution. Coordinating resources is a part of the action planning phase of the nursing consultation process. In a content-oriented interaction pattern, resource coordination may entail accessing needed resources on the consultee's behalf. When the nursing consultation process is guided by a process consultation interaction pattern, coordinating resources means working with the consultee to both identify needed resources and how to obtain them. Coordinating resources is illustrated in the following examples:

- A nurse consultant accesses a portable fetal monitor so that a home health care agency can conduct nonstress tests on homebound women who have high-risk pregnancies.
- A nurse consultant works with the staff of a home health care agency to help them identify needed equipment and possible equipment vendors and funding sources for starting an in-home nonstress testing program.

Process-Oriented Consultation Roles

In contrast to task-oriented nurse consultant roles, process-oriented roles are more facilitative than directive in nature. Process-oriented nurse consultant roles focus on helping con-

sultees accept and take responsibility for problem situations and for ongoing problem-solving activities. These nurse consultant roles are most apparent when the nursing consultation process is being guided by a process consultation interaction pattern. There are, however, two process-oriented nurse consultant roles that can be identified in almost all nursing consultation relationships.

Joint Problem Solving

Nurse consultants who are engaged in joint problem solving combine their expertise and professional resources and form a partnership with a consultee to respond to a problem situation. In this capacity, a nurse consultant acknowledges the insight and information a consultee can contribute to the nursing consultation process as well as encourages a consultee to identify alternative problem explanations and solutions. In a purchase of expertise interaction pattern, the nurse consultant acts as a joint problem solver by verifying a consultee's assessment of the problem situation. Thus, joint problem solving is incorporated into problem diagnosis and intervention selection activities. When a doctor–patient/prescriptive interaction pattern is being applied, joint problem solving is most apparent during assessment activities when the nurse consultant relies on information from the consultee to formulate a valid problem diagnosis. Joint problem solving occurs on a more continual basis when a process consultation interaction pattern is being applied.

Process Counseling

Process counseling involves helping a consultee perceive, understand, and act on the interpersonal and intergroup behaviors that are contributing to a problem situation (Lippitt & Lippitt, 1986). The goal of a nurse consultant who is engaged in process counseling is to support the improvement of the human dynamics within a problem setting. To achieve this aim, the nurse consultant helps consultees clarify the meaning of their words and explore the factors that contribute to problematic behavior. The following scenario illustrates process counseling:

Consultee: The nurses in this clinic aren't performing as effectively as they were when we were in our old clinic site.

Nurse consultant: What do you mean by "not as effectively"? (Clarifying communication)

Consultee: Well, I mean they don't help each other out. It's like everyone is only interested in their own tasks. There's no teamwork.

Nurse consultant: How has the move affected their work roles? Can you think what this behavior might mean? (Helping consultee explore reasons for intergroup behavior)

Universal Consultation Roles

Providing expertise, presenting information, role modeling, and providing leadership are four "universal" roles that occur throughout every nursing consultation relationship. These roles are often superimposed on the other nursing consultation roles that are being enacted.

Providing Expertise

In many ways, "expert" is viewed as synonymous with "consultant." It is no surprise, then, that providing expertise is superimposed on most other nurse consultant roles; if a nurse consultant is not perceived as having specialized knowledge or skills, it is unlikely a consultee would request the consultant to help in solving a problem. As the different interaction patterns for nursing consultation illustrate, consultees seek content as well as process expertise from nurse consultants.

The nurse consultant's role in providing expertise deserves particular qualification because novice nurse consultants can be easily seduced by the label of "expert" as well as

the authority and social and professional prestige that tends to accompany that label. Furthermore, some consultees may be lulled into a false sense of security or complacency by a consultant's "aura of expertise." As useful as this perception may be for establishing credibility and gaining psychological entry, relying on the role of expert to the exclusion of all other roles can foster dependency on the part of the consultee rather than facilitate the development of problem-solving skills. The nurse consultant needs to be aware that while consultation, by its very nature, incorporates the expert role, actually providing expertise is only appropriate to the degree that doing so helps a consultee learn to resolve the problem situation.

Presenting Information

The task of presenting information, like providing expertise, occurs in all phases of the nursing consultation process. A nurse consultant must continually present and share information so that a consultee can be an active participant in the problem-solving process. Typical situations in which nurse consultants are presenting information include:

- Presenting information that has been gathered during fact finding
- Presenting conclusions about a problem's cause that have been developed while enacting the role of diagnostician
- Presenting information while providing education
- Presenting problem-solving alternatives that have been brainstormed during the process of joint problem solving
- Presenting impressions about a group's interactions when engaged in process counseling

Role Modeling

Effective nurse consultants consciously and unconsciously role model problem-solving competencies throughout the nursing consultation process. In a sense, role modeling can be considered a form of educating. Role modeling includes demonstrating the skills and qualities used by a successful consultant. As a form of "teaching by showing," role modeling can be a powerful strategy for teaching problem-solving skills because it enables consultees to see how specific actions, such as different ways of collecting and presenting information, influence reactions and problem-solving results.

Providing Leadership

The fourth universal nurse consultant role is providing leadership in problem solving. Nurse consultants provide this leadership by ensuring that the phases and tasks of the nursing consultation process are completed and, if necessary, repeated. Providing leadership also entails ensuring that the consultant and consultee carry out the tasks that need to occur if a specific nursing consultation interaction pattern is to be effective. It is important to recognize that providing leadership does not mean taking over the nursing consultation process. Rather, providing leadership can be thought of as a "total quality management" strategy for ensuring that the consultee's needs are met and the consultation problem has the best chance of being resolved.

Choosing Among Consultation Roles

Effective nurse consultants are able to choose the appropriate role for each step of a problem situation and implement those roles in a balanced way that respects the norms and standards of the consultee and client system. Most nurse consultants, while aware of the many roles they play during the consultation process, have preferred ways of solving problems. Nurse consultants who work repeatedly and successfully with a limited range of prob-

lem issues may be tempted to implement roles in a similar fashion in all problem situations. Moreover, nurses may be asked to consult about a specific problem because of their reputation for performing specific roles effectively. The danger of relying on personal preferences and what has worked before is that doing so overlooks the unique qualities of each consultee and problem situation. Factors that the nurse consultant should consider when choosing a nursing consultation role include the consultee's confidence and level of skill within the consultation process, time constraints, and issues related to trust, teamwork, and acceptance (Ulschak & SnowAntle, 1990). These factors and their implications for role choice are summarized in Box 5-2.

Consultee Skills and Confidence

The roles that a nurse consultant enacts tend to change as the relationship with a consultee develops. At the beginning of a consultation relationship, the consultee may be in a relatively dependent relationship with the nurse consultant. During this time, more directive consultative roles are often needed. As a nursing consultation relationship evolves, however, consultees acquire problem-solving skills and generally gain confidence. As this growth occurs, less directive roles become appropriate.

Time Constraints

The urgency of a consultation problem is often a driving force behind a nurse consultant's decision to use a more or less directive role when interacting with a consultee. Because nondirective, process-oriented roles tend to require more time, these roles are generally not effective in problem situations in which time is limited. Task-oriented roles, however, are particularly appropriate for urgent situations. Consider, as an example, the scenario of a budget crisis at a downtown shelter for homeless women: If funds are not secured within a

BOX 5-2   CHOOSING AMONG CONSULTATION ROLES

The choice of a nursing consultation role is largely determined by the consultee's level of skill and confidence, time constraints, and issues related to trust, teamwork, and acceptance.

Factor	Role Considerations
Consultee skills and confidence	Low skills and confidence—use a more directive role. As skills and confidence are acquired, roles can become less directive.
Time constraints	Urgent situation—consider task-oriented roles.
	Nonurgent situation—consider process-oriented roles.
Trust	Nurse consultant has low trust in consultee—time factors determine whether task- or process-oriented roles should be used.
	Consultee has low trust in nurse consultant—build trust by effectively implementing a task-oriented role or by including consultee in problem-solving activities.
Teamwork	Teamwork present or desired—consider process-oriented roles.
Acceptance	Not important—consider task-oriented roles.
	Important—consider process-oriented roles.

week, the shelter will need to close. While enacting process-oriented roles might help the consultee learn how to keep a budget crisis from recurring, these roles would likely take too long to implement to solve the immediate crisis. Instead, task-oriented, directive roles such as coordinating resources, solution advocacy, and directing intervention implementation are indicated.

Trust

The level of trust between the consultee and nurse consultant is another issue to consider when selecting a nursing consultation role. Trust is present between a nurse consultant and consultee when there is rapport and a sense of mutual respect and credibility. The absence of trust can create a "Catch-22" situation in nursing consultation.

In problem situations in which the nurse consultant has a low level of trust in the consultee's problem-solving abilities or contributions to the problem-solving process, the nurse consultant may need to enact a task-oriented role (such as fact finding) if any progress is to be made in resolving the consultation problem. On the other hand, if there is time to use a process-oriented role such as joint problem solving, the nurse consultant may be able to gain trust in the consultee's problem-solving abilities.

In situations where the consultee has low trust in the nurse consultant, successful implementation of a task-oriented role, such as providing education, can enhance the consultee's perception of the nurse consultant's credibility and help build trust. Once initial trust has been established, the nurse consultant can more effectively implement a process-oriented role. At the same time, however, a consultee who has little trust in a nurse consultant may become very resistant to the problem-solving process when a directive, task-oriented role such as diagnosing or advocacy is used. Enacting a process-oriented role can help the consultee build trust in the nurse consultant's intentions and abilities. Trust, therefore, should not be the only criterion used for choosing a nurse consultant role, but should be considered with other factors in the problem situation.

Teamwork

A further consideration for a nurse consultant when choosing a role is teamwork—both as a norm within the client system and as a desired outcome of the nursing consultation relationship. A teamwork-oriented consultee makes it more feasible for the nurse consultant to use a process-oriented role such as joint problem solving. If enhanced teamwork is a goal of the nursing consultation relationship, as is the case in many problem situations involving human dynamics issues, process counseling would be appropriate, either alone or in combination with another consultative role such as providing education.

Acceptance

Finally, the nurse consultant needs to assess how important it is for the consultee to accept the problem solution. If the consultee's acceptance of the problem-solving strategy is not important (as in the earlier example of the shelter with a budget crisis where it is the outcome rather than how it is achieved that is important), directive and task-oriented nurse consultant roles are appropriate. On the other hand, if consultee acceptance of a problem solution is important (e.g., using position cuts or fees for service as the strategy to prevent a recurring clinic budget crisis), more facilitative and process-oriented roles are likely to be effective.

SKILLS BASE FOR NURSING CONSULTATION

Nursing consultation requires a broad skills base. Nurse consultants need technical competence to perform the task-oriented roles needed during each phase of the nursing consultation process. If these roles and technical skills are to be implemented effectively, nurse consultants also need human process and communication skills. Box 5-3 outlines the technical and human process skills base needed for effective nursing consultation.

Technical Competencies

Technical competencies are the task-oriented skills needed to complete the phases of the nursing consultation process. These competencies can be grouped into two categories: diagnostic skills and problem-solving skills.

Diagnostic Skills

The diagnostic skills needed by nurse consultants include the ability to select and implement data-gathering approaches that are appropriate for both assessment and evaluation purposes. Effective data gathering requires knowing what information is needed and how to access it; it also requires a broad understanding of the issues related to a presenting problem—that is, an appreciation of multicausality, or systems-thinking—so that important sources and pieces of information are not overlooked. A nurse consultant working with a community, for example, would demonstrate competence in diagnostic skills by looking beyond the obvious cause of the problem and considering the interrelationships of political, social, and economic variables that are present within the community (Balik, 1998).

Another set of diagnostic skills needed by a nurse consultant is problem conceptualization. Skill in conceptualizing problems involves the ability to assimilate and synthesize an extensive quantity of information in order to come to conclusions about a problem's cause (Cohen &

BOX 5-3   TECHNICAL AND HUMAN PROCESS SKILLS BASE FOR NURSING CONSULTATION

Technical competencies: Task-oriented skills needed to complete the phases of the nursing consultation process.

Diagnostic Skills

- Assessment approaches and techniques
- Appreciation of multicausality
- Data analysis and interpretation
- Problem conceptualization

Problem-Solving Skills

- Collaboration
- Goal setting
- Ability to establish priorities
- Designing, implementing, and modeling interventions
- Mobilizing resources
- Motivating and instilling confidence
- Political astuteness
- Imagination
- Risk taking

Human process competencies: "People-oriented" skills needed to gain consultee acceptance of the consultation process and its resultant changes.

Communication Skills

- Sending messages
- Receiving verbal and nonverbal messages
- Formal information presentation skills
- Ability to give and receive feedback

Interpersonal Skills

- Building, maintaining, and terminating relationships
- Group management skills
- Ability to manage conflict and hidden agendas
- Ability to manage resistance
- Ability to manage dependency
- Negotiation skills

Murri, 1995). Problem conceptualization requires skills in both analyzing and interpreting assessment and evaluation data.

Problem-Solving Skills

Nurse consultants use problem-solving skills to help consultees formulate goals, establish priorities, and implement problem solutions. Problem solving requires proficiency with a range of interventions such as program planning, educating, and team building. Effective nurse consultants are able to design, implement, and model a variety of problem-solving strategies. Chapter 11 discusses problem-solving strategies in detail; team building is addressed in Chapter 12.

Problem solving also requires the ability to translate an idea for a possible problem solution into practice (Cohen & Murri, 1995). This means that the nurse consultant must be able to set the stage for successful implementation of a problem-solving strategy by mobilizing resources and by motivating and instilling confidence into consultees. Effective problem solving requires a nurse consultant to be comfortable working at all levels of a client system to effect change, which, in turn, requires political astuteness. Imagination and risk taking are other useful problem-solving skills.

Human Process Competencies

Human process competencies are the "people-oriented" skills needed by nurse consultants to work effectively with individuals and groups in problem-solving situations. Human process competencies reflect the "how" component of nurse consultant–consultee interactions. Competence in human process skills facilitates consultee acceptance of the nursing consultation process and the change it produces. Process competencies include communication and interpersonal skills.

Communication Skills

Communication skills are essential for maintaining the momentum of the consultation process and sustaining consultee motivation and loyalty (Cohen & Murri, 1995). Effective nurse consultants are proficient at both sending and receiving messages. When sharing assessment and evaluation findings with consultees, nurse consultants need proficiency in formal information presentation skills, that is, writing and speaking. Throughout the nursing consultation process, nurse consultants must be skilled at listening, nonverbal attending, expressing empathy, questioning, clarifying, summarizing, and giving and receiving feedback.

Interpersonal Skills

Effective nurse consultants know how to create, maintain, and terminate relationships with both individual and group consultees. Nurse consultants must be able to put people at ease and build trust. This requires skills in establishing rapport and credibility and using humor appropriately. Specific interpersonal skills needed by nurse consultants are skills in group management and negotiation.

Group management skills needed to be an effective nurse consultant include the ability to keep group members focused on the task at hand, manage conflict, manage hidden as well as formal agendas, and balance consultee needs for autonomy and direction. Other relationship-oriented human process skills needed by nurse consultants include knowing when to confront and when to listen, understanding and managing the dynamics of resistance, and recognizing and managing excessive dependency in oneself as well as in consultees (Kurpius, Fuqua, & Rozecki, 1993). These human process skills are essential for working with individual as well as group consultees.

Negotiation, the process of getting what one wants from others, is an interpersonal skill that is often needed in several phases of the nursing consultation process. Implementing process-oriented nurse consultant roles such as joint problem solving may also require negotiation skills. As an example, a nurse consultant may need to negotiate the parameters of staff nurse involvement (e.g., will they be paid) in education sessions that are to be part of a problem solution. Effective negotiation requires communication skills, understanding the consultee's point of view, flexibility, and a willingness to take risks. Effective negotiation also includes the ability to separate the consultee from the problem issue, explore the consultee's interest, focus on common interests rather than on position, and generate multiple problem definitions and problem solutions (Fisher & Ury, 1981).

KNOWLEDGE BASE FOR NURSING CONSULTATION

The roles that are used by nurse consultants and the skills that are needed to implement these roles suggest the need for nurse consultants to have a broad knowledge base. Nurse consultants need to know about the purposes and phases of nursing consultation. Knowledge of indirect or supportive areas is also needed for effective nursing consultation. The outline of the knowledge base for nursing consultation in Box 5-4 reflects the consensus of several writers (Balik, 1998; Barron & White, 2000; Dougherty, 1995; Monicken, 1995). The technical knowl-

---

BOX 5-4   KNOWLEDGE BASE FOR NURSING CONSULTATION

Technical knowledge: Content that promotes understanding of nursing consultation relationships and the nursing consultation process.

- The nursing process
- The nursing consultation process
- Interaction patterns for nursing consultation
- Systems theory
- Organizational theories and structures
- Community health theories
- Models of health promotion
- Change theory
- Principles of group dynamics
- Power
- Leadership theory

General knowledge: Supportive content that varies according to the nursing consultation setting, the interventions selected, and the nature of the problem.

- Specialized clinical knowledge
- Adult learning theory
- Conflict resolution
- Cultural diversity
- Knowledge about current models of health care delivery
- Knowledge about health care financing

edge areas that are listed in the box reflect content that is foundational to an understanding of the nature of nursing consultation relationships (e.g., change theory and group dynamics) and typical nursing consultation problem settings (e.g., systems theory and organizational theories). General knowledge areas include content that supports a nurse's practice of the consultant role and the nursing consultation process in specific situations.

PERSONAL ATTRIBUTES FOR NURSING CONSULTATION

Effective nurse consultants have more than technical expertise, process skills, and a broad knowledge base. They also have personal and professional qualities and competencies that enhance their implementation of the nursing consultation process. These attributes are summarized in Box 5-5.

Personal Qualities

Nurse consultants often find themselves working with a variety of clients in a wide range of settings. Interacting effectively with individual and group consultees in diverse settings requires the ability to communicate personal qualities such as empathy, warmth, respect, acceptance, and concern (Barron & White, 2000; Ulschak & SnowAntle, 1990).

BOX 5-5   PERSONAL ATTRIBUTES FOR NURSING CONSULTATION

- Ability to listen and empathize
- Ability to communicate warmth, acceptance, and concern
- Self-direction
- Flexibility
- Tolerance for ambiguity
- Ability to share control with others
- High threshold of frustration
- Charisma
- Credibility
- Poise
- Vision
- High energy level
- Passion for problem solving
- Ability to engage in self-examination
- Professionalism
- Good judgment
- Self-awareness
- Sense of humor
- Personal and professional growth orientation
- Respect for confidences
- Clear sense of responsibilities
- Ability to respect and uphold contractual obligations
- Willingness to be evaluated

Nurse consultants also need to be self-directed and flexible. They need to be able to tolerate ambiguity and a lack of control. In other words, nurse consultants must be comfortable in situations in which problem causes and "best" solutions are not readily apparent. They must be comfortable with sharing problem-solving and decision-making activities with consultees, even when they would rather solve the problem on their own. Nurse consultants must be able to accept the right of a consultee to act or not act on their recommendations; this requires a high threshold of frustration and the ability to tolerate rejection. Nurse consultants who are personally charismatic and who readily demonstrate their credibility are able to construct a power base for their consultation recommendations (Cohen & Murri, 1995).

Poise, vision, a passion for problem solving, and boundless reserves of energy are other personal attributes needed for successful nursing consultation (Metzger, 1993). Finally, effective nurse consultants have the ability to engage in self-examination and reflection about skills and knowledge areas that need further development (Barron & White, 2000).

Professionalism

This final set of attributes needed for effective nursing consultation enables the nurse consultant to be identified as a professional. One such attribute, judgmental competency, is the ability to make decisions about appropriate courses of action in a specific consultation relationship (Brown, 1993). Another important competency of effective professional nurse consultants is having a clear understanding of their responsibilities and obligations as a nurse consultant. For example, client well-being should not be sacrificed for the sake of fostering consultee independence in problem solving.

Effective nurse consultants have a high level of self-awareness. That is, they know and respect the limits of their expertise and skills. They refer to or consult with other professionals as necessary. Effective nurse consultants also maintain a personal and professional growth orientation so that they are continually updating and expanding their expertise and repertoire of intervention skills. Effective professional nurse consultants respect confidences but are also able to make appropriate judgments about the limits of confidentiality. Professional nurse consultants recognize their responsibilities to honor contractual agreements and are willing to have their performance as a nurse consultant evaluated.

DEVELOPING KNOWLEDGE AND SKILLS FOR CONSULTATION

There is a prevailing yet mistaken belief that a nurse can become an effective nurse consultant without any deliberate education or training. Many nurses, and consultees for that matter, believe that the only thing needed to be effective as a nurse consultant is content expertise or specialized information (Brown, 1993). While it is true that consultation is a functional role into which many nurses evolve as they acquire experience, content expertise, and confidence (Monicken, 1995), it is also true that the different competencies required for effective nursing consultation are best acquired through different types of learning experiences. The knowledge base needed for effective nursing consultation can be effectively acquired through didactic (classroom) learning activities. Skills-base competencies can be acquired in laboratory settings and through structured application exercises such as videotaping and critiquing one's interviewing and presentation skills. The judgmental competencies needed for effective nursing consultation are best acquired through supervised practice experiences (Brown, 1993).

Foundational knowledge and skills for effective nursing consultation can be acquired or enhanced through a variety of formal and informal means. Academic courses and continuing education workshops are two of the more formal or structured ways of gaining theoretical knowledge. A less formal and structured way of updating knowledge is reading in both the professional and popular press topics related to personal and organizational development, current trends in one's specialty area, and health care in general. Networking, special interest groups, and general and specialty professional organizations are additional opportunities available to most nurses for enhancing their knowledge base for effective nursing consultation.

Consultation skills and judgmental competencies can be expanded and refined by actively seeking out feedback about one's performance as a consultant. Supervised practice experiences can often be developed in return for providing nursing consultation services on a volunteer basis, especially in community service agencies. These experiences can offer opportunities to practice and receive feedback on foundational nursing consultation skills such as problem identification, educating, giving presentations, developing action plans, interpersonal communication, and evaluation.

Finally, self-assessment tools, self-reflection, and peer review processes can be used to develop insight into the personal and professional qualities one brings to a nursing consultation situation.

CHAPTER SUMMARY

Nurse consultants interact with consultees in a variety of roles. These roles require many different skills, as well as a broad knowledge base. Effective nursing consultation is built on choosing the consultative role that is most appropriate for the problem setting and applying it to the nursing consultation process.

Effective nursing consultation requires personal qualities and professionalism. While some of the competencies needed for effective nursing consultation can be acquired and developed through experience and professional maturation, a variety of formal and informal learning opportunities can also be used to build and enhance the knowledge, skills base, and personal attributes needed for effective nursing consultation.

APPLYING CHAPTER CONTENT

1. Review the emergency service merger scenario presented in Chapter 2. Analyze the nurse consultant's actions in each phase of the nursing consultation process. Identify the knowledge, skills, and personal qualities underlying each role.
2. Review the skills, knowledge, and personal attributes for effective nursing consultation that are identified in Boxes 5-3, 5-4, and 5-5 of this chapter. Identify areas of personal weakness. Also identify strategies you might use to further develop these areas.

References

Balik, R. (1998). The impact of managed cared and integrated delivery systems on registered nursing education and practice. In E. O'Neil & J. Coffman (Eds.), *Strategies for the future of nursing* (pp. 41–63). San Francisco: Jossey-Bass.

Barron, A., & White, P. (2000). Consultation. In A. Hamric, J. Spross, & C. Hanson (Eds.), *Advanced nursing practice: An integrative approach* (2nd ed.) (pp. 217–243). Philadelphia: Saunders.

Brown, D. (1993). Training consultants: A call to action. *Journal of Counseling and Development, 72,* 139–143.

Cohen, W., & Murri, M. (1995). Managing the change process. *Journal of AHIMA, 66*(6), 40–47.

Dougherty, A. (1995). *Consultation: Practice and perspectives in school and community settings* (2nd ed.). Pacific Grove, CA: Brooks-Cole.

Fisher, R., & Ury, W. (1981). *Getting to yes: Negotiating agreement without giving in.* Boston: Houghton-Mifflin.

Kurpius, D., Fuqua, D., & Rozecki, T. (1993). The consulting process: A multidimensional approach. *Journal of Counseling and Development, 71,* 601–606.

Lippitt, G., & Lippitt, R. (1986). *The consulting process in action* (2nd ed.). San Diego, CA: University Associates.

McDougall, G. (1987). The role of the clinical nurse specialist consultant in organizational development. *Clinical Nurse Specialist, 1*(3), 133–139.

Metzger, R. (1995). *Developing a consultation practice.* Newbury Park, CA: Sage.

Monicken, D. (1995). Consultation in advanced practice nursing. In M. Snyder & M. Mirr (Eds.), *Advanced practice nursing: A guide to professional development* (pp. 183–195). New York: Springer.

Ulschak, F., & SnowAntle, S. (1990). *Consultation skills for health care professionals.* San Francisco: Jossey-Bass.

THE CONTEXT
OF NURSING
CONSULTATION

6

Understanding Communities

We are capable of creating wonderful and vibrant communities when we discover what dreams of possibilities we share. (Wheatley & Kellner-Rogers, 1998)

 KEY CONCEPTS:

community, organization, open system, culture, power, frame

 KEY TERMS FOR YOUR SEARCH ENGINE:

community (or organization) and culture, community (or organization) and power, open systems theory, nursing and theory

INTRODUCTION

Entering a new setting can be overwhelming, particularly when you have a specific task to accomplish in only a limited period of time. Think of the last time you entered an unfamiliar setting; perhaps you were starting a new job or returning to school. Think, too, how much easier it would have been to enter this setting if you had some sense of what the setting was *really* like. Because all settings are complex, ambiguous, and full of conflict, it is easy for a newcomer to experience frustration, cynicism, powerlessness, and failure (Bolman & Deal, 1991). Nurse consultants work with, on behalf of, and within communities and experience these feelings every time they begin a new consultation relationship. For nurse consultants, understanding a com-

munity can both alleviate these feelings of frustration and facilitate a successful consultation outcome.

Recall, from Chapter 2, that a community is a group of people who not only share time and space, but also share a history, language, culture (in the broadest sense of the word), sense of purpose, interests, and responsibilities. In fact, a community is shaped more by the interactions and quality of relationships among its members than by the geography they share (Anderson & McFarlane, 2000). Based on this definition, an organization, a neighborhood, a unit within a hospital, a community agency, a school, a support group, or persons who share the same diagnosis can be considered a community.

In a nursing consultation relationship, a community can be the consultee, the client, or the problem setting. Regardless of the role a community plays in a specific consultation situation, understanding the characteristics, or "personality," of the community increases the likelihood that the consultation relationship will be efficient and effective. Without this understanding, a nurse consultant may attribute problems to the wrong cause or develop an action plan that is incomplete or simply incompatible with the characteristics of the community. In fact, without this understanding, a nurse consultant may never even accomplish psychological entry. (Psychological entry was defined in Chapter 3 and is discussed in depth in Chapter 9.) Savvy nurse consultants can also capitalize on a community's characteristics to enhance a nursing consultation relationship. For nurse consultants, the ability to understand a community and answer the question "What *really* is going on here?" is an essential skill.

The content in this chapter is a combination of (a) traditional organizational theory content that has been "translated" to apply to communities and (b) community health nursing concepts. This makes sense both because organizations are one type of community and because needs and opportunities for nursing consultation are moving out of organizational settings and into communities. It is beyond the scope of this chapter to present all theories and perspectives on communities. Instead, the focus of this chapter is providing enough practical information to enable nurses to function professionally and effectively as consultants with, for, or within a community. This focus is consistent with the goal of this text: teaching and promoting the specific knowledge and skills of nursing consultation as a framework for working with communities. The references at the end of the chapter are excellent resources for reading more about the nature of communities and organizations.

This chapter begins by presenting open systems theory as an overarching description of communities and how they function. Next, culture and power, two key attributes of communities that are particularly important in nursing consultation relationships, are discussed. The final section of this chapter introduces the concept of "frames" as a means of both synthesizing the characteristics of a community and gaining additional perspective on a community. As you read this chapter, think about the following questions:

- How do a community's characteristics affect the nursing consultation relationship? Think specifically about the effect of a community's characteristics on a nurse consultant's access to information, choice of interaction pattern, and selection of a problem solution.
- What are your own beliefs and biases about communities? What implications might these have for your practice of nursing consultation?

COMMUNITIES AS OPEN SYSTEMS

Open systems theory is a broad-based perspective on organizations that is derived from attempts to understand biological events (Dougherty, 1995). Open systems theory views organizations as living organisms striving to adapt and respond to their environments, and having varying degrees of success in doing so.

An open systems perspective is the one used most frequently by consultants (Ridley & Mendoza, 1993). Open systems theory also undergirds several nursing theories, such as those of Imogene King, Betty Neuman, and Sister Callista Roy. The perspective cuts across all other organizational perspectives and is generally considered the best perspective available for conceptualizing an organization as a complex and dynamic whole. Because organizations are one type of community, this perspective is equally helpful for understanding communities.

Features of Open Systems

Open systems are characterized by internal and external environments that shape the "personality" of the system. Open systems are also characterized by a set of attributes or functional components, including subsystems that interact with one another to help the system respond to its environments and accomplish its goals. Finally, open systems have a set of properties or "behaviors" that describe how their subsystems interact and how the system as a whole interacts with its environments. Each of these features of open systems, as they apply to communities, will be discussed in turn.

Open System Environments

An open system has both internal and external environments.

Internal Environment. An open system's internal environment is comprised of its population, subsystems, and culture. The population of an open system (i.e., a community's residents) is considered its core (Anderson & McFarlane, 2000). The population's demographics, values, beliefs, and history have a major influence on the community's culture and power structure (both of which are discussed in later sections of this chapter), goals, problems, and problem-solving resources and preferences. Members of a community form groups such as families, neighborhoods, and worksites. They are also members of the community's various subsystems, each of which contributes in its own way to the community's overall well-being. Community subsystems are described in a separate section of this chapter.

A community's populations can also be conceptualized as an energy field (Helvie, 1998) that affects and is affected by the energy exchanges that occur among the community's subsystems and between the community and its external environments. As an energy field, a community's residents determine the community's activity, vigor, resilience, capabilities, and capacity to do the work of maintaining its health and achieving its goals.

External Environments. As systems, communities are embedded in two layers of environment. The *task environment* is the external conditions that affect a community's functioning on a day-to-day basis (Harrison, 1994). Examples of components of a community's task environment includes its physical location (e.g., climate and geography), availability of needed resources (including funding and manpower), collaborative partners, regulators (such as tax laws, zoning policies, pollution controls), and funding sources. The *general environment* is the more removed external conditions that have either ongoing and long-term or infrequent effects on a community and its task environment. The general environment includes influences such as social trends, the economy, the legal system, the general state of scientific and technologic knowledge, and social institutions such as Medicaid or the family (Harrison, 1994).

Attributes of Open Systems

Open systems have a set of tasks or responsibilities they must fulfill if the system is to survive and thrive. Another attribute of open systems is its arrangement of subsystems.

Outputs. Outputs are the products, services, or ideas that result from the interactions of a system's residents with its internal and external environments. Outputs are sometimes thought of as a system's reason for existence (Harrison, 1994). The output of a hospital is health care services, the output of a school is education, and the output of a community neighborhood is safety and security for its residents. A system's outputs must be of sufficient quantity and quality and must be needed by its external environments.

Inputs. Inputs are the resources a system needs from its environments to create its outputs. Inputs can be raw materials, people (i.e., human resources), financial resources, information, and legal authorizations. If a system is to survive, inputs must be accessible, available in the needed quantity, and have the needed characteristics.

Technology. Technology refers to how a system transforms inputs into outputs. In a hospital, technology refers to the procedures and services offered by the hospital. In a school, technology would include teaching strategies and educational technology. In a neighborhood, technology would include the strategies used by the neighborhood to promote the safety, security, and general well-being of its residents.

Goals. Goals are future states sought by a system's dominant decision makers (Harrison, 1994). Health may or may not be the primary goal of a system; however, it is always at least an intermediary goal because it is an important resource that affects a system's ability to meet its ultimate goal (Anderson & McFarlane, 2000). Every community defines health in its own unique way. An organization might define health in terms of financial well-being or market share. A neighborhood might define health in terms of its crime rate. A city might define health in terms of population growth. Community theorists define community health as an efficient range of adaptability, balanced energies, and the ability to engage in effective problem solving (Helvie, 1998). A healthy community is able to respond to its own developmental needs as well as those of its members, cope with system and member "breakdowns," and modify itself to meet its own changing needs (Anderson & McFarlane, 2000).

Behavior and Processes. A community's behavior and processes are the prevailing patterns of behavior, interactions, and relations among its members. These behaviors and processes include activities such as cooperation, conflict, communication patterns, power relations, information gathering, decision making, and problem solving.

Structure. The final generally recognized attribute of a system is its structure. A system's structure is the enduring relationships among its members and the means by which these relationships are maintained (Harrison, 1994). Thus, a community's structure includes how its members organize or arrange themselves into subsystems to pursue the community's goals, as well as the policies, procedures, and processes that direct how these groupings of a community's residents interact with one another and carry out their tasks. Eight different subsystems are usually recognized in a community: physical environment, education, safety and transportation, politics and government, health and social services, communication, economics, and recreation (Anderson & McFarlane, 2000). Figure 6-1 depicts the attributes of an open system.

Properties of Open Systems

In addition to having the attributes previously described, open systems are characterized by a set of "properties" or behavioral characteristics.

First and foremost, the internal and external components of an open system are interrelated and influence one another through a bidirectional exchange of energy (Bolman & Deal, 1991; Fuqua & Kurpius, 1993; Harrison, 1994; Helvie, 1998). This means that the health of a community is influenced by its population and internal environments as well as by its external environments. Conversely, community and population activities affect the health of the environment (Anderson & McFarlane, 2000). Developments in one part of a system can, thus, have far-reaching effects. For example, new regulations (external environment) about air quality could affect bus service (safety and transportation subsystem) and access to preventive health services. This could result in a decrease in community productivity because of poorer health among the community's population. In turn, this decreased productivity could decrease

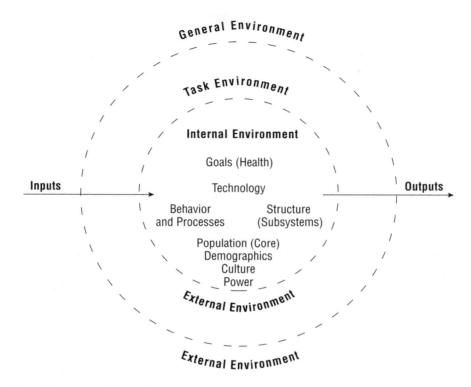

Figure 6-1   Attributes of Open Systems.
These attributes of an open system (such as a community) define its personality, describe the system's tasks and responsibilities, and identify factors that explain its operating style.

the revenue available for funding social and health services at the very time there is likely to be more of a demand for these services.

A second property of open systems, closely related to the first, is their hierarchical arrangement (Bolman & Deal, 1991; Harrison, 1994). Thus, every component of an open system is at once a supersystem or environment for the subsystems or components it contains and a subsystem for the systems in which it is embedded. In a hierarchy of systems, a neighborhood community would be a supersystem in relation to families and a subsystem in relation to a city.

The interrelatedness of a system's components gives rise to the third property of open systems: A system is more than and different from the sum of its parts (Bolman & Deal, 1991). The nature of a community as a whole is a product of the relationships among its population and with its environments. A bereavement support group, for example, is a product of the group's members and their histories and personalities, where and when the group meets, and the resources (e.g., time, information, leadership) available to the group.

A fourth property of an open system is its ability to be somewhat selective about what it imports from and exports to the environment. In fact, communities survive because they have more energy concentrated inside than they exchange with their environments (Helvie, 1998). If a community takes in too much energy from its environment (e.g., state funding for social service programs), it can become dependent on the environment for survival. On the other hand, if a community lets out too much energy, it can become energy depleted and lack the reserves needed to respond to crisis situations.

The ability to selectively exchange energy with its environments accounts for the fifth property of open systems: Open systems are capable of "negative entropy." This means that an open system can grow and survive rather than decline and die, if it is able to work out a mutually beneficial relationship with its environments (Bolman & Deal, 1991). The capacity of negative entropy is illustrated in health care when a small rural hospital responds to the changing needs and demographics of its external environment by changing its services—adding long-term care beds, for instance—rather than closing its doors.

A sixth property of open systems is that they are constantly in a state a dynamic equilibrium. More specifically, an open system strives to maintain a steady state in environments that are constantly changing (Bolman & Deal, 1991). Change can be reactive and in response to a problem, or it can be anticipatory and aimed at improving conditions before problems arise (Harrison, 1994). The well-being of a community depends on its ability to adapt to its environments and manage its subsystems (Helvie, 1998).

The final property that characterizes an open system is "equifinality." Because systems are comprised of highly interactive components, many paths can lead to the same result (Fuqua & Kurpius, 1993). This means that communities have options in terms of how they achieve their goals and maintain a steady state. For example, if it is not feasible to address teen gang activity and increase community well-being by imposing a curfew and working through the government and politics subsystem, it may be possible to achieve the same result by working through the recreational subsystem.

Box 6-1 summarizes the properties of open systems.

Implications for Nursing Consultation

A systems perspective is useful to nurse consultants because it encourages consideration of all parts of a community, as well as their

BOX 6-1   THE PROPERTIES OF OPEN SYSTEMS

- The internal and external components of an open system are interrelated and influence one another through a bidirectional exchange of energy.
- Every system is a hierarchical arrangement of subsystems and supersystems.
- A system is more than and different from the sum of its parts.
- System components communicate selectively with their environments.
- Open systems are capable of negative entropy; that is, they have a survival and growth orientation.
- Open systems strive to maintain a dynamic equilibrium; they engage in both reactive and anticipatory change.
- The property of equifinality means a system has options for achieving its goals and maintaining a steady state; that is, in an open system, many paths can lead to the same result.

interactions and level of functioning. Because problems are viewed as part of a complex chain of possible events and interactions, a system perspective helps a nurse consultant more accurately diagnose the cause of a community's problem. A system perspective (i.e., "systems thinking") reminds a nurse consultant that "there is no outside" and that the community and the cause of its problems are part of a single system (Senge, 1990).

Systems thinking also helps a nurse consultant develop more effective interventions for resolving a consultation problem. Because of the interaction or chain of influence that exists among a system's subsystems, different consultation interventions may accomplish the same end results. If one proposed intervention is unacceptable to a consultee or is not feasible for the community, a systems perspective allows the nurse consultant to consider other interventions that might accomplish the same goal. As Senge (1990) points out, systems thinking "shows that small, well-focused actions can sometimes produce significant, enduring improvements if they are in the right place."

Furthermore, systems thinking facilitates the development of more effective problem solutions because it forces a nurse consultant to consider how a specific problem-solving strategy will affect other parts of the community. Anticipating how a problem solution will affect the various subsystems in a community decreases the likelihood that the consultation process will be disrupted because of adverse "side effects."

A final advantage of a systems perspective of communities is that during the evaluation phase of the nursing consultation process, it encourages the nurse consultant to look for a variety of possible indicators of success. Recognizing that success can be demonstrated in multiple ways increases the likelihood that a community will realize enhanced well-being as a result of the consultation relationship. This is because most nursing consultation relationships will have a positive effect somewhere in the system, even if the original nursing consultation problem is not completely resolved. For example, as a result of the nursing consultation relationship, a community may mobilize resources in its political subsystem that continue to be active once the crisis phase of a problem (e.g., deaths among a city's homeless during a cold spell of weather) is over, even if a problem (e.g., homelessness) remains.

Box 6-2 gives guidelines for assessing a community as an open system.

CULTURE AND COMMUNITIES

Culture is a key feature of an open system's internal environment. Culture is more than ethnicity or membership in a specific subgroup, although different groups (e.g., defined by ethnicity, income, employment, etc.) may have their own culture. A community's culture is the pattern of values, beliefs, patterns of thinking, actions, and artifacts that define for its members who they are and how they are supposed to do things (Bolman & Deal, 1991). These patterns reflect the basic assumptions that the community has developed over time as it has learned how to interact with its environments. A community's culture represents its accumulated wisdom. This wisdom is continually being renewed, altered, and recreated as new members enter the community.

A community's culture serves several purposes. First, culture functions as a type of behavioral control. It does this by implicitly mandating, allowing, and prohibiting certain behaviors. A strong culture operates as an informal system of rules that spells out how people are supposed to act most of the time. A second purpose served by a community's culture is integration. Culture fosters a sense of identity, thus creating "buy-in" to the community's goals and operating decisions. A

BOX 6-2   LOOKING FOR PROBLEM CAUSES: AN OPEN SYSTEMS PERSPECTIVE

Explanations for a community's problems can often be identified by gathering the following information about its components:

Environment

- Affiliation and ownership: Associated benefits and constraints
- Physical and social surroundings
- Recent or anticipated changes

Outputs

- Quantity
- Quality
- Responsiveness to consumer needs and desires

Inputs

- Availability
- Quality
- Access issues: Timeliness, seasonal variation
- Cost—does high price of inputs strain other parts of the system?
- Reserves and their liquidity

Technology

- Cost
- Efficiency: Accidents, waste, downtime

Goals

- Official goal statements
- Plans for achieving goals—are they realistic?
- Budget patterns and their consistency with goals
- Consistency of strategies with goals, resources, and culture

Behavior and Processes

- Communication patterns
- Decision-making practices

Structure

- Arrangement of the system: Subsystems, units, levels of hierarchy
- Control mechanisms: Policies, procedures, rewards, punishments, communication

community's culture also provides a framework that helps its members uniformly interpret situations they encounter. As an example, an organization's culture influences the extent to which a potentially threatening event, such as a power shortage or budget crisis or the shutdown of a public clinic, is perceived as an overwhelming and unsolveable problem or as an opportunity for creativity and growth.

Reading a Community's Culture

"Reading" or assessing a community's culture involves gathering clues and drawing conclusions about the cultural meaning of these clues. Because clues can be interpreted in many ways and can contradict one another, it is important to validate the accuracy of any conclusion about a community's culture with its members. It is equally important to forgo the temptation to assume specific cultural attributes (i.e., stereotype) on the basis of such superficial characteristics as a community's predominant ethnicity.

Assessing a community's culture is complicated by the fact that much of its culture operates on an unconscious level and is taken for granted by both the community as a whole and its members. Consequently, a nurse consultant must rely on observing symbolic artifacts (tangible, visible indicators of an organization's culture) for clues about the community's beliefs, values, and assumptions (Hughes, 1990; Kuh, 1993). Cultural artifacts can be material, verbal, or behavioral in nature.

Material Artifacts
Material artifacts are physical indicators of a community's culture. An organization's logo or seal is one example of a material artifact. The inclusion of a cross, for example, on the logo of many health care organizations communicates the traditional association of providing health care with benevolent, charitable, and altruistic motivations (Hughes, 1990). How a community uses space is another material artifact. Yards with high fences versus open gathering spaces may suggest a community value of privacy as opposed to openness (or may suggest safety concerns). The dress and appearance of a community's residents is a third example of a material artifact. This indicator may provide clues about the tolerance of diversity and individualism within the community. Furnishings, decor, bulletin boards, and the like, especially in public buildings, can communicate community values such as pride, care for others, and being oriented toward the future versus the past. The pattern of ethnicity in a community could also be considered a material artifact in that it suggests certain attributes such as the value of time, present versus future orientation, response to outsiders, and so on.

Verbal Artifacts
Examples of verbal artifacts include the written materials (brochures, signage, etc.) a community makes available to outsiders. A community's promotional materials are particularly revealing verbal artifacts as they reflect what the community wants the public—and its members—to believe are its values and beliefs (Kuh, 1993).

Community myths and legends are additional verbal artifacts. Myths and legends are stories that have developed about a community and its history and residents; these stories may or may not be true. Myths help to establish, maintain, and explain certain behaviors and material artifacts within the community. Myths also legitimize certain behaviors, mediate contradictions, communicate unconscious wishes and conflicts, and anchor an organization to its past. Myths often include heroes that personify a community's values and provide role models.

Behavioral Artifacts

Behavioral artifacts include rituals as well as standard community practices. Rituals are systematic routines of day-to-day life. They show what is expected and therefore decrease uncertainty and anxiety among a community's members, especially during times of transition. Rituals also function to socialize new community residents and stabilize the community as a whole (Bolman & Deal, 1991). Rituals communicate values about such things as use of time, productivity, and priorities. Other behavioral artifacts that can provide clues about a community's culture include how the community greets strangers, forms of address, how people spend their time, and how people interact with one another (humor, celebrations, sharing work, sharing food, etc.).

Behavioral artifacts can be evaluated in terms of their consistency with what the community communicates about its culture by means of verbal and material artifacts. When behavioral artifacts conflict with other artifacts, behaviors should be considered the more reliable indicator of the community's culture.

Box 6-3 summarizes the guidelines for assessing a community's culture.

Implications for Nursing Consultation

A nurse consultant who is aware of a community's culture is able to better understand the hidden and complex parts of the community's life. She or he is also less likely to be puzzled, irritated, and anxious when unfamiliar and seemingly irrational behavior is encountered (Schein, 1992).

Knowledge about a community's culture provides a nurse consultant with information about what is permissible when implementing a consultation relationship. Communities vary, for example, in terms of beliefs about how permissible it is to ask for help in solving problems. This cultural belief affects both when in the problem cycle a nurse consultant is likely to be contacted (at the prevention, early intervention, or crisis stage) and the nursing consultation interaction pattern that is most likely to be acceptable to the community. A process consultation interaction pattern, for instance, requires a culture of open-

---

BOX 6-3   GUIDELINES FOR ASSESSING A COMMUNITY'S CULTURE

- Observe artifacts:
  Material artifacts: Use of physical space, furnishings, residents' appearance and attire
  Verbal artifacts: Public relations materials, signage, myths
  Behavioral artifacts: Rituals, standard community practices, interactions among residents and with outsiders
- Consider as many artifacts as possible since some might have more than one possible meaning or may contradict other artifacts.
- Use inductive reasoning (drawing general conclusions from specific observations) to form a cultural profile of the community.
- Verify this profile with residents of the community.
- Refine impressions and gather more information as needed.

ness and assuming personal responsibility for problems and solutions.

Sensitivity to a community's culture enables a nurse consultant to tailor interventions and recommendations to the norms and values of the community. For example, if privacy is a value, assessment and evaluation findings are not likely to be accepted if they are presented in a public forum. Likewise, if self-sufficiency is a priority, a problem solution that is dependent on external funding or resources may not be acceptable. When a nurse consultant's interactions and interventions ignore, or are in direct conflict with, a community's culture, they are likely to create tension, resistance, and frustration for everyone involved in the nursing consultation relationship. As a result of this, the underlying nursing consultation problem will remain unresolved.

Finally, awareness of a community's culture makes good "business sense" for a nurse consultant. A nurse consultant is always a guest in a problem setting, and cultural awareness and sensitivity can decrease the discomfort and feelings of awkwardness often associated with visitor status. Cultural awareness and sensitivity also facilitate gathering needed information, establishing rapport and credibility, and generating an acceptable and successful action plan.

POWER IN COMMUNITIES

Like culture, power is a feature of an open system's internal environment. Power is shaped by a community's culture, its needs, and the characteristics of both its population and external environments.

In a classic and frequently used definition, Yukl (1989) defines power as the capacity to influence someone else's behavior and attitudes. Power is reflected in the ability to get things done. Every member of a community, including a nurse consultant,

has some kind of power. The ability to decipher who in a community has what kind of power helps a nurse consultant identify groups and individuals who can either facilitate or act as barriers to the nursing consultation relationship.

Sources of Power

Generally, two possible sources of power are recognized: positional and personal. These two sources or determinants of power can interact in complex ways. In many cases, it is difficult to determine the sources from which an individual or group derives power. Nonetheless, it is important for a nurse consultant to be able to identify the nature of the power being exercised in a situation since power dynamics and reactions to them are a common cause of community problems.

Positional Power

Positional power is derived from the opportunities that come with an individual's position or formal role within an organization or community (Yukl, 1989). Positional power is usually associated with being a member of the "upper" part of a community's hierarchy. However, members of the "lowerarchy" (Bolman & Deal, 1991) have their own types of positional power.

Formal authority is the most familiar type of positional power and belongs to community members who are in officially sanctioned leadership or management positions. Individuals who have formal authority are entitled to make requests and binding decisions, as well as exercise control to the extent that those under their authority have the duty to obey. Because authority is not associated with an obligation to return favors, it is acceptable as a form of power for day-to-day community functioning. Authority is accepted, however, only when the person or group exercising it is perceived by members of the lowerarchy to be a legitimate occupant of their position of authority.

An individual's position within a community is also associated with control over rewards and punishments. Reward power is effective only when the promised reward is actually bestowed and is perceived as fair exchange for the request that is being made. Coercive power (related to control over punishments) is effective only when it is applied to a small proportion of followers under conditions perceived to be legitimate by the majority of them (Yukl, 1989).

Other specific types of power associated with being a member of a community's upper hierarchy include control over resources and information, ecological control, and orchestration power. Information control is a particularly important type of positional power because individuals who are able to access information also have the ability to distort it and control its distribution.

Individuals in gatekeeper and boundary positions within a community also have positional power. These individuals interact directly with the community's external environments or liaison with other community subsystems on a day-to-day basis. Because of this, they have a certain degree of control over resources and information. Think, for example, of the control an office receptionist has over the number of patients (resources) seen by a health care provider during any given day.

Members of a community's lowerarchy have their own types of positional power. The lowerarchy determines whether and how tasks are actually carried out (implementation power). Members of the lowerarchy also possess "helpless power," the right to expect assistance from individuals who are in a position to render it (Friedman, 1992). Homeless persons, for example, have helpless power in that they have the socially agreed upon right to receive assistance and resources from a community's health and social services subsystem and the general public. Helpless power can become manipulative and problematic when the part of the community that is being asked for help is already drained of resources. Finally, members of the lowerarchy have a certain amount of reward and punishment power. For example, workers can reward their supervisors (enhance the supervisor's image) by doing good work. They can also "punish" their supervisors by giving them unfavorable evaluations.

Personal Power

Personal power is derived from an individual's personal characteristics such as knowledge, special skills, persuasiveness, and the ability to establish rapport, trust, and friendships. Personal power can be possessed by any member of a community. Personal power is important because it can substitute for, enhance, or help an individual acquire positional power.

Expert power is personal power that is derived from an individual's possession of specialized knowledge and skills (i.e., expertise) and the fact that others need this knowledge and skill. Expert power is effective only to the extent that it is recognized and perceived as credible and reliable by others.

Charisma is power that is derived from "emotional attractiveness" (Yukl, 1989). An individual with charisma exudes vision, enthusiasm, and strong convictions, and is able to gather followers through the use of persuasive speaking skills. Charisma enables an individual to build coalitions. Charisma is also associated with the ability or opportunity to define a group's beliefs and values.

The abilities to establish rapport, trust, and friendships are additional types of personal power. Friendship and trust facilitate coalition building, as well as create loyalty and a willingness in others to return favors.

Box 6-4 summarizes the different types of power associated with position and personal qualities.

BOX 6-4   SOURCES OF POWER

Positional Power

Positional power is derived from an individual's position or role within a community. Positional power includes the following types of power:

- Formal authority: The right to make requests and binding decisions
- Control over resources: The ability to access needed community resources
- Control over rewards and punishments: The ability to bestow rewards and impose punishments
- Control over information: The ability to access, distribute, and distort information
- Ecological control: Control over the community's internal physical environment and the organization of work
- Orchestration power: The right to organize and plan tasks
- Implementation power: The ability to determine whether and how tasks are carried out
- Helpless power: The right to expect assistance

Personal Power

Personal power can be possessed by any member of a community and can substitute for, enhance, or help an individual acquire positional power. Personal power includes the following types of power:

- Expertise: Power derived from the dependence of others on an individual for special advice or assistance
- Charisma: Power derived from "emotional attractiveness" and persuasive skills
- Friendship: Power that creates a desire of others to please
- Trust and rapport: Power that facilitates coalition building

Sources: Bolman, L., & Deal, T. (1991). *Reframing organizations: Artistry, choice, and leadership.* San Francisco: Jossey-Bass; and Yukl, G. (1989). *Leadership in organizations* (2nd ed.). Englewood Cliffs, NJ: Prentice Hall.

Assessing Power in a Community

A nurse consultant needs to be able to identify who has what types of power within a community. This information gives the nurse consultant the opportunity to mobilize and create partnerships with individuals in the community who are able to gather followers and cooperation from others.

To a large extent, a nurse consultant needs to piece together information from a variety of observations and reports (including reports of community members) in order to determine who within a community has what kind of power. Symbols of power, such as office location and furnishings or location of an individual on an organizational chart, often correspond to positional power. Job descriptions and titles (e.g., associate versus assistant) also are traditional symbols of positional power. However, it is a mistake to assume that the individual with the symbols of power has the true power within the community. Assigning or delegating tasks, for instance, may suggest authority but may also reflect simple tradition.

The ability to set a community's goals and determine what issues are addressed may be a more accurate indicator of real power. Power outcomes, such as who wins or has the final say, and decision-making processes (such as consensus or compromise and who agrees with whom) also tend to be accurate indicators of who has real influence within a community. Compromise, for example, may indicate the ability of the lowerarchy to overrule the hierarchy. Consensus reflects the ability to form coalitions and most likely results from personal rather than positional power.

Box 6-5 lists questions for assessing power in communities.

Implications for Nursing Consultation

Recognizing and understanding power dynamics can help a nurse consultant explain many community problems. For example, conflict can occur in a community when a member of the lowerarchy who has personal power threatens the power of someone in a position of formal authority. Efficiency problems might be attributable to a person in a boundary position who is exercising inappropriate control over resources. Finally, low morale or a lack of community cohesiveness might be traced to problems with a lack of information. A nurse consultant could respond to these problems that are related to a community's power dynamics in the following ways:

- Help the person in a position of formal authority acquire personal skills that will enhance his or her positional power
- Clarify roles and responsibilities in relation to control over resources
- Enhance the timeliness and availability of information

An understanding of power dynamics also enables a nurse consultant to recognize and capitalize on the power associated with the consultant role. Because the nursing consultation relationship is a time-limited one, nurse consultants lack any positional power of their

BOX 6-5   QUESTIONS FOR ASSESSING POWER IN COMMUNITIES

- Who do organizational charts or a community's charter identify as being in positions of power?
- Who is in boundary positions? How much control do they have over information and other scarce resources?
- With whom are traditional symbols of power associated?
- Who gives the "orders"?
- Who wins or has the final say?
- Who controls decision-making processes?
- Who sets agendas?
- Who agrees or compromises with whom?

own. The nurse consultant's power is derived instead from a combination of personal qualities and the ability to recognize and become aligned with persons in the community who have positional power and can legitimize the nursing consultation relationship.

Nurse consultants are most frequently asked to work with a community to address a problem because of their perceived expertise, and for this reason it is important for nurse consultants to understand the limitations of expert power. Expert power is effective only to the extent that consultees lack the knowledge and skills needed to solve a problem on their own. Thus, as a nursing consultation relationship progresses and consultees gain more skill in managing their own problems, expertise becomes less effective as a source of power for maintaining the nursing consultation relationship. (However, as Chapter 14 discusses, consultee skill in managing the consultation problem on their own can be a signal to begin the disengagement phase of the nursing consultation relationship.) Moreover, expert power can be initially intimidating to a consultee, especially if it increases the consultee's feeling of inadequacy. Because of these limitations of expert power, a nurse consultant needs to cultivate other forms of personal power, such as charisma, friendship, and trust, in order to establish and maintain an effective working relationship with a client system. Finally, nurse consultants need to learn how to supplement their personal power by building coalitions with the individuals in a community who have different types of positional power.

THE CONCEPT OF FRAMES

Open systems theory explains organizations in terms of interacting components. While this is one explanation for how organizations and communities work and what makes them effective or ineffective, it is not the only explanation. In fact, viewing a community from only an open systems perspective fails to acknowledge the other beliefs, assumptions, and motivations that can account for its behavior. A more complete picture of a community can be gained by viewing it from additional vantage points or "frames" (Bolman & Deal, 1991).

A *frame* can be thought of as a window on the world or a lens that helps bring the world into focus. Each of us—and every community, as well—has a personal frame that we use to make judgments and determine how to get things done. A frame, then, can be thought of as a preferred perspective.

The major schools of organizational thought can be consolidated into four frames, each of which focuses on a different dimension of an organization. Superimposing these frames on an open systems perspective of a community increases the nurse consultant's ability to appreciate the complexity of community life. This, in turn, increases the likelihood that a nurse consultant will accurately diagnose a community's problem and generate meaningful, feasible, and acceptable problem solutions.

The Structural Frame

The structural frame emphasizes the link between the formal roles and relationships within a community (the structural component of an open system) and the community's ability to achieve its goals (Bolman & Deal, 1991). Communities that view themselves through a structural frame create structures to fit their environments. For example, a community may establish rules, policies, task forces, and hierarchies. These communities tend to experience problems when their structures fail to fit the situation. Their preferred way of resolving problems is "restructuring": developing new policies, procedures, and governing systems.

The Human Resource Frame

This frame emphasizes the interdependence between a community and its members. It recognizes that communities are inhabited by individuals with unique needs, abilities, beliefs, and attitudes (Bolman & Deal, 1991). Communities that operate through a human resource frame maintain that the key to their well-being is a good fit between the needs of the community as a whole and the needs of its residents. Conversely, when there is a poor fit between the community and its residents, one or both will suffer: Individuals will be exploited or will seek to exploit the community, or both (Bolman & Deal, 1991). Thus, the human resource frame emphasizes the importance of the relationship between the open system components of behavior and processes and human resource inputs (including satisfaction) on one hand, and technology, goals, and structures on the other.

Communities with a human resource perspective try to solve their problems by changing the community's form (behavior and processes, structure) in such a way that enables people to contribute to the community and feel good about what they are doing. Offering education and training, adding more services, and changing the community's reward structure are examples of consultation interventions that are consistent with the human resource frame.

The Political Frame

The political frame views communities as "arenas" in which groups compete for power and scarce resources (Bolman & Deal, 1991). This frame attaches particular importance to both the structural and behavior/process components of an open system. The political frame emphasizes that conflict is a fact of life because of differences in the needs and perspectives of a community's various members. The political frame asserts that community well-being is the result of the community's ability to effectively negotiate, build coalitions, bargain, and compromise with its residents and subsystems and with its external environments. Communities working from a political frame may experience problems because power is either concentrated in the wrong places or is so broadly dispersed that nothing gets accomplished. Problems are solved by changing the power dynamics in the community.

The Symbolic Frame

The final frame identified by Bolman and Deal (1991)—the symbolic frame—emphasizes the importance of a system's culture. The symbolic frame differs from the other frames because it asserts that communities are not rational and that community leaders have only a limited ability to create community well-being through power, processes, or structures. The symbolic frame views communities as cultures driven by images and rituals rather than by rules and authority. From a symbolic perspective, a community will experience problems when "actors play their parts badly, symbols lose their meaning, and ceremonies and rituals lose their potency" (Bolman & Deal, 1991). This frame asserts that communities can best address their problems by rebuilding their culture.

Box 6-6 summarizes the key attributes of these four organizational frames.

Implications for Nursing Consultation

The capacity to view a community through multiple frames enhances a nurse consultant's ability to accurately diagnose a community's problems and arrive at effective problem solutions. In contrast, a single frame captures only a part of a community's picture. Because each frame has its blind spots and biases, no single

BOX 6-6   FRAMES: ALTERNATIVE VIEWS OF COMMUNITIES

The Structural Frame

- Emphasis: Rules, policies, managerial hierarchy, division of labor
- Problem explanations: Poor fit between a system's structural components and its environment and technology
- Preferred problem solutions: Restructuring
- Open systems components reflected in frame: Structure, environments, technology

The Human Resource Frame

- Emphasis: Interdependence between a community and its residents
- Problem explanations: Poor fit between the needs of the community as a whole and the needs of its residents
- Preferred problem solutions: Change the community's structure and processes to meet resident's needs
- Open systems components reflected in frame: Inputs (human resources), technology, goals, behavior and processes, structure

The Political Frame

- Emphasis: Conflict, power
- Problem explanations: Power concentrated in the wrong places or too widely dispersed
- Preferred problem solutions: Change power dynamics; negotiate, compromise, build coalitions
- Open systems components reflected in frame: Behavior and processes, structure

The Symbolic Frame

- Emphasis: A community's culture and its symbolic rather than rational nature
- Problem explanations: Symbols lose their meaning, rituals lose their potency, "actors play their parts badly"
- Preferred problem solutions: Rebuild or reinforce the community's culture
- Open systems components reflected in frame: Behavior and processes, structure

---

frame is comprehensive enough to make a community truly understandable or manageable. The following examples demonstrate a nurse consultant using only a single frame to approach the problem of low morale in a public health department. Note how a "single-frame approach" can limit the scope of a problem solution.

- *Structural frame:* "As the city and the department have grown, nurses' responsibilities have become blurred. Frequently, it is unclear which unit within the department is responsible for what. This is causing stress and conflict. You need to restructure. Let's start by drawing a new organizational chart. Then we'll tackle policies and procedures."

BOX 6-7   LOOKING FOR PROBLEM CAUSES: USING MULTIPLE FRAMES

Structure-Oriented Questions

- What is the community's structural arrangement (subsystems, levels of hierarchy)?
- How is the community's structure maintained?
- Is the community's structure "in sync" with its internal and external environments?
- What effects does the community's structure have on its cohesiveness and ability to interact with its environment (procure inputs, dispense outputs)?

Human Resource–Oriented Questions

- To what extent do people feel a part of the community?
- To what extent are members' needs met by the community?
- How could processes and structures be changed so that needs are better met?

Political-Oriented Questions

- What are the resources that are scarce in this community?
- How are problems related to scarce resources handled (conflict, compromise, negotiation)?
- Who is best able to obtain scarce resources? How do they do this? What conflicts does this create?

Symbolic-Oriented Questions

- What is the community's identity? How is this identity communicated? Is the identity clear? Is it universally shared?
- What values are reflected in the community's identity? Are these the values really held by the community and its residents?
- How is the community's identity reinforced (symbols, rituals, and so forth)? Are these strategies effective?
- How could the community's structure and behavior and processes be altered to strengthen its culture and symbolic dimension?

- *Human resource frame:* "You are ignoring the nurses' needs to feel autonomous and valued. Let's put together some workshops on communication and look at some sort of an incentive system."
- *Political frame:* "The real problem is that the medical director and county health board have too much power and the staff nurses

and community residents have too little. We need to bring these parties together to negotiate and compromise."
- *Symbolic frame:* "Rapid growth has caused the department to lose its identity. Its values have also become unclear—is it environmental health or population health or services to individuals that is of primary inter-

est? Let's try to revitalize the department's sense of identity and purpose. We'll start by designing a new logo."

In contrast, the nurse consultant who uses all four frames and open systems theory to approach this problem might respond as follows:

This is a complex problem. As the city has grown, the department has had to grow, and roles and relationships have changed. The addition of more staff has also changed the department's culture and power structure. Old ways of doing things and relating don't work anymore. We need to make sure we address all of these problems. Otherwise, we will only put a band-aid on the problem and the band-aid will fall off in a couple of days. Let's start by meeting with the staff to find out what they identify as the key issue. Then we will hold a town hall meeting for the community. We'll go from there . . ."

In summary, the nurse consultant who can view a community through multiple frames has a more flexible and comprehensive approach to problem solving. Hence, problem solutions are more likely to be meaningful and feasible and have longevity. Moreover, a nurse consultant who can help a community to see itself through multiple frames is teaching the community valuable self-assessment and self-help strategies.

Box 6-7 provides examples of questions a nurse consultant can use to approach a community and its consultation problem from multiple frames.

CHAPTER SUMMARY

Nurse consultants work with, on behalf of, and within communities. How a nurse consultant looks at a community and how much is understood about what is *really* going on within the community determines how successful the nursing consultation relationship will be. Viewing a community through multiple frames (including open systems theory), being aware of its culture, and understanding its power structure can help the nurse consultant gain entry to, as well as problem solve more effectively with, the community. If ignored, these key characteristics of a community can act as barriers to effective nursing consultation. On the other hand, the nurse consultant who is aware of a community's unique characteristics and their relationship to a specific problem situation can at least accommodate and, possibly, mobilize these characteristics and individualize a problem solution to increase the effectiveness of the consultation relationship.

APPLYING CHAPTER CONTENT

1. Use an open systems perspective to diagram your neighborhood. Identify who within this system has what kind of power. What types of consultation problems are likely to arise in this system? How would the components of this system act as facilitators and barriers to the nursing consultation process?

2. Examine promotional materials from your community or from several community health-oriented agencies. What do these materials communicate about the community or agency's culture? Is the culture conveyed by these verbal artifacts consistent with material and behavioral artifacts you have observed?

3. Consider the frames that were discussed in this chapter. Which frame do you think your neighborhood uses to see itself? Can you identify any current health-related problems in your neighborhood that are related to this frame? Which frame do you find most appealing? How might this influence your effectiveness as a nurse consultant?

References

Anderson, T., & McFarlane, J. (2000). *Community as partner: Theory and practice in nursing* (3rd ed.). Philadelphia: Lippincott.

Bolman, L., & Deal, T. (1991). *Reframing organizations: Artistry, choice, and leadership.* San Francisco: Jossey-Bass.

Dougherty, A. (1995). *Consultation: Practice and perspectives in school and community settings* (2nd ed.). Pacific Grove, CA: Brooks-Cole.

Friedman, M. (1992). *Family nursing: Theory and practice* (3rd ed.). Norwalk, CT: Appleton & Lange.

Fuqua, D., & Kurpius, D. (1993). Conceptual models in organizational consultation. *Journal of Counseling and Development, 71,* 607–618.

Harrison, M. (1994). *Diagnosing organizations: Methods, models, and processes* (2nd ed.). Thousand Oaks, CA: Sage.

Helvie, C. (1998). *Advanced practice nursing in the community.* Thousand Oaks, CA: Sage.

Hughes, L. (1990). Assessing organizational culture: Strategies for the external consultant. *Nursing Forum, 25*(1), 15–19.

Kuh, G. (1993). Appraising the character of a college. *Journal of Counseling and Development, 71,* 661–667.

Ridley, C., & Mendoza, D. (1993). Putting organizational effectiveness into practice: The preeminent consultation task. *Journal of Counseling and Development, 72,* 168–177.

Schein, E. (1992). *Organizational culture and leadership* (2nd ed.). San Francisco: Jossey-Bass.

Senge, P. (1990). *The fifth discipline: The art and practice of the learning organization.* New York: Currency-Doubleday.

Wheatley, M., & Kellner-Rogers, M. (1998). The paradox and promise of communities. In F. Hesselbein, M. Goldsmith, R. Beckhard, & R. Schubert (Eds.), *The community of the future* (pp. 9–18). San Francisco: Jossey-Bass.

Yukl, G. (1989). *Leadership in organizations* (2nd ed.). Englewood Cliffs, NJ: Prentice Hall.

Human Dynamics in Community Groups

It is evident that health in this country cannot be improved by the mere provision of health services, but needs to be based on principles of equity, participation, and involvement of communities in making decisions about health care. (Anderson & McFarlane, 2000)

 KEY CONCEPTS:

task roles, personal roles, counteractive influence, groupthink, team

---

 KEY TERMS FOR YOUR SEARCH ENGINE:

community and dynamics, groupthink

INTRODUCTION

Being a member of a group can be stressful. "Have I been accepted?" and "What am I supposed to do?" are just two of the many questions that group members frequently have. Working with a group to help its members accomplish a specific task can also be stressful. Nurse consultants frequently work in this capacity with groups of consultees or on behalf of client groups such as communities. Indeed, a premise of a community perspective in health is that "Partnerships between community members and health professionals are critical for collaborative decision-making in order to improve health" (Anderson & McFar-

lane, 2000). Questions that nurse consultants need to be able to answer when implementing the nursing consultation process with a group include "What really is happening here?" "Why do people behave the way they do?" and "What can I do about it?"

Working with a group to problem solve and implement change has both advantages and disadvantages. On the one hand, groups have greater cumulative knowledge and diversity of perspective, as well as more time and energy than individuals. Community partnerships work because they integrate ideas, people, and resources, in both the problem-solving and intervention implementation process, from the community's perspective (Anderson & McFarlane, 2000). Groups, therefore, can be very creative, productive, and stimulating.

On the other hand, groups have certain liabilities. They can be stagnant and conformist. Too often, groups overrespond to social pressures or allow personal goals or needs of group members to undermine the group's purpose (Bolman & Deal, 1991). In fact, too often groups are "antiholistic" (Robbins & Finley, 1996), and optimal group productivity is rarely attained because of faulty social processes (Oyster, 2000). A nurse consultant working with a group must be able to understand group dynamics and intervene to facilitate effective functioning of the group if the nursing consultation relationship is to be successful.

A group's dynamics have a decisive influence on the work it is able to accomplish. The dynamics observed in groups reflect issues related to group members' roles and functions, group norms, intragroup cooperation and cohesiveness, and the exercise of influence within the group (Bolman & Deal, 1991; Goodstein, 1978; Oyster, 2000). How these issues affect both individual group members and the group as a whole can be observed in a group's communication and decision-making processes. These issues and the ways in which group members respond to them, both individually and collectively, constitute a group's dynamics.

Much has been written in nursing literature about group dynamics. Most of these discussions have either a mental health (nurse as

therapist) or management (nurse as supervisor) perspective. The nurse consultant–consultee relationship is, in contrast, a peer relationship; this influences the group dynamics that will be observed and has implications for appropriate interventions.

This chapter begins with an overview of group characteristics, group behavior, and explanations of group behavior. The discussion that follows centers around what a nurse consultant can learn from observing a group. The chapter then focuses on two different group situations that a nurse consultant will likely encounter: building a work group and working with an established group. The final section of the chapter discusses teams as a specific type of group. Some questions to think about as you read this chapter are:

- What is your own preferred role in a group? What implications might this have when you work with a group as a nurse consultant?
- What would be the advantages and disadvantages of working with a group of consultees as an internal and external nurse consultant?
- Does any one nursing consultation interaction pattern seem most appropriate for situations in which the consultee is a group?
- What different nursing consultation roles and skills are needed for working with individuals and groups? Which of these are strengths and weaknesses for you?

UNDERSTANDING GROUP BEHAVIOR

Understanding groups and group behavior is facilitated by an understanding of communities. Because groups are microcosms of larger communities, they share all of the same problems seen in larger communities: interpersonal friction, emotional outbursts, confusion,

competing agendas, power struggles, conflict, and disputes over resources and values. Groups also face the same structural issues as communities: how to divide responsibilities and how to integrate diverse activities into a unified whole (Bolman & Deal, 1991). Finally, like a community, any group may (and usually does) serve more than one purpose at a time. In fact, a group may serve a different purpose for different group members (Sampson & Marthas, 1990). Understanding a group's behavior—its dynamics—is facilitated by understanding the forces that influence group behaviors, group functions, levels of behavior in groups, and the relationship between interactions and influence in groups.

Forces that Influence Group Behavior

Groups mirror communities that are open systems. (Chapter 6 discusses characteristics of open systems in detail.) Groups consist of subsystems—dyads, triads, and individuals—and are embedded in the suprasystem or environment of the larger community. A group's behavior, then, is influenced by the community of which it is a part, as well as by the characteristics of its members (Harrison, 1994).

Consider an outreach clinic that is sponsored by a church (i.e., a faith community). The clinic's functioning is influenced by the characteristics of the larger community and the church, as well as by the characteristics of the people who work in the clinic and the people who use the clinic's services. Characteristics of the church that could influence the clinic's functioning include its governing structure and style (viewing itself through a human resource rather than structural frame), size, mission, goals, values, beliefs about the relationship between spirituality and health, and policies. Provider (group member) characteristics that might influence the clinic's behavior and functioning are the mix of workers (nurse practitioner, physician, physician's assistant, etc.), years of work experience, individual personalities (e.g., mix of type A and type B personalities), and individual spiritual belief systems.

Consider, as a second example, how a neighborhood action committee would be influenced by both its environment (urban, suburban, or rural) and group member characteristics (such as age, gender, ethnicity and related culture, how long they have lived in the neighborhood). Because of the way in which a group's members interact and influence one another, a group, like a community system, is more than and different from the sum of its parts. A single clinic or neighborhood group, then, is something unique in and of itself and more than just a collection of individuals.

Like communities, groups are influenced by norms and culture. As discussed in Chapter 6, culture is not always easy to identify, but it has a strong influence on the perceptions, feelings, and behaviors of a group's members. A group's culture is reflected, in part, by its norms. Norms are assumptions and expectations about behavior that is appropriate or inappropriate in a specific situation (Oyster, 2000; Schein, 1988). An example of norm-driven behavior would be a community's practice of dealing with its problems by forming task forces rather than waiting for assistance and intervention from the city. This practice reflects norms of trust, autonomy, and perhaps efficiency. In a support group, referring to each member by only their first name could reflect a norm of informality.

Other group and community characteristics that influence, and in fact enhance, group behavior and effectiveness include the following:

- Cooperation and a sense of cohesiveness among group members and between the group and its parent community
- Honest communication that cuts across the community's sectors and levels of hierarchy
- A group norm that supports productivity
- Participative supervision that is both task oriented and supportive of individual effort and learning (Harrison, 1994).

Cohesiveness is a group characteristic that deserves special mention because it can have both positive and negative effects on a group's behavior. When group cohesiveness is high, group members express security, solidarity, mutual liking, and positive feelings about the group's purpose as well as its routine tasks (Janis, 1982). High cohesiveness is also associated with higher levels of self-esteem among individual group members, increased member participation, increased acceptance of goals, and increased productivity (Oyster, 2000). Cohesiveness, however, can also have a "darker" side. Cohesiveness can cause group members to develop mutual dependency rather than autonomy and to emphasize preserving the group without attention to the work (such as problem solving) that is at hand (Janis, 1982). This can result in the phenomenon of "groupthink." Groupthink is discussed in a later section of this chapter.

Group Functions

An effective group is able to accomplish its task or purpose, meet the needs of its members, and respond to its environment. "Group functions" are the sets of activities in which a group must engage to meet these three demands.

Task Functions

Task functions are goal-oriented activities. Initiating is the first task function in which a group must engage. Initiating involves stating the problem and goal, making tentative proposals about how the goal might be pursued, and identifying factors such as time and money constraints that might affect goal accomplishment (Schein, 1988). A community often engages in initiating before contacting a nurse consultant for help with problem solving. Initiating may also occur during initial contact with a nurse consultant, or may continue throughout the entry and problem identification phases of the nursing consultation process. Other task functions include

gathering and communicating information that will facilitate problem identification and action planning.

Internal Maintenance Functions

Internal maintenance functions are activities in which group members engage for the purpose of building and maintaining "group harmony" or good interpersonal relations, and repairing damaged relationships (Goodstein, 1978). Maintenance functions need to occur on an ongoing basis in any group. However, because members of groups that are just forming are frequently preoccupied with their own personal needs and the process of group building, maintenance functions are often more pronounced in established groups in which some "relationship repair work" needs to take place before the group can engage in task functions. If maintenance functions are not carried out, a group member who is angry or hurt or who feels left out can be lost as a resource to the group or can act to sabotage the group's activities (Schein, 1988).

Boundary Management Functions

Because every group exists in a larger community environment, one of a group's key tasks is to manage its relationships with its environment (Schein, 1988). Boundary management activities center on accessing information and other resources from the environment and defining the group's niche or purpose in relationship to its environment.

Specific activities related to each of a group's functions are described in Box 7-1. As you study the list of specific activities related to each group function, think how these activities might apply to a task force that a nurse consultant is facilitating for a local school. (In this scenario, the task force is the consultee. The client is the school. Students, their parents, and teachers would all be stakeholders.) Task functions that this group would need to

BOX 7-1   GROUP FUNCTIONS

An effective group is able to accomplish its purpose, meet the needs of its members, and respond to its environment. "Group functions" are sets of activities in which a group must engage in order to meet these demands.

Task Functions

These functions help a group pursue its goal:

- Initiating: Stating the problem, making proposals about how it might be resolved
- Information and opinion seeking
- Information and opinion sharing
- Clarifying and elaborating: Testing the adequacy of information and improving the quality of proposed problem solutions
- Summarizing: Reviewing what is known (or unknown) and what has been decided
- Consensus testing: Assessing readiness to make a decision

Internal Maintenance Functions

These functions focus on keeping the group intact and keeping group members happy and productive:

- Gatekeeping: Ensuring that all members have an opportunity to contribute to the group
- Supporting: Ensuring that members feel included and accepted
- Harmonizing and compromising: Intervening to reduce destructive disagreements
- Diagnosing, standard setting, and standard testing: Remedial measures such as airing problems and looking at the group rules and processes that are used when the group appears to be breaking down
- Energizing: Keeping the group moving forward toward its goals

Boundary Management Functions

These activities focus on a group's relationship with its environment:

- Boundary defining: Establishing the group's identity
- Scouting: Seeking information about the environment that could have an effect on the group
- Technology gatekeeping: Bringing the group information it needs to be able to perform its tasks
- Translating: Ensuring that information is understood
- Negotiating: Ensuring the group gets the resources it needs from its environment
- Guarding: Maintaining integrity of the group by determining what information it will share with its environment
- Patrolling: Looking for information leakage
- Entry and exit management: Bringing in and releasing members

Sources: Harrison, M. (1994). *Diagnosing organizations: Methods, models, and processes* (2nd ed.). Thousand Oaks, CA: Sage; Oyster, C. (2000). *Groups: A user's guide.* Boston: McGraw-Hill; and Schein, E. (1988). *Process consultation, volume I: Its role in organization development* (2nd ed.). Reading, MA: Addison-Wesley.

undertake include initiating activities that center around defining the nursing consultation problem (fear and grief after the recent death of a popular teacher due to an act of violence on the school's grounds) and possible solutions (a support group, increased safety measures, etc.). Before the consultees (i.e., the task force) can decide on the most appropriate intervention, however, they need to gather information to more clearly identify the problem. Specifically, they need to determine whether their fear is a normal or "exaggerated" reaction and whether the school's normal security measures actually failed. They also need to gather information and opinions about possible problem solutions. Information sharing, clarifying, and consensus testing need to follow before a support group can be decided on as the "best" problem solution.

Once the support group is established, group members' efforts focus on ensuring that the group is meeting the needs of all members. Internal maintenance activities such as gatekeeping, encouraging, harmonizing, and compromising assume primary importance. All group members need to feel able to share their concerns and ask for as well as give support.

Boundary management functions would be important to this task force because the group operates in a highly emotional environment. Even if the school's reaction to this event is determined to be exaggerated and it is determined that a lapse in security did not contribute to the event, the task force as well as the support group and other stakeholders need to be kept informed (through scouting, technology gatekeeping, and translating) about new policies and procedures that could affect the school environment. These changes could either increase or alleviate their stress. The members of the task force will engage in guarding and patrolling when they decide what information to share with the support group, the media, teachers, students, and parents.

Levels of Behavior in Groups

Members of groups engage in both formal and informal levels of behavior (Oyster, 2000). The formal level of behavior is a rule-centered, task-oriented level of behavior whereas the informal level is a personal level of behavior. The informal level of behavior is a more subtle, implicit level of behavior that focuses on group maintenance and the personal needs of group members (Oyster, 2000). At any one time, group members may be working on the group's tasks—but never working only on the group's tasks; they are also working on whatever personal and social needs are important to themselves as individuals at that point in time. In groups, then, individual behavior is shaped largely by a personal agenda of needs and values, such as competition, control, self-protection, and autonomy (Sampson & Marthas, 1990).

Because group members are always functioning at these two levels of behavior, each group member has two roles: a task role and a personal role. A group member's task roles are assigned responsibilities that need to be carried out in order for the group to accomplish its task (Goodstein, 1978). In a support group, task roles for group members might include "attender at meetings," "active listener," and "sharer of concerns." A group member's personal roles are roles that are assumed for personal comfort and satisfaction. Examples of personal roles and needs include leader, follower, listener, talker, being liked, and being valued. The right set and assignment of task roles helps a group to accomplish its task and make optimal use of each member's talents. If group members are unable to fulfill their desired personal roles, their dissatisfaction can distract, disrupt, or destroy the group because they are unwilling or unable to take on their task roles (Bolman & Deal, 1991; Oyster, 2000).

The concepts of two levels of behavior and group members' personal needs are important for nurse consultants because surface, observed behavior is often inadequate for fully under- standing group interactions. For example, per- sonal needs and agendas often help explain the way in which a group member interacts with the group leader (who is often the nurse con- sultant in a nursing consultation situation) and with other group members. As described in Box 7-2, how an individual interacts with the group's leader may reflect needs and issues related to authority, dependency, freedom, and individuality. Interactions with other group members may reflect needs and issues related to intimacy, sexuality, envy, giving, and privacy (Sampson & Marthas, 1990).

BOX 7-2   UNDERSTANDING GROUP MEMBERS' BEHAVIOR: PERSONAL AGENDAS AND INTERPERSONAL INTERACTIONS

In any group, individuals take on personal as well as task roles. The personal roles a group member assumes reflect a personal agenda of needs and issues. Personal roles are wanted for personal comfort and satisfaction. The needs and issues that drive personal roles can often be inferred from an individual's way of interacting with the group leader and other group members.

Interactions with Group Leaders

Need or Issue	Possible Behavior
Authority	Challenges group leader's knowledge, opinions, and right to make decisions
Dependency	Unquestionably obeys group leader; tries to establish a coalition with the leader; asks for unneeded assistance
Freedom/Autonomy/ Power	Disregards task role; makes statements such as "Let me do it my way"
Individuality	Calls attention to self through interaction with and comments to group leader

Interactions with Other Group Members

Need or Issue	Possible Behavior
Intimacy and friendship	Shares personal thoughts; excessive friendship overtures
Sexuality	Provocative posturing and/or comments
Envy	Criticizes others' ideas and actions; calls attention to own ideas and actions
Giving	Offers physical and material assistance (this often seems to occur in exchange for gestures of friendship)
Privacy	Reluctance to share personal thoughts and ideas with group members

Source: Sampson, E., & Marthas, M. (1990). *Group process for the health professions* (3rd ed.). Albany, NY: Delmar.

Influence in Groups

Just as all members of a community (including the nurse consultant) have some type of power, all group members exert influence of one kind or another over the group's functioning. This influence is a result of the way in which a member interacts with others in the group (Schoonover-Shoffner, 1989). Depending on how a group member interacts with others in the group, influence can be promotive, disruptive, or counteractive.

Promotive influence occurs when a member's behavior facilitates progress of the group toward its goals. Examples of promotive behavior include providing helpful suggestions ("In other situations, I've seen this work . . . "), and encouraging and participating in brainstorming. However, most groups are characterized by more disruptive than promotive interactions (Schoonover-Shoffner, 1989). Disruptive influence is exerted when behavior inhibits a group's movement to a decision or its goals. Pressure tactics, giving wrong information, and drawing incorrect conclusions from information are examples of behavior that can have a disruptive influence. Counteractive influence negates or neutralizes disruptive interactions and restores a group's movement toward its goals. Exposing and correcting misinformation is an example of an interaction that would have a counteractive influence.

A nurse consultant who is working with a group needs to create an environment where group members feel safe engaging in behaviors that will have a productive or counteractive influence. The nurse consultant, as the implied group leader, also needs to role model promotive and counteractive influence behaviors. Strategies a nurse consultant can use to exert and role model promotive and counteractive influence are identified in Box 7-3.

BOX 7-3 PROMOTIVE AND COUNTERACTIVE INFLUENCE STRATEGIES FOR NURSE CONSULTANTS

Promotive influence strategies facilitate a group's progress toward its goals. *Counteractive influence* strategies neutralize disruptive group interactions and restore a group's movement toward its goals. The following strategies represent both promotive and counteractive influence strategies for nurse consultants:

- Agree on decision-making guidelines and criteria that will be used to make decisions.
- Establish norms and guidelines for brainstorming activities.
- Ask for a "recheck" of questionable information.
- Don't deal with the source (person) or the nature of the wrong information, assumptions, or ideas; instead, point out questionable features and ask the group to reexamine the idea's acceptability.
- Point out fallacies and concerns using "I" language ("I am concerned because . . .").
- Be prepared to limit the interactions and contributions of disruptive group members; do this by focusing on functions or actions rather than on personal faults.
- Do your homework ahead of time so that you know the issues related to the problem.

Source: Schoonover-Shoffner, K. (1989). Improving work group decision-making effectiveness. *Journal of Nursing Administration, 19*(7), 10–16.

LEARNING FROM OBSERVING GROUPS

A nurse consultant can learn much about a group's norms and power structure by simple but focused observations. This information can help the nurse consultant gain psychological entry into a group and can help build coalitions for problem solving. Group communication and decision making are two of the most important and accessible processes that can be observed.

Observing Group Communication

Communication includes the spoken word as well as facial expressions, gestures, physical posturing, tone of voice, and timing (Oyster, 2000). A single message can convey facts, feelings, perceptions, and innuendoes. Of particular interest to a nurse consultant are the dynamics and interpersonal interactions that accompany the verbal dimensions of communication; these behaviors are most likely to reveal a group's norms and power structure. Box 7-4 summarizes questions that can be used to guide observation of a group's communication processes. Key issues and observations are discussed in depth below.

Observation 1: Who Communicates? How Often? For How Long?

Answers to these questions reveal not only who the group's informal leader is, but also reveal members' needs for inclusion, individuality, and privacy. These observations can actually be charted and summarized to indicate how much of the total available "talk time" is taken up by each group member (Schein, 1988). Frequently, these observations reveal that members who have been labeled as quiet and nonparticipatory have actually been talking, but no one has been listening. These observations, therefore, can

---

BOX 7-4   OBSERVING GROUP COMMUNICATION

A nurse consultant can use the following questions as a guide for observing group communication:

- Who communicates? How often? For how long?
- Who speaks but is apparently never heard?
- Who is included in the communication network?
- Who communicates with whom?
- Who talks after whom? Who interrupts whom?
- Who is never allowed to complete their thoughts?
- Does an interruption represent support ("Attaboy") or challenge ("Yes, but . . .")?
- Whose words seem to have especially heavy impact?
- What communication styles are observed? How do these seem to affect others in the group?
- What does the total communication picture reveal about a group's norms and values?

Source: Schein, E. (1988). *Process consultation, volume I: Its role in organization development* (2nd ed.). Reading, MA: Addison-Wesley.

also answer the question, "Who speaks but is apparently never heard?"

Observation 2: Who Is Included in the Communication Network? Who Communicates with Whom?

To make these observations, a nurse consultant must watch a speaker's body language and eyes since a target of communication is not always addressed by name. These observations can be recorded on a matrix that has the names of group members on both the horizontal and vertical axes. A check mark can be placed in the appropriate cell on the matrix grid each time a communication event occurs (Schein, 1988).

Often, group members will speak first to members of the group from whom they expect resistance to an idea. This enables the speaker to determine whether the "toughest hurdle" to an idea can be passed before moving on to a problem solution. The nurse consultant may want to follow this lead of who to talk to first when presenting information (especially controversial information) to the same group. These observations can also reveal subgroups and coalitions within a group.

Observation 3: Who Talks After Whom? Who Interrupts Whom?

These observations provide information about perceptions of status and group norms regarding attention to status. Usually, group members of higher rank or power or those with higher perceived status feel free to interrupt a member of lower perceived status. Thus, individuals who are never allowed to complete their thoughts are generally recognized as less powerful and less important by a group.

Occasionally, a group member with lower status will interrupt a member of higher status. While this might be acceptable if a group has a norm of openness, it is more likely to represent a challenge to the influence of the group member who has been interrupted (Schein, 1988). Thus, interrupting a person of higher status may indicate a strong negative reaction to that person's words and what they imply in terms of behavioral expectations. Note that *never* being interrupted can sometimes indicate a total disregard for a message rather than respect for power and status.

In addition to observing patterns of interruption, a nurse consultant should observe the "patterns of triggering" represented by the interruption (Schein, 1988). Interruption can be supportive ("Attaboy!") or can represent a desire to undo a decision ("Yes, but . . ."). In general, it takes three "Attaboys" to undo the damage caused by a single "Yes, but" (Schein, 1988).

Observation 4: What Communication Styles Are Observed? What Effects Do They Have?

This observation focuses on tone of voice, use of gestures, and delivery styles (e.g., humorous or assertive). While these behaviors tend to reveal the sender's underlying personality more than anything else, they are also important because of the effect they can have on other members in the group. For example, do group members become defensive or are they put at ease? These behaviors can also reflect the sender's personal needs for control, individuality, and/or inclusion.

Observation 5: What Does the Total Communication Picture Reveal About a Group's Norms and Values?

In making this final observation, a nurse consultant considers the meaning of a group's communication processes as a whole. A nurse consultant should try to infer the following specific norms and values because of their potential influence on the nursing consultation relationship: authoritarianism versus democracy and participation, openness versus privacy, group cohesiveness versus individualism, and dependence versus self-confidence and autonomy.

Observing Group Decision-Making Processes

Group decision making involves combining the preferences of individual members into a group choice (Schoonover-Shoffner, 1989). A group's decision-making processes reveal sources of influence within the group, values about individual contributions and openness, and norms about participation. More importantly for a nurse consultant, a group's decision-making processes may help explain poor morale, lack of cohesiveness, lack of group effectiveness, and other problems that can interfere with goal accomplishment.

A group is more likely to attain its goals when its decision-making processes allow all members to have their say and argue openly for what they believe. In contrast, if there is manipulation, compromising just to settle things, smoothing over and ignoring biases and conflicting information, or the forcing of a decision by those in authority, decision-making outcomes (and group dynamics) are more likely to be negative (Goodstein, 1978). The five patterns of decision making observed most frequently in groups are: decision by lack of response (or default), decision by authority, decision by minority, decision by majority rule, and decision by consensus.

Decisions by default, authority, or minority rule occur most frequently in groups that discourage openness and participation. In groups with these norms, speaking up and opposing a decision is negatively labeled as "blocking." In these groups, there are strong pressures on group members to remain silent (Schein, 1988). The danger of using one of these processes for decision making is that decisions often end up being made on the basis of inaccurate or incomplete information. Admittedly, decision by authority is a highly efficient way of making a decision and is appropriate in crisis

situations such as a natural disaster that completely immobilizes a community. Whether decision by authority is effective, however, depends on the extent to which adequate information about the problem and possible solutions have been solicited before the decision is made.

Decision by majority is popular because it implies a value of democracy within a group. The danger of voting and operating on the basis of majority rule, however, is that it creates coalitions of winners and losers. Unless the losers feel that they have been really listened to before voting, they can become preoccupied with "winning the next round" rather than implementing the group's decision.

Decision by consensus does not mean unanimity. Rather, consensus means that everyone in a group has had an opportunity to openly share concerns and influence the decision (Oyster, 2000). Consensus reflects a "sense of the group" rather than voting to demonstrate majority agreement (Schein, 1988). While consensus is the most time-consuming process for reaching a decision, groups that make decisions on the basis of consensus usually make higher-quality decisions because the process allows consideration of all information and all opinions. Consensus also avoids the creation of winners and losers. Groups that make decisions by consensus frequently request nursing consultation for help with the efficiency of their decision-making processes.

ISSUES RELATED TO BUILDING A GROUP

Nurse consultants often work with groups that are coming together for the first time in a working relationship. In this situation, group-building activities need to begin during the gaining entry phase of the nursing consultation process. Group-building activities can take place as the nurse consultant establishes physical entry and works to gain psychological entry into the consultee group and client system. (*Note:* Group-building activities and group-maintaining activities, which are discussed in the next section, are different from team-building activities, which are discussed in Chapter 12.)

Building a group is a stressful process because members are simultaneously bombarded with a variety of tasks, roles, and interpersonal demands. The beginning of a group, in particular, is marked by member anxiety related to uncertainty and apprehension about both individual acceptance within the group and group expectations. The question of "How good of a group member will I be?" causes a sense of "I-ness" to prevail during the process of group building. This self-centered behavior reflects various concerns that any new group member could be expected to experience. A nurse consultant needs to attend to these concerns so that group members will be able to pay attention to each other and the task at hand.

Human Dynamics in New Groups: "I-ness"

The behavior of group members during the group-building process can be explained by the underlying emotional issues and anxieties that an individual must resolve before comfort is established in any new situation. Each member of a new group needs to resolve issues related to identity, control, balancing personal and group needs, and acceptance and intimacy (Schein, 1988). Until group members' roles and relationships are sorted out, the group will not be productive and anything that is produced will not be of high quality (Oyster, 2000).

Issue 1: Identity

Each group member needs to answer the question "Who am I to be in this group?" This issue centers around determining members' task roles. Until this issue is resolved, group members demonstrate poor listening skills, anxiety, inattention, and a lack of concern for others.

Issue 2: Control, Power, and Influence

This issue addresses group members' questions about "How much power will I have and how should I express it?" Group members try to resolve these issues by testing each other and experimenting with the effectiveness of different forms of influence, such as expertise and charisma. Concerns about power can cause inconsistency in group members' behavior as they try to sort out the most effective way of relating to each other. If the nurse consultant insists on a tight task schedule and fails to allow time for power concerns to be resolved, "testing" behavior will continue and delay work on the group's task.

Issue 3: Individual Needs and Group Goals

This issue concerns group members' anxieties about balancing their own needs with the needs of the group as a whole. Specifically, group members have anxiety about "Will the group's goals meet my own needs?" Preoccupation with this issue can cause an individual to develop a "wait and see" attitude rather than be an active participant in group activities. If too many group members take this attitude, the group never gets moving.

The danger with this issue is that the nurse consultant or another group member may try to rescue the group by using authority to set an agenda and formulate goals. This has the effect of creating dependency in the consultee group rather than fostering the development of problem-solving skills.

Issue 4: Acceptance and Intimacy

The questions behind this issue are "Will I be liked and accepted by the group?" and "How open will we need to be with each other?" This issue is a source of tension until the group establishes working norms about intimacy and individual members resolve their concerns about acceptance. Group members often respond to these issues by exhibiting charisma and by looking for another group member with whom they can agree and form a supportive alliance. This tendency can create dependency as well as foster the development of coalitions that emphasize meeting group members' personal and social needs rather than the group's task needs.

Strategies for Nurse Consultants

Because group members are preoccupied with their own feelings during the group-building process, they are less able to listen to each other and solve group problems. A nurse consultant needs to clarify and acknowledge the personal needs of group members during the group-building process and legitimize members' testing and coping behaviors. A nurse consultant also needs to help the group understand the dynamics that are occurring so that they can confront and respond to each other's concerns, rather than just react to each other's behavior. Helping group members establish group norms and resolve concerns about their identity with the group are additional strategies that are useful during the group-building process.

A nurse consultant can decrease the anxiety of group members by helping them establish group norms ("how we want to do things") early in the group-building process. For example, the group may need help in coming to a consensus about norms and expectations for participation, listening, interrupting, confidentiality, and formality of a group's processes. Groups also need to decide on acceptable decision criteria. A nurse consultant can facilitate group members' involvement in establishing these norms by asking them how they would like to see the group operate. Developing these norms and rules can help resolve group members' concerns about power and intimacy within the group.

Group members may also need help in resolving their concerns about identity. As a helping strategy, a nurse consultant may assist group members in identifying what specific roles and responsibilities they want to assume within the group and what contributions they think they bring to the group. A specific strategy a nurse consultant can use to help group members negotiate roles and responsibilities is responsibility charting. A responsibility chart (Bolman & Deal, 1991) identifies who is going to do what tasks in a group and how the person responsible for a particular task will relate to other group members in regard to that task. Figure 7-1 is an example of a responsibility chart for a consultee group of representatives from a variety of community social and health service agencies who are working with a nurse consultant to plan a community's first health fair.

A responsibility chart decreases group members' anxieties about what they are expected to do in a group in terms of helping that group meet its goals. If group members are active participants in developing the responsibility chart, they can address issues related to balancing their own needs with those of the group. Group involvement in developing a responsibility chart also facilitates the development of trust and cohesion early in the group-building process.

ISSUES RELATED TO MAINTAINING A GROUP

To some extent, it is easier to work with an established group than with a group that is coming together to problem solve for the first time. Established groups tend to have norms that are understood and have become integrated into the group's way of interacting. Established groups also tend to have developed ways of accommodating members' personal roles without compromising the overall functioning of the group. Because these tasks

Tasks	Group Members				
	Chairperson	Treasurer	A	B	C
Establish program/ agenda	R	C	C	C	C
Select date/time	A	C	R	I	I
Make facilities arrangements	A	C	I	R	I
Publicity	C	I	I	I	R
Solicit vendors and displayers	I	I	I	R	R
Act as on-site facilitator	R	I	C	I	I
Solicit financial sponsorship	C	R	I	R	I
Track expenses/ pay bills	A	R	I	I	I

Key:
R = Individual who is responsible for a task or decision (this person should be identified first)
A = Individuals who need to approve the actions of R
C = Individuals whom R needs to consult before making a decision
I = Individuals who need to be kept informed by R

Figure 7-1   Example Responsibility Chart for a Community Consultation.
This example responsibility chart illustrates tasks and responsibilities related to planning a health fair. The responsibility chart identifies who is responsible for a specific task and how other group members relate to this task. The nurse consultant works with the group to identify the person designated as "R" first. The nurse consultant remains available to the group for further problem-specific consultation, but is typically not involved in ongoing consultation about the implementation of each task.

have been accomplished, the climate of an established group can be more trusting and supportive than that of a group that is coming together in a working relationship for the first time. Members of established groups tend to be less overtly anxious than members of new groups. They are also more willing to take personal and collective risks. Established groups are characterized by a sense of "we-ness" rather than "I-ness," and by collective work toward the group's goal. The disadvantage of working with an established group, however, is that the group may have developed dysfunctional and unproductive ways of interacting. If this is the case, a nurse consultant will need to undertake group-building processes before problem solving can get under way.

Nurse consultants often work with established groups of consultees to help them solve a community-wide health-related problem. For example, a nurse consultant might work with a group of school nurses to help handle a head lice epidemic (client = school system). In another situation, a nurse might provide consultation to a group of day care providers about meeting the health care needs of toddlers who are infected with HIV and dealing with parents' concerns about having their children in a facility with an HIV-infected child.

Human Dynamics in Established Groups: Groupthink

The same cohesiveness that can make working with an established group productive can also get the group into trouble. Established groups that are excessively cohesive can become careless in their boundary management and information-gathering activities. They can also develop a sense of omnipotence and overestimate their own power and morality. This tendency causes established groups to sometimes engage in excessive risk taking. Finally, excessive cohesiveness may lead a group to develop informal norms about preserving an appearance of group harmony at all costs. Whenever the group needs to make a decision, these norms may function as a hidden agenda. The potential side effects of this type of cohesiveness can result in "groupthink" (Janis, 1982).

Groupthink is the term that has been coined to describe a deterioration of mental efficiency, reality testing, and moral judgment that can result from in-group pressures and cohesiveness. This same phenomenon has also been referred to as the *Abilene Paradox:* a willingness of group members to set aside their individual preferences and opinions to accommodate the perceived majority will (Robbins & Finley, 1996). When groupthink occurs, a group's drive for cohesiveness and unanimity overrides group members' judgment as well as their motivation to consider the range of possible solutions to a problem (Janis, 1982). In other words, groupthink occurs when a desire for conformity saps diversity and individual judgment. Groupthink results in poor-quality decisions. Indeed, near-catastrophes, such as the Cuban Missile Crisis, and actual catastrophes, such as the explosion of the space shuttle Challenger, have been attributed to groupthink.

Cohesiveness of the extreme type that results in groupthink is particularly likely to develop when a group perceives itself to be facing an "enemy." The first clue that this dangerous type of cohesiveness might be developing is a group's development of a stereotyped and dehumanizing image of the source of their perceived threat. An example of this would be a community group blaming an apparent shortage of flu vaccine on the "money-hungry and insensitive" pharmaceutical industry. As these groups become cohesive, they also tend to develop extreme ideas about how the threat should be handled. These ideas are more extreme and involve more risk taking than what members would be inclined to do on their own. What develops is, in a sense, a type of "mob mentality."

Group cohesiveness sets the stage for the development or operation of the other conditions also associated with groupthink. Group cohesiveness causes a group to insulate itself from its environment and miss opportunities to take advantage of information that might challenge their decisions. Leaders of tightly cohesive groups tend to become partial to group members who conform to the majority view; this has the effect of preventing minority members from expressing their doubts. Finally, cohesiveness sets the stage for groupthink by discouraging norms that require methodical procedures and criteria for decision-making tasks (Janis, 1982). The outcome of groupthink is poor-quality decisions. Figure 7-2 summarizes the conditions associated with groupthink.

Strategies for Nurse Consultants

A key task for nurse consultants who are working with established groups in a problem-solving relationship is preventing groupthink. Nurse consultants need to work with established groups to maintain the positive aspects of cohesiveness such as increased group member security and productivity. At the same time, nurse consultants need to work to prevent cohesiveness from becoming dysfunctional by enforcing effective decision-making processes and reinforcing (or helping a group

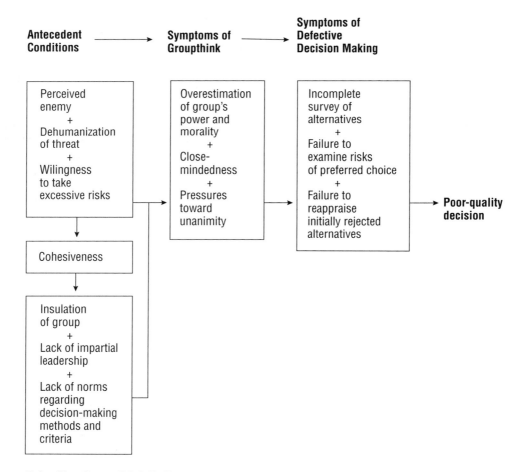

Figure 7-2   The Groupthink Pathway.
Groupthink is a result of excessive group cohesiveness that develops in response to the perception of an extreme external threat ("the enemy"). Group members develop a type of cohesiveness that encourages increased risk taking, incomplete information gathering, and a drive for group unanimity that overrides effective decision-making processes. The outcome of groupthink is poor-quality decisions.

develop) norms about impartiality, listening, and information seeking.

One specific strategy a nurse consultant can help a group implement to protect against groupthink is that of developing a process for monitoring group compliance with decided-upon decision-making processes. This can be done by assigning to each member the formal roles of critical evaluator and "devil's advocate" (Janis, 1982). This strategy creates the expectation that group members will voice concerns they have about a proposed decision and removes the stigma that might otherwise be associated with being a critic and dissenter. Finally, a nurse consultant can role model the behaviors of both "critical evaluator" and "impartial leader" to the group. Additional strategies nurse consultants can use to prevent groupthink are identified in Box 7-5.

TEAMS: A SPECIAL KIND OF GROUP

Teams, particularly interdisciplinary teams, have become an increasingly popular component of strategies for solving the types of complex problems that abound in today's health care environment. A team is a specific type of group that is distinguished by a collaborative effort ("teamwork") and a collective perspective. More specifically, teams are small groups of people with "complementary skills who are committed to a common purpose, performance goals, and approach for which they hold themselves to be mutually accountable" (Katzenbach & Smith, 1993). In contrast, traditional work groups may be characterized by teamwork, but they lack a collective perspective. Instead, traditional work groups interact to help each individual member perform

BOX 7-5   STRATEGIES FOR PREVENTING GROUPTHINK

The following are various strategies a nurse consultant can use to prevent groupthink:

- As the group leader, avoid stating personal preferences and try to be impartial; merely introduce the problem and the resources and limitations relevant to its solution.
- Educate the group about the phenomenon of groupthink.
- Establish and enforce norms regarding mutual responsibility.
- Discourage the practice of trying to "score points" in a power struggle.
- Role model the solicitation and acceptance of criticism.
- Assign the role of "critical evaluator" to each group member.
- Assign one member the role of devil's advocate.
- Break a group into several subgroups, each with its own leader.
- Prevent insulation by seeking the reactions of outsiders to the group's decision; invite outsiders to meetings in order to provide another perspective on the problem and possible solutions.
- Encourage consideration of the impact of the group's decision on stakeholders in the problem situation.
- Hold a "second chance meeting" before implementing the decision; review problem-solving options as well as their advantages and disadvantages.

Source: Janis, I. (1982). *Groupthink* (2nd ed.). Boston: Houghton-Mifflin.

more effectively. Table 7-1 summarizes additional differences between work groups and teams.

The Usefulness of Teams

Teams are useful whenever a specific objective requires collective work and the integration of multiple skills, perspectives, and experiences. In fact, a demanding performance challenge tends to naturally create a team (Katzenbach & Smith, 1993). The usefulness of incorporating a team approach into solving complex problem situations that are likely to recur is related to several innate characteristics of teams. First, the complementary skills and perspectives of team members increases the likelihood that a problem solution will fit the client system's needs and resources. Second, teams tend to develop communication patterns that facilitate present as well as future problem solving. Teams also derive effectiveness from team members' trust and confidence in each others' abilities. For these reasons, teams are often the best way to integrate problem solving across structural boundaries (units and hierarchies) of an organization. A team approach fosters the development of long-term problem-solving skills that will be dispersed throughout the client system once the nursing consultation relationship has terminated. In other words, teams naturally integrate performance and learning. Finally, team effectiveness is related to a sense of "safety in numbers." That is, a team is not as threatened by taking risks and changing as are individuals who are left to fend for themselves (Katzenbach & Smith, 1993).

Transforming Work Groups into Teams

Because teams are potentially useful in solving many nursing consultation problems, nurse consultants need to know how to create and work with teams. Transforming a work group into a team, or creating a team "from scratch," requires that a nurse consultant have a knowledge of "team basics" as well as demonstrate abilities to build team performance and function as a temporary team leader.

Team Basics

Team basics are the structures and processes that enable a group to function as a team. Team basics are size, skills, common purpose, common approach, and accountability (Katzenbach & Smith, 1993).

TABLE 7-1. WORK GROUPS VERSUS TEAMS

Characteristic	Work Group	Team
Leadership	Strong, clearly focused	Shared
Accountability	Individual	Individual and collective
Purpose	Same as the community's	Specific and unique to the group
Work style	Emphasis on efficiency: Discuss, decide, delegate	Characterized by open discussion and problem solving: Discuss, decide, do real work together
How effectiveness is judged	Influence on members	Collective work products

Source: Katzenbach, J., & Smith, D. (1993). *The wisdom of teams: Creating the high performance organization.* New York: HarperBusiness.

Size. Teams range in size from 2 to 25 members (the ideal size is said to be 12). Teams of more than 25 members tend to get bogged down by logistics (such as meeting times) and because of difficulty reaching agreement on specifics. Larger groups also have a tendency to become hierarchical in nature and develop individual rather than collective performance goals.

Skills. Three types of skills need to be represented among team members: technical or functional expertise related to the consultation problem (such as familiarity with the needs of a certain population group), problem-solving and decision-making skills, and interpersonal skills. Team members, therefore, should be selected on the basis of their skills and skill potential, not their personality. Sometimes, however, it makes sense to choose an individual as a team member for political reasons. Team members with skill potential will usually develop needed skills as the team evolves.

Common Purpose. Teams are defined by a common purpose that is shaped in response to demands from actual or potential internal or external environmental changes (such as budget cuts at a free clinic). This common purpose must be linked to specific performance goals (e.g., "Find ways to reduce operating costs by 20 percent within two months"). Clear goals help a team maintain its focus and structure small steps and "small wins" toward an overall problem solution. The achievement of small wins provides feedback to a team that is moving in the right direction.

Common Approach. Teams work only to the extent that they use a single, unified approach to making decisions while working as a group. Teams also need to agree on time commitments for both individual and group tasks.

Accountability. Teams are characterized by mutual accountability. More specifically, team members need to hold themselves accountable for their individual contributions to the team while they hold one another accountable for members' collective contributions to the team. In addition, the team as a whole needs to hold itself accountable for the overall results.

Building Team Performance

A work group needs more than the structures and processes that comprise team basics if it is to function as an effective team. Teams also need energy, enthusiasm, and dedication to the project (e.g., achieve a 20 percent budget cut), client needs related to the project (such as maintaining quality care), and the team itself (Peters, 1987). Nurse consultants can build team performance by instilling "caring, daring, and sharing" (Peters, 1987)—that is, creating an environment of mutual support and open and honest communication, encouraging risk taking and a sense of adventure, asking the "hard" questions, and creating commonly held objectives as well as a clear sense of how everyone fits in as a team member.

Specific strategies a nurse consultant can use to build team performance are identified in Box 7-6. Notice from this list that "building team performance" is a more comprehensive concept than is "team building." Team building commonly refers to efforts to establish cooperation and comfort among the members of a group. Chapter 12 discusses team building as a universal consultation intervention.

The Nurse Consultant as Temporary Team Leader

Because the nursing consultation relationship is a temporary one, a nurse consultant's ultimate goal is to ensure that a team becomes either self-directed or led by one of its members. However, nurse consultants

BOX 7-6   STRATEGIES FOR BUILDING TEAM PERFORMANCE

A nurse consultant can use the following strategies to build team performance:

- Establish the urgency and direction of the team's purpose.
- Pay particular attention to first meetings and actions ("first impressions count"); be clear and attentive to members' thoughts and responses.
- Set clear standards of behavior: Attendance, discussion, confidentiality, task participation, constructive confrontations, end-product orientation.
- Give the team credibility by enforcing behavioral expectations.
- Set upon and seize a few immediate performance-oriented goals and tasks.
- Challenge the team regularly with fresh facts and information (this redefines and enriches the team's understanding of its purpose).
- Spend a lot of time together, especially at the beginning (this creates camaraderie and solidarity).
- Exploit the power of positive feedback, recognition, and reward.
- Establish a measurement and reward system that fosters a sense of cohesion and unity.
- Engage in ongoing team building (this facilitates discovery of personal abilities and the abilities of others as well as builds and restores trust).

Sources: Katzenbach, J., & Smith, D. (1993). *The wisdom of teams: Creating the high performance organization.* New York: HarperBusiness; and Peters, J. (1987). *Thriving on chaos: Handbook for a management revolution.* New York: HarperCollins.

often find it necessary to assume a temporary role as team leader during the process of establishing team basics and building team performance. To a large extent, team leadership is taking a course of "disciplined action" and helping a work group adjust its attitudes and behaviors so as to develop a team perspective.

The primary task of a team leader is to keep the team's purpose, goals, and approach meaningful and relevant. Team members usually do not want leaders to go beyond this, and can become resentful if they attempt to do so (Katzenbach & Smith, 1993). A team leader's other key task is to manage outside relationships on behalf of the team, including securing needed resources and removing obstacles to team functioning. To be effective as a team leader, then, a nurse consultant needs to balance patience and action. Strategies for effective team leadership are presented in Box 7-7.

Challenges Related to Working with Teams

Teams are hard work. Developing and maintaining a team takes time, energy, and organizational commitment. Moreover, even once teams are up and running, they can develop dysfunctional behaviors and "get stuck." In order to maximize the advantages a team approach can bring to a problem situation, a nurse consultant needs to be able to respond to two challenges: biases related to teams and teams that have lost their effectiveness.

BOX 7-7   STRATEGIES FOR EFFECTIVE TEAM LEADERSHIP

A nurse consultant can use the following strategies to be effective as a team leader:

- Keep the team's purpose, goals, and approach meaningful and relevant.
- Build commitment and confidence among team members (this needs to be aimed at both individual members and the team as a whole).
- Help the team strengthen its mix and level of skills by providing role modeling and task-specific training.
- Manage the team's relationships with outsiders, including removing community obstacles to team functioning.
- Create opportunities for other team members.
- Do real work with the team—be a team member as well as leader:
- Do not blame or allow specific individuals to fail.
- Never excuse shortfalls in team performance.
- Keep your leadership temporary; help the team become self-managing and/or facilitate the development of team leadership skills in a permanent team member(s).

Source: Katzenbach, J., & Smith, D. (1993). *The wisdom of teams: Creating the high performance organization.* New York: HarperBusiness.

Biases Related to Teams

Nurse consultants encounter individual and community biases that can lead to both the overuse and underuse of teams. Some consultees see a team approach as the only way to solve problems. However, teams are not a solution for all problems and, if misapplied, can be wasteful (of both time and resources) and disruptive. As discussed earlier, teams are useful when solving a problem requires collective work and the integration of multiple skills, experiences, and perspectives. If a performance goal can be met through a sum of individual responsibilities and contributions, however, a traditional work group can get the job done and can often do so more effectively (Katzenbach & Smith, 1993).

Communities can also have mindsets that discourage the use of teams, even when a team approach would clearly be the most effective. A community may, for example,

have a cultural norm of individual rather than group accountability. A community with this norm might equate group accountability with "no accountability." A nurse consultant can confront this bias by educating the consultee about the nature of team accountability and how it can be reinforced through a performance-oriented reward system.

Another bias that can discourage the use of teams is the belief that teams are costly and time consuming. A nurse consultant needs to confront this belief by acknowledging that while teams do take time to develop, they usually pay off in the long run. The long-term benefit of a team approach is that it will be useful for solving future community problems. Skills that will be used for future problem-solving situations are learned by members dispersed throughout the entire community, rather than limited to one sector or hierarchical level.

BOX 7-8   WHEN TEAMS "GET STUCK"

Teams that have lost their effectiveness and become "stuck" frequently exhibit the following symptoms:

- Loss of energy
- Sense of hopelessness
- Lack of purpose and identity
- Cynicism and mistrust
- Finger pointing and personal attacks

A nurse consultant can use the following strategies to help a team become "unstuck":

- Revisit "team basics"—size; skill mix, level, and potential; clear and meaningful purpose, clear and unified approach; collective and individual accountability
- Go for small wins
- Inject new information and approaches
- Seek outside facilitation and help
- Change the membership of the team

Source: Katzenbach, J., & Smith, D. (1993). *The wisdom of teams: Creating the high performance organization.* New York: HarperBusiness.

Teams that Have Lost Their Effectiveness

Teams are prone to the same dysfunctional behaviors as any other group: not listening, idea killing, personal attacks, apathy, anarchy, and groupthink (Peters, 1987). When teams develop these behaviors, team functioning can break down and the team "gets stuck" (Katzenbach & Smith, 1993). When a team becomes stuck, it loses its effectiveness. Teams that are stuck are characterized by a loss of energy, a sense of hopelessness, a lack of purpose and identity, cynicism and mistrust, and finger pointing and personal attacks.

A nurse consultant needs to respond to the challenge of a "stuck team" by first ensuring that all the team basics are present. Strategizing for small wins and providing new information can also help revitalize a team. If these efforts fail, outside facilitation or a change in membership may be needed. A change in membership (particularly adding new members) is usually considered a last resort, because it often means the team-building efforts will need to be repeated; this can create frustration for ongoing members (Katzenbach & Smith, 1993). Box 7-8 summarizes symptoms of "stuck teams" and strategies for helping them become "unstuck."

CHAPTER SUMMARY

Working with groups and teams can be productive and stimulating as well as confusing and frustrating. Nurse consultants are frequently asked to problem solve with groups of consultees and form problem-solving teams. To work effectively with a group or team, a nurse consultant must understand and know how to respond to group dynamics.

Understanding both the needs of individuals within groups and the significance of observations about a group's communication and decision-making processes helps a nurse consultant avoid overreacting or underreacting to a group's behavior. Awareness of problems that can arise in groups and teams, such as groupthink and getting stuck, and the ability to address these problems are essential skills for nurse consultants. These skills facilitate effective problem solving and a successful nursing consultation relationship.

APPLYING CHAPTER CONTENT

Make arrangements to observe two meetings of the same group or view a videotape of a meeting. (Many communities broadcast their city council meetings over cable television; this could be videotaped and viewed in class.) Complete the observation guide in Box 7-9 and then answer the following questions:

1. What were the group's goals? Were these consistent with the group's mission?
2. Was the group more concerned with task, internal maintenance, or boundary management functions?
3. What decision-making processes did the group use? Were they effective?
4. Was there any evidence of groupthink?
5. What can you infer about group norms, personal needs of group members, and the group's power structure?
6. Would you describe this group as a working group or a team?
7. How would you interact with this group in a (nursing) consultation relationship?

What strengths would this group bring to a nursing consultation relationship? What problems do you anticipate might arise?

References

Anderson, E., & McFarlane, J. (2000). *Community as partner: Theory and practice in nursing* (3rd ed.). Philadelphia: Lippincott.

Bolman, L., & Deal, T. (1991). *Reframing organizations: Artistry, choice, and leadership.* San Francisco: Jossey-Bass.

Goodstein, L. (1978). *Consulting with human service systems.* Reading, MA: Addison-Wesley.

Harrison, M. (1994). *Diagnosing organizations: Methods, models, and processes* (2nd ed.). Thousand Oaks, CA: Sage.

Janis, I. (1982). *Groupthink* (2nd ed.). Boston: Houghton-Mifflin.

Katzenbach, J., & Smith, D. (1993). *The wisdom of teams: Creating the high performance organization.* New York: HarperBusiness.

Oyster, C. (2000). *Groups: A user's guide.* Boston: McGraw-Hill.

Peters, T. (1987). *Thriving on chaos: Handbook for a management revolution.* New York: HarperCollins.

Robbins, H., & Finley, M. (1996). *Why change doesn't work.* Princeton, NJ: Peterson's.

Sampson, E., & Marthas, M. (1990). *Group process for the health professions* (3rd ed.). Albany, NY: Delmar.

Schein, E. (1988). *Process consultation, volume I: Its role in organization development* (2nd ed.). Reading, MA: Addison-Wesley.

Schoonover-Shoffner, K. (1989). Improving work group decision-making effectiveness. *Journal of Nursing Administration, 19*(7), 10–16.

BOX 7-9   GROUP OBSERVATION GUIDE

Group being observed:

Stated mission of group:

Date and time of observation:

Nature of meeting observed (routine, emergency, etc.):

Frequency of meetings:

Date of last meeting:

Agenda (attach, if available):

Composition of group (members and "official" roles):

1.	7.
2.	8.
3.	9.
4.	10.
5.	11.
6.	12.

Communication Processes (Summary)

1. Who talked the most? What was the content of their talk?

2. Who talked but was apparently never heard?

3. Who tended to speak to whom? What is the significance of this?

4. Who interrupted whom? What did these interruptions signify?

5. What was the general communication style used by this group? What effect did this have?

6. What was the total communication picture of this group?

Communication Processes

Target of Communication

Group Member (Initiator)	1	2	3	4	5	6	7	8	9	10	11	12	General Content of Talk	Communication Style	Attentiveness of Others
1.															
2.															
3.															
4.															
5.															
6.															
7.															
8.															
9.															
10.															
11.															
12.															

Key: √ = communication event   I+ = supportive interruption   I- = negative interruption

Group Decision-Making Processes
1. What decision-making processes did the group use?
    Default
    Authority
    Minority rule
    Majority rule
    Consensus
2. Who appeared to be the key decision maker?

Risk Factors and Evidence for Groupthink
1. Was there a perception of an "enemy"?
    Yes (identify):
    No
2. Was there dehumanization of the perceived enemy?
    Yes (identify label used):
    No
3. How would you describe the level of group cohesiveness?
    Low   Medium   High   Extreme
4. Was the group willing to take excessive risks?
    Yes (describe):
    No
5. Did the group overestimate its power and morality?
    Yes (example):
    No
6. Did the group seem insulated?
    Yes   No
7. What was the nature of the group's leadership?
    Partial (example):
    Impartial
8. Was there evidence of close-mindedness?
    Yes (example):
    No
9. Were there pressures toward unanimity?
    Yes (example):
    No
10. Did the group engage in a survey of alternatives?
    Yes   No
11. Was there an examination of risks related to preferred choice?
    Yes   No
12. Was there consideration of the effects of the preferred choice on stakeholders?
    Yes   No
13. Was there reappraisal of initially rejected alternatives?
    Yes   No
14. Was there a presence of critical evaluation, a devil's advocate?
    Yes   No

8

Change in Communities

Change is one of the most reliably constant phenomena in the world. (Tiffany & Lutjens, 1998)

 KEY CONCEPTS:

ambivalence, resistance, reluctance, force-field analysis

 KEY TERMS FOR YOUR SEARCH ENGINE:

change theory, communities (or organizations) and change

INTRODUCTION

Change is the only constant in health care today. Individual health care providers and health care organizations are operating in an environment that is demanding increasingly complex changes at an increasingly rapid pace. More than 10 years ago, it was estimated that organizations, in general, need to "restructure" about every two years in order to keep up with the demands of the marketplace (McDougall, 1987). Most likely, this time frame is even shorter for today's health care organizations. For nurses and other individual health care providers, health care consumers, and communities, the rapid pace of change at the organizational and policy level of health care means that change must also occur at the personal level: New ways of thinking and doing must be learned in order to maintain the highest possible level of well-being. In particular, health care providers are finding that partnerships with communities and their members are increasingly important

strategies for fostering both individual and population health. As emphasized in Chapter 2, nurse consultants have key roles to play in these partnerships, and can make key contributions with this new community perspective of health and health care.

So, how does change fit into the nursing consultation process? First of all, nurses are often asked to help communities solve health-related problems that arise because of changes in internal or external environmental factors. Second, by definition, nursing consultation involves working with consultees to solve actual or potential problems related to a client's (i.e., community's) health status or health care delivery issues. "Solving problems" implies needing to learn to do something differently—in other words, changing one's way of thinking and/or behaving. Thus, change and the dynamics of change are pervasive themes in all nursing consultation relationships.

A request for nursing consultation means either that something is wrong now for a community or that the community's equilibrium is threatened in some way. In effect, then, a request for nursing consultation is a request for change. The fact that change is needed or desired, however, doesn't mean that it will be easy to accomplish. Furthermore, just because a problem needs to be solved (either reactively or proactively) doesn't mean that the community and its members will embrace the opportunity to change (Brack, Jones, Smith, White, & Brack, 1993).

Change occurs on two levels: the situational/mechanical and the personal/emotional. A nursing consultation relationship will be successful only if both levels of the change experience are managed effectively. For nurse consultants, then, an understanding of the dynamics of change is essential knowledge.

This chapter begins by discussing the "mechanics" of change, or how change evolves from its first rumblings to its stabilization as the new status quo. Next, the discussion turns to common emotional responses to change and the methods used to manage these responses. The final section of this chapter presents "changemaker" skills for nurse consultants: assessing a consultee's perspective of change, actualizing change, and communicating about change. As you read this chapter, consider the following questions:

- How will a community's culture affect the change process?
- What types of power will facilitate versus act as a barrier to change?
- How might the dynamics of change differ for communities that emphasize a structural, human resource, political, and symbolic frame?
- How might the dynamics of change differ with the use of different nursing consultation interaction patterns?
- What are your personal feelings about and typical reactions to change? What implications might these have for your practice of nursing consultation?

THE MECHANICS OF CHANGE

Change is the intentional movement from a current situation (the nursing consultation problem) to a futuristic, more desirable one (the goal) (Fuqua & Kurpius, 1993). Change has three identifiable stages that, while overlapping and frequently occurring very rapidly, are conceptually distinct. The "mechanics of change" are the situational events and nursing consultation tasks within each of these stages that must be accomplished if a change is to be accomplished by a community. A nurse consultant must be aware of these stages because each stage has its own set of dynamics and requires different nursing consultation roles and skills.

The stages and mechanics of change that are presented in this section—unfreezing, moving, and refreezing—are based on Kurt Lewin's (1947, 1951) classic model of change. Lewin's model, while written over 50 years ago, remains elegant in its simplicity and is the most popular explanation of how change occurs (Tiffany & Lutjens, 1998). It is also the model on which more recent (and complex) explanations of how change occurs at both the individual and organizational levels are founded.

Unfreezing

It is during the change stage of "unfreezing" that a consultee first becomes aware of a problem and is motivated to change. Unfreezing represents an awakening to a new reality and a willingness to disrupt the status quo and disengage from the past (Anderson & McFarlane, 2000). There is recognition that the current way of doing things is no longer acceptable (Kanter, Stein, & Jicks, 1992). Unfreezing, then, indicates a community's belief that the outcome of change will be better than the present situation (Brack et al., 1993). Lewin (1951) identifies three conditions that must be present if unfreezing is to occur: disconfirmation, guilt or anxiety, and psychological safety.

Disconfirmation

Disconfirmation occurs when a community perceives that the current situation is just not good enough anymore (Lewin, 1951). There is evidence that expected or desired outcomes are not happening or are threatened. Consider, as an example, a community (the client) that has found out that there is an excessive rate of dental caries among its children. In response to this finding, the county health district is recommending that the community fluoridate its drinking water. A task force of community members (the consultees) has been appointed to work with a nurse consultant to get the community to act on this recommendation. In this scenario, awareness of failure to meet a health goal (e.g., optimum dental health) is an intrinsic indicator that the community needs to engage in change. An external indicator that might provide disconfirmation to the community would be a policy that makes a community eligible for state funding of dental health programs if its drinking water is fluoridated. Whether its source is internal or external, disconfirmation indicates that a problem is either present or looming on the horizon and serves as the initial stimulus for undertaking change. This causes unfreezing to begin.

Guilt and Anxiety

Guilt or anxiety is the second condition that must be in place for unfreezing to occur. A community must feel guilty that a goal is not being met or anxious that a value is being vio-

lated (Lewin, 1951). In other words, if unfreezing is to occur, disconfirmation must be about something that is important to the consultee. Because change means a disruption of the status quo, unfreezing doesn't always happen readily, and disconfirmation must be accompanied by guilt or anxiety. For example, a marked increase in dental caries may not trigger a community reaction until it is linked to other, more serious health problems and increased health and dental care expenditures at the community level.

Psychological Safety

Disconfirmation and guilt or anxiety are enough to get a community to begin to "melt" or think about making a change. However, the "big thaw" will not occur unless a third condition, psychological safety, is present (Lewin, 1951). Psychological safety means the problem-solving environment will allow "face" or self-esteem to be maintained while help is being sought. In many nursing consultation situations, by the time a nurse consultant has been contacted, a community has already experienced disconfirmation and feels anxious and/or guilty about performance or an outcome. A nurse consultant must begin to create psychological safety at the time of initial contact. Failure to create psychological safety can cause a community to freeze back up before the nursing consultation problem has been solved. As discussed later in this chapter, failure to create psychological safety is associated with resistance to change.

There is no easy formula for creating psychological safety. The key, however, is to keep a community from feeling humiliated and losing face or self-esteem (Schein, 1987). The nurse consultant must help the community and its consultees feel worthwhile as individuals or a community even though current goals are not being met. In other words, a community or consultee needs to feel specific performance or outcome-related guilt in order for unfreezing to occur, but not at the risk of feeling worthless as an individual person or community. After all, the community knows there is a problem if help has been sought and doesn't need reminding that the problem exists, but rather needs to be given confidence that the problem is solvable.

Reassurance and supportive comments also help to create psychological safety. Communities often need to know that their problem is within the "normal range" or has been experienced by others before they can accept responsibility for working on it. If a problem is seen as too big and its intervention too complex, the "complexity syndrome" can set in and become an excuse for abandoning change efforts (Brack et al., 1993). A nurse consultant should offer reassurance that similar problems have been successfully resolved by others. Sometimes, former consultees with whom the nurse consultant has successfully worked on a similar problem can help to provide this reassurance. Often, consultees simply need to hear that the situation is under control and is not unusual. This "saves face" by communicating that the consultee is not "abnormal" or "bad" because of the problem.

Moving

Moving is the second stage of change. In this stage, change is under way and a community is making the transition from what is known and comfortable to a new way of thinking and doing. Moving means embracing a vision of a new future and uniting behind the steps necessary to achieve that future (Kanter et al., 1992).

Moving requires cognitive restructuring or developing a new mindset. Cognitive restructuring can only take place, however, once unfreezing has occurred and the community is open to viewing a situation in a different way. Cognitive restructuring involves searching for new viewpoints or information about a situation. The two most common strategies for gathering the data needed for cognitive restructuring are identification and scanning.

Cognitive Restructuring Through Identification

Identification involves becoming aligned with a role model and taking on the role model's point of view. Identification is a relatively quick way of gaining a new viewpoint and provides a certain amount of comfort to the consultee because less time is spent "in limbo" looking for a problem solution. The limitation of identification as a means of cognitive restructuring is its narrow scope: Only one alternate viewpoint is accessed.

Often, consultees identify with the nurse consultant as a role model. This is most likely to happen when the purchase of expertise model is used to guide a nursing consultation relationship, or when a nurse consultant has other sources of personal power such as charisma. When identification is used as the means to facilitate cognitive restructuring, a nurse consultant should link consultees to appropriate role models in their environment. Communities that have successfully resolved a problem similar to that of the consultee are particularly appropriate choices for role models. For example, a community that is undertaking an educational campaign in regards to water fluoridation could be linked with a community that has already successfully implemented fluoridation of its water supply.

Cognitive Restructuring Through Scanning

Scanning is a second strategy that a community can use to obtain information that will help it with cognitive restructuring. Because scanning involves seeking information from a variety of sources (peers, the Internet, workshops, etc.), this strategy is more thorough than identification as well as more likely to produce a new perspective that really fits the community's needs, culture, and constraints. However, scanning is a slower means of acquiring information and, therefore, unsuitable for urgent consultation situations.

Refreezing

Refreezing is the final stage of change. Refreezing has occurred when a community has integrated a new point of view into both its self-concept and its relationships with others (Schein, 1987). It means that the "new rules of behavior" (Helvie, 1998) have become a part of the system. Refreezing means that new attitudes, practices, and policies have been put into place and are the new status quo (Kanter et al., 1992). Refreezing occurs as a result of "internal sorting." That is, a community discards old and inappropriate habits and attitudes and develops and takes on new ones (Bridges, 1991).

A nurse consultant can facilitate refreezing by helping a community evaluate the effectiveness of the implemented change and by making revisions as needed. A nurse consultant can also facilitate refreezing by ensuring that system supports needed to maintain a change are in place. Examples of system supports frequently needed to support change are financial and human resources, vision, skills, enthu-

siasm, equipment, positive feedback, and reward structures. In some cases, in order to facilitate refreezing in one sector of a community, the nurse consultant will need to help other sectors of the community unfreeze in terms of their relationship to and perceptions of the consultee (Helvie, 1998). In a scenario in which community residents have become educated in regard to fluoridation issues, for example, dentists (and other health care providers) may need to learn new ways of interacting with health care consumers who have acquired more education and, perhaps, more political skills.

The Mechanics of Change and the Nursing Consultation Process

While the theme of change permeates the entire nursing consultation relationship, the different stages of the change process coincide with different stages in the nursing consultation process (see Figure 8-1). Disconfir-

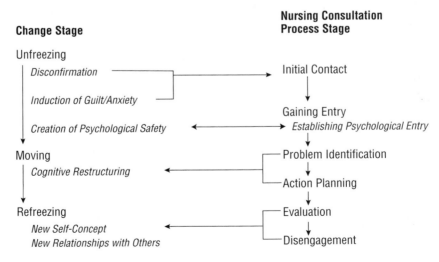

Figure 8-1   The Mechanics of Change and the Nursing Consultation Process.
Change is a pervasive theme in nursing consultation relationships. The different stages of change coincide with the different stages and tasks of the nursing consultation process. The two biggest mistakes in nursing consultation and trying to facilitate change are: attempting to introduce change before unfreezing has occurred, and a lack of attention to issues and conditions needed in order for refreezing to occur.

mation and guilt/anxiety are often in place by the time a community makes initial contact with a nurse consultant. These conditions need reinforcement throughout the entire gaining entry phase of the nursing consultation process so that the community doesn't back down from problem-solving efforts. The creation of psychological safety needs to begin with initial contact and must be well under way before a nursing consultation contract can be agreed on. However, concern with creating psychological safety continues throughout the entire nursing consultation relationship and change process.

Once unfreezing has occurred, moving can get under way. The change stage of moving coincides with the problem identification and action planning stages of the nursing consultation process. Cognitive restructuring occurs during these stages as problem explanations and solutions are explored. Refreezing should be detected during the evaluation phase of the nursing consultation process and signals that it is appropriate to begin the disengagement phase. The continuity supports that are established during the disengagement phase help to ensure that refreezing will be permanent.

EMOTIONAL RESPONSES TO CHANGE

Change is difficult. It helps. It hurts. It helps and hurts at the same time. Change is inevitable. We ignore change at our own peril. (Tiffany & Lutjens, 1998)

Change occurs on two levels: the situational/mechanical level and the personal/emotional level. While Lewin's description of the mechanics of change is helpful for understanding how change occurs, it fails to address the emotions that individuals (i.e., consultees) experience in response to change. Unless the emotions that accompany change are addressed, the change process itself will

become stuck and a community's problem will remain unsolved.

"Transition" is the psychological process people go through to come to terms with the personal/emotional level of a new situation (Bridges, 1991). Unless transition occurs, implementing and maintaining change will be difficult. Because any change requires resources and energy from within an individual (the consultee) as well as the larger community, the nurse consultant must be able to deal consciously and constructively with the emotions and psychological transition that accompanies change (Perlman & Takacs, 1990; Schoolfield & Orduna, 1994). Even when a problem solution or change is as seemingly concrete as adding fluoride to a community's drinking water, it is consultees'—and a community's—knowledge, attitudes, beliefs, and values that are the real targets of change (Haffer, 1986; Helvie, 1998). On an individual level, then, change means three things: recognizing a deficit, giving something up, and learning something new. These demands can create feelings of ineffectiveness, loss of control, confusion, conflict, and loss of meaning (Bolman & Deal, 1991). What change means on an individual level explains the emotional responses that tend to be associated with change: ambivalence, resistance, and grief.

Ambivalence

Ambivalence is a natural response to change (Lippitt & Lippitt, 1986; Ulschak & SnowAntle, 1990). Consultees representing a community might welcome the novelty of change or the improvement a change promises and be exhilarated by the challenge of change but, at the same time, question whether expectations are realistic and timing is right. A community and consultees may also feel ambivalent toward the nurse consultant as an agent of change. The nurse consultant can be seen as both necessary and hostile to the community: As much as the community would like its problem solved, it would also like to maintain much of the status quo (Price & Reiss-Brennan, 1990).

Ambivalence causes a community to alternate between feeling optimistic and pessimistic about the change process. Ambivalence often results in one of two responses: ignoring concerns and losses and rushing ahead with change, or keeping things as they are and replaying the past (Bolman & Deal, 1991; Bridges, 1991). Both of these responses are counterproductive to the nursing consultation process. The first ignores the need for psychological transition and the second simply abandons problem solving.

Managing Ambivalence

A nurse consultant must be able to manage ambivalence if transition and change are to be successful. The first step to managing ambivalence is simply bringing it out into the open and communicating its legitimacy. These actions alone can help decrease the likelihood of a counterproductive response to ambivalence (Lippitt & Lippitt, 1986). A nurse consultant also needs to remain objective and avoid becoming defensive when consultees voice doubts about a proposed change. Instead, doubts and negative comments should be used as cues to verify the soundness of a proposed action plan.

Another strategy for responding to ambivalence is to have consultees list their questions and doubts about a proposed change in one column and their positive feelings about the change in another. The nurse consultant can then help consultees brainstorm about what can be done to respond to doubts as well as what can be done to support positive feelings (Lippitt & Lippitt, 1986). In this way, ambivalence can be used as a resource for enhancing the likelihood of a more successful and long-lasting change effort. Box 8-1 summarizes strategies for managing ambivalence about change.

Resistance

Any community has good reason to resist change. Change is associated with the discomfort of giving up the familiar. Unlearning current ways of doing things implies doing something wrong and, therefore, threatens face (Schein, 1987). Furthermore, learning something new creates a period of uncertainty, feelings of incompetence, and a temporary decrease in effectiveness. Learning something new, in other words, causes the expert to once again become a novice.

Resistance also occurs because change can disrupt the structural arrangements of a community. During the moving stage of the change

---

BOX 8-1   MANAGING RESPONSES TO CHANGE: AMBIVALENCE

Ambivalence occurs because any change has costs as well as potential benefits. Strategies a nurse consultant can use to manage ambivalence include:

- Publicize it—"There seems to be some ambivalence . . ."
- Normalize it—"Ambivalence is a normal response to change . . ."
- Use it as an opportunity to check the soundness of the action plan—"What doubts do you have about this change? How could these doubts be addressed?"

process, there can be a lack of clarity about who has authority, who is supposed to do what, and how to relate to each other (Bolman & Deal, 1991). This creates instability and confusion and causes feelings of powerlessness and insecurity.

Finally, change can be resisted for ideological reasons. Some consultees or a community as a whole may truly believe that a change is misdirected and that the current situation or another alternative is better than the proposed change. For other consultees, a proposed change may violate important values or community/organizational principles. For example, consultees involved in a fluoridation education project may resist these efforts because of fundamental beliefs about the role of government in relation to health issues. Box 8-2 identifies other reasons for resisting change.

Managing Resistance

Too often, resistance is used as an excuse by a consultant for neglecting to reach out and understand people who are only reluctant to change (Smith, 1996). Because resistance (or reluctance) is an expected response to change, nurse consultants must be skilled at managing resistance if a consultation relationship is to be successful. Key strategies for managing resistance are validating emotions, providing information and support, and dealing with bargaining.

Nurse consultants need to confront resistance by validating its underlying emotions, while still holding consultees accountable for their performance (Schoolfield & Orduna, 1994). For example, a nurse consultant can empathize with consultees about their feelings of insecurity and incompetence in regard to providing community education about fluoridation, but still communicate the expectation that quality work will be done. If consultees are to be held accountable for standards of performance while a change is being implemented, however, they must be given what they need to feel competent and secure (Bolman & Deal, 1991). Too often, the response to resis-

---

BOX 8-2   REASONS FOR RESISTANCE

- Loss
- Too much uncertainty
- Surprises: No preparation or background information
- Confusion and interruption of routines
- Loss of face: Looking "stupid" for past actions
- Concerns about competence to deal with the new ways
- More work: Meetings, learning, and so forth
- Past resentments: Memories of negative change experiences
- Real threats: Job loss and so forth
- Inertia: Too comfortable doing things the old way
- Uncertainty about the personal payoff versus costs of change
- Low energy: Too many changes happening too fast
- Ripple effects: There is never only one change

Sources: Kanter, R., Stein, B., & Jicks, T. (1992). *The challenge of organizational change.* New York: Free Press; and Robbins, H., & Finley, M. (1996). *Why change doesn't work.* Princeton, NJ: Peterson's.

tance is a lecture about productivity. Instead, the nurse consultant can help decrease consultees' feelings of powerlessness and uncertainty by using such strategies as providing information and feedback, controlling rumors, teaching needed skills, providing needed material and psychological support, and encouraging involvement in change decisions.

Typical questions that consultees have about change are identified in Box 8-3. These questions underscore the importance of communication in overcoming resistance to change. Consider the information and supports that might be needed to overcome resistance to a proposal for water fluoridation: The consultees responsible for community education could be expected to have questions and need information about the risks and benefits of fluoridation and costs involved. They might also need assistance in developing effective teaching strategies.

Bargaining is a resistance tactic that is used frequently by consultees. What consultees try to do during bargaining is offer compromises that will bargain away the proposed change. A nurse consultant needs to address bargaining by first considering that it might be a valid reaction to the nurse consultant's attempt to implement a change that would either be a

poor fit with a community and its problem or would possibly create new problems (Brack et al., 1993). If this explanation for bargaining is ruled out, a nurse consultant should respond to bargaining by focusing on the needs of the consultee that are threatened by the change (e.g., security and feelings of competence) and exploring how these needs can be met (e.g., with information or training) without compromising the desired change outcome (Perlman & Takacs, 1990). If bargaining is a reaction to a genuine difference in values, a nurse consultant should try to persuade the consultee to give the change a try, and then evaluate and reconsider. Box 8-4 summarizes strategies for managing resistance to change.

Grief

Grief is the third common emotional response to change. Grief occurs because change involves the loss of old, established, comfortable ways as well as one's old role and identity. Because change involves loss, a grieving process needs to take place so that the past is let go of and the change can be embraced (Schoolfield & Orduna, 1994). In change situations, the grief response consists of the classic grief reactions: denial, anger, bargaining, depression, resigna-

BOX 8-3   TYPICAL QUESTIONS ABOUT CHANGE

- How do we get from here to there?
- What is involved in this change process?
- Who will do what and how will they do it?
- What do we have to learn that we don't already know?
- When will we start to see results?
- How will we be kept informed of progress?
- What is expected of me and of the community as a whole?
- Is this change the only one planned, or is it just one of many?
- Is the community truly committed to this idea?

Source: Robbins, H., & Finley, M. (1996). *Why change doesn't work.* Princeton, NJ: Peterson's.

BOX 8-4   MANAGING RESPONSES TO CHANGE: RESISTANCE

Consultees resist change because it is associated with feelings of incompetence, ineffectiveness, and confusion. Resistance can also occur when change conflicts with personal values. Strategies a nurse consultant can use to manage resistance include:

- Validate the underlying emotions of the resistance while still demanding accountability.
- Keep communication open: Listen, solicit and give feedback, and provide information.
- Give consultees the material and psychological support they need to feel competent and secure.
- Realign and renegotiate policies and roles to make them supportive of expected new behaviors.
- Explore the possibility that bargaining may indicate a proposed change is a poor fit for the community.
- Respond to bargaining by negotiating a "trial" or "pilot" of the proposed change that will be followed by evaluation and reconsideration.

---

tion, openness/acceptance, and reemergence (Perlman & Takacs, 1990).

Denial and Anger

The first stage of the grief response, denial, often takes the form of denying that a problem actually exists. In other cases, ambivalence and active resistance may signal denial. To some extent, denial is an unavoidable part of the unfreezing process. Just as unfreezing must occur, denial must be resolved before moving toward change can get under way.

When consultees or a community realize that change is going to proceed and the status quo is going to be disrupted, anger often occurs. In this stage of the grief process, consultees tend to glorify the past and exaggerate the problems of the present. Others—the nurse consultant and persons in supervisory positions, in particular—become the target of anger and are blamed for the difficulties of the change process.

Bargaining, Depression, and Resignation

Bargaining occurs as a resistance tactic once change efforts are under way or perceived as inevitable. Once the change is, in fact, under way and accompanying feelings of incompetence, ineffectiveness, and powerlessness become a reality, depression follows. When resistance tactics are recognized as being ineffective by a consultee, resignation occurs. During this phase of the grief process, there is usually compliance with a change, but no enthusiasm for it. The challenge for a nurse consultant is to transform compliance into commitment so that change will continue (refreeze) once the nursing consultation relationship has ended.

Openness/Acceptance and Reemergence

The final stages of the grief response coincide with the refreezing stage of the change process. Openness/acceptance occurs when consultees accept the personal implications of change and rearrange their values and self-concept to accommodate the change. Reemergence, the last stage in the classic grief response process, signifies that refreezing has occurred and the change is integrated fully into consultees' ways of interacting within the community. Reemergence means that the past has been let go of both emotionally and intellectually. Reemergence (and refreezing) means that consultees have redefined their roles and identity in relationship to the nursing consultation problem and the community. Figure 8-2 illustrates the relationship between the grief process and the mechanics of change.

Managing Grief

Nurse consultants need to understand that completion of the grief process is necessary if a change is to be successful and long lasting. Failure to allow a grief response results in change that is only short-lived because losses have not been adapted to or acknowledged. Rather than managing grief in the sense of eliminating it, a nurse consultant needs to facilitate a community's movement through the various stages of grief by helping consultees accept and adapt to the losses and role changes associated with the change. Managing grief requires acknowledgment, empathy, and patience. What a community has lost even temporarily as a result of change needs to be acknowledged. The past and emotions associated with this loss need to be respected.

Patience and support are also needed as a community adapts to the loss of an old identity and the taking on of a new identity. Finally, rituals can be used to help a community achieve closure with its past and recognize the future (Bridges, 1991).

Box 8-5 summarizes grief management strategies for nurse consultants. As you review these strategies, consider how they might be applied to this chapter's change scenario of adding fluoride to a community's drinking water. Some of the losses experienced by the consultees who are involved in the preliminary community education activities could be loss of their traditional role as caregiver (replaced by the role of educator) and loss of a certain type of relationship with the larger community. These losses require adaptation and the taking on of a new professional identity. All of these losses can also result in a typical grief response on the part of the consultees. A nurse consultant working with the consultees in this scenario needs to acknowledge these losses and put supports (such as education) in place that will promote adaptation to new roles. The community as a whole will need to be patient as the role changes for the consultees result in changes in the usual

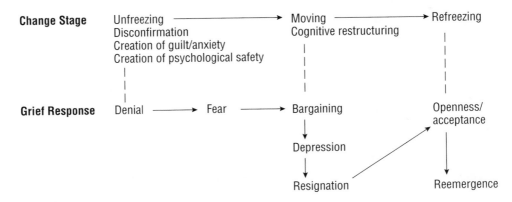

Figure 8-2   Change and Grief.
Grief accompanies change because change entails loss. The classic grief reactions of denial, anger, bargaining, depression, resignation, openness/acceptance, and reemergence can be observed as the stages of change unfold.

BOX 8-5   MANAGING THE EMOTIONS OF CHANGE: GRIEF

Grief is a normal reaction to change because change means the loss of comfortable habits, as well as familiar ways of interacting, thinking, and behaving. Change also means the loss of actual or symbolic roles and identities. Passage through the stages of grief is necessary if change is to be successful and long lasting. Managing grief means facilitating passage through the stages of grief rather than trying to eliminate it. Grief management strategies for nurse consultants include:

- Acknowledge what has been lost
- Respect the past
- Have empathy for what the loss means to those involved (consultees)
- Put supports in place to facilitate adaptation to both the loss and new identity
- Have patience
- Use rituals to bring closure to the past and recognition to the future

Sources: Bridges, W. (1991). *Managing transitions: Making the most of change.* Reading, MA: Addison-Wesley; and Perlman, D., & Takacs, G. (1990). The 10 stages of change. *Nursing Management, 21*(4), 33–38.

services they offer. Accomplishment of the change (implementation of the fluoridation system) could be acknowledged with "rituals" such as newspaper and television news features.

CHANGEMAKER SKILLS FOR NURSE CONSULTANTS

As discussed in Chapter 1, change agency is fundamentally different from nursing consultation. In order to differentiate the two, Kanter, Stein, and Jicks (1992) use the term *changemaker* to describe a consultant's role in the change process. Nurse consultants fulfill the specific changemaker roles of strategist and implementor. In the strategist role, a nurse consultant identifies a problem, creates a vision, and identifies feasibility issues related to the proposed change. In the implementor role, the nurse consultant manages the day-to-day process of change and ensures that the

supports needed for the change are in place. The specific changemaker skills that the nurse consultant needs in order to fulfill these roles are the abilities to assess a consultee's perspective of change, actualize change, and communicate about change.

Assessing Consultees' Perspective of Change

Say the word "change" to any randomly selected group and you will likely get three different responses. Some throw up their hands and say, "God, not again." Others say, "Well, it's about time." The third group will simply throw up. (Robbins & Finley, 1996)

A community's perspective of change has implications for the roles a nurse consultant will need to assume during the nursing consultation relationship. A community's perspective of change also determines the types of barriers that may be encountered as change strategies are being developed and implemented. Understanding a community's perspective of change helps a nurse consultant anticipate the ways in which change may be experienced by the community and its members, including the consultees. Understanding a community's perspective of change also helps a nurse consultant select the intervention strategies and interaction style that will most effectively facilitate problem solving and subsequent change. Change is generally viewed by communities in one of three ways: as something needed to achieve a goal, something needed in order to solve a problem, or something that "just happens" (Hansen, 1995). Box 8-6 presents questions a nurse consultant can ask to determine a consultee's perspective of change.

Change as Choice

When a community views change as a choice, it is often undertaken proactively rather than reactively; it may even be pursued aggressively. Communities and consultees who view change as choice see change as tolerable, if not desirable. Communities with this perspective view change as a means to achieve a goal (such as improved community well-being). They also tend to view change as a linear, orchestrated process and, therefore, respond well to carefully orchestrated change activities where change can be experienced as a series of steps and stages. Since these communities often plan change in anticipation of environmental events, they are ideal candidates for a process consultation interaction pattern.

BOX 8-6   ASSESSING A COMMUNITY'S PERSPECTIVE OF CHANGE

Change is generally viewed by a community in one of three ways: as something undertaken by choice in order to attain a goal, something to become involved in only when a problem needs to be solved, or something that is an inevitable necessity and "just happens." Questions a nurse consultant can ask to determine a community's perspective of change include:

- What triggers change for the community?
  Goals?
  Problems?
- How does the community respond to pressure about change?
  Proactively or reactively?
  Aggressively, passively, or with resistance?
  With a time crunch?
- What is valued as the outcome of change?
  Improved health?
  Security?
  Stability and equilibrium?
- What does change look and feel like as it is occurring?
  Steps and stages?
  Chaos, confusion, and panic?
  Patterned transition in growth?
  Lurches and stumbling?

A potential challenge of working with communities who undertake change proactively is getting them to slow down. Communities with this perspective of change are sometimes so enthusiastic that they rush through a change process without allowing time for the needed psychological and cultural transition to occur. In this situation, the nurse consultant needs to function as a process advocate (this consultation role was decribed in Chapter 5) so that critical elements of the change process are not overlooked.

Change Only if Necessary

A community that views change as something that is undertaken only when a problem needs to be solved tends to view change as troublesome and unpredictable, and as something that "has to be done." From this perspective, a community's need to change is often triggered by input and output problems such as the inability to secure needed resources (such as funding) or to satisfy needs of its members. The desired outcome of this type of change is increased security. For these communities, change is often reactive and occurs under a time crunch.

A nurse consultant is likely to encounter increased resistance from consultees who have this perspective of change. Even though these communities recognize that they have a problem to solve, they perceive themselves (perhaps accurately) as having little choice in regard to change. A community in this type of situation often experiences change as chaos, confusion, and panic.

Nurse consultants often find themselves assuming the role of troubleshooter for communities that have a problem-oriented view of change. In these situations, the purchase of expertise or doctor–patient interaction patterns tend to be the most effective and, in fact, are sometimes necessary. A goal of a nurse consultant working with consultees who view change from this perspective is to help them learn to engage in environmental

monitoring and more proactive forms of change.

Change "Just Happens"

The third perspective that a community may have about change is that change is something that "just happens." Change is viewed by these communities as inevitable and inherent to the process of evolving with their environments. A community with this perspective of change may undertake change proactively or may seek nursing consultation and change when it is experiencing problems with equilibrium and stability (e.g., health issues). Grief, ambivalence, resignation, and passive resistance are common responses of communities that have this perspective of change. These communities tend to experience change as a patterned transition in growth, but also as a process that occurs with lurches and stumbling.

Nurse consultants working with communities that view change as an inevitable necessity need to encourage community involvement in the change process. In these situations, nurse consultants often find a process consultation interaction pattern to be a necessary and effective means of creating ownership of a problem solution and its resultant change.

Actualizing Change

The costs of failed change attempts are high. Loss of energy, loss of trust and credibility, loss of respect, anger, increased stress, poorer health for a community and its members, and a decreased willingness to take risks are just a few of the outcomes of change failures (Robbins & Finley, 1996). Change can fail for any number of reasons (see Box 8-7), many of which a nurse consultant can prevent by attending to the dynamics of the nursing consultation process and by managing the emotional responses to change. Two additional strategies a nurse consultant can use to ensure that a proposed change is actually

BOX 8-7   WHY CHANGE FAILS

- The wrong idea
- The right idea but the wrong time
- The wrong reason
- Lacks authenticity
- Reality contradicts the change
- Loss of perspective (mission, values, etc.)
- Wrong leader
- The change is only for the sake of change
- The community isn't prepared or convinced about the need for change
- The community gets carried away by change: "The sin of excess"
- The community doesn't get carried away enough
- Bad luck: Unforeseen environmental events

Source: Robbins, H., & Finley, M. (1996). *Why change doesn't work.* Princeton, NJ: Peterson's.

implemented are force-field analysis and creating ownership of change.

Force-Field Analysis

Force-field analysis (Lewin, 1951) is a classic and time-tested strategy nurse consultants can use to help consultees as well as a community as a whole identify and visualize factors in a problem situation that could act as either barriers or supporters of change. Force-field analysis can also be used to assess the "rightness" of a community's decision to proceed with a specific change.

In force-field theory, a system's current state is conceptualized as reflecting an equilibrium in which two sets of forces are visible: restraining forces or factors that act to maintain the status quo, and driving forces or factors that encourage movement away from the status quo and support a proposed change (Lewin, 1951). Driving and restraining forces can be environmental/situational or personal/emotional factors. These forces vary in their degree of intensity or importance.

Equilibrium or the status quo exists as long as these two sets of forces—the "force field"—

are in balance. According to force-field theory, there are three basic interventions a nurse consultant can use to induce change: add driving forces, eliminate or reduce restraining forces, or do some of both. Changing the balance of driving and restraining forces introduces a state of disequilibrium and provides the disconfirmation needed to get a change under way ("unfreezing"). Disequilibrium remains as long as a change is in progress. Once goals have been accomplished or "refreezing" has occurred, a system returns to a state of equilibrium under new conditions.

Force-field analysis is most useful when carried out collaboratively by the nurse consultant and the consultees. Consultees can help identify relevant drivers and restrainers as well as estimate their intensity. Consultees can also help identify which forces are most important and feasible to act on to encourage movement away from the status quo. Figure 8-3 depicts what a force-field analysis might look like, in this case, completed by a group of individuals involved in a fluoridation task force.

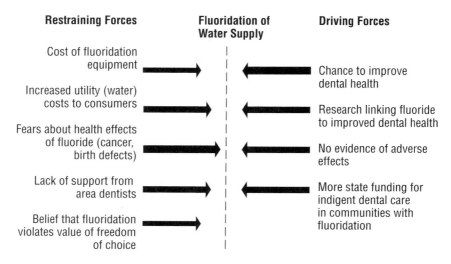

Figure 8-3   Force-Field Analysis for Fluoridating a Community's Drinking Water.
This force-field analysis is from the perspective of community members who have been assigned to a task force to implement a plan to fluoridate a community's drinking water. In this force field, fear is the strongest restraining force and the opportunity to improve the community's health status is the strongest driving force. In this scenario, the nurse consultant needs to develop interventions that will address the restraining force of fear if the fluoridation plan is to gain community support. The driving force of increased state funding for indigent dental care, which would be a part of the fluoridation "package," can be emphasized to help gain acceptance for this change.

Creating Ownership of Change

A second change-actualizing skill that nurse consultants need is that of creating ownership of change. To create ownership of change, a nurse consultant needs to help consultees and the community see themselves as beneficiaries rather than victims of change (Cohen & Murri, 1995). This can be accomplished by painting a picture of what the change will be like and engaging the community's imagination in further developing this vision. Ownership of change is facilitated when a community has a strong sense of being a part of the change process and its outcome (Price & Reiss-Brennan, 1990). A community as a whole and consultees, as representatives of the community, should be encouraged to play with a proposed problem solution or "change idea" and modify it as needed to fit both their own needs and those of the community. Encouraging consultee involvement in this way communicates a valuing of both the consultee as an individual and the expertise he or she is contributing to the change situation. Change (problem-solving) strategies will more likely be accepted, implemented, and long lasting when community members are involved in every step of the problem-solving process.

Because change is resisted less when a community is actively engaged in the change process, establishing a sense of "we-ness" and unity ("We're all in this together") is essential for creating ownership of change. Unity and ownership of change is facilitated when consultees feel supported, both administratively and emotionally, for exposing themselves to the possible personal risks associated with involvement in a change effort. Nurse consultants need to persuade a community to give consultees the time and resources needed to make the change and show measurable success.

Sometimes unity and ownership of change can be fostered by first implementing the change in a pro-change sector of the community and by building supportive coalitions. Once this "pilot group" demonstrates success, their results can be broadcast throughout the community. Members of the pilot sector can then be used to work with the remaining sectors in the community to decrease their resistance or reluctance to change. This strategy creates unity and ownership of change by its "snowball effect" of involvement and success.

Finally, any change must be consistent with the needs and culture of a community if it is to be owned by the community and its members. Change that violates cultural norms will most likely be resisted, rejected, or sabotaged. Box 8-8 summarizes strategies for creating ownership of change.

Communicating About Change

The importance of communication in the change process has been mentioned a number of times throughout this chapter. How-ever, communication is frequently impeded during the change process by several forces:

- A community's belief that change is a waste of time due to previous negative change experiences
- False familiarity ("We've been through this before")
- Fear
- The rumor mill
- "Sloppy execution" of communication: incomprehensibility, abstraction, complexity, and clichés (Hammer & Stanton, 1995)

Facilitating change demands two sets of communication skills: selling change and talking through the change process.

Selling Change

Change is an act of the imagination. Until the imagination is engaged, no important change can occur. (Robbins & Finley, 1996)

Until a community is sold on a change, it will be resistant, or at least reluctant, to expose itself to the costs associated with change. A key to selling change is creating a vision of

BOX 8-8   CREATING OWNERSHIP OF CHANGE

Strategies a nurse consultant can use to create ownership of change include the following:

- Help the community see itself as a beneficiary rather than as a victim of change.
- Involve community members in creating the change vision and in developing problem-solving/change strategies.
- Create a sense of "we-ness" and unity about the change effort and what it involves.
- Ensure administrative and emotional support for undertaking the change.
- Use a pilot group to demonstrate the change; broadcast their success and let them "teach" the next group.
- Be sure that proposed changes are consistent with the needs, constraints, and culture of the community.

Source: Robbins, H., & Finley, M. (1996). *Why change doesn't work.* Princeton, NJ: Peterson's.

how the change will look and feel, both while it is under way and once it is accomplished. To sell change, a nurse consultant must first "segment the audience" (Hammer & Stanton, 1995). This means a nurse consultant first recognizes that different groups in a community will be affected by a change in different ways and then personalizes the change message given to each group in terms of timing, media, and emphasis. To continue with the example of adding fluoride to a community's drinking water, the community would need to hear that fluoridation will mean improved dental health—and no health risks. Dental care providers may need to hear that fluoridation may actually result in increased demand for their services because of an increase in funding for indigent dental care that will be associated with fluoridation. Selling change is also facilitated by using multiple voices (e.g., both providers and consumers of dental care) and multiple channels of communication;

this increases the likelihood that each listener will find a speaker to whom they can relate.

Talking Through the Change Process

Closely related to change-selling skills, but having a different focus, are the communication skills that a nurse consultant needs to use on an ongoing basis to guide consultees through the change process. Specific attention needs to be given to reinforcing the "core message" of the change process:

- Purpose: Why we must go through this; the scope and scale of the change
- Process: How it will be accomplished, including the governing process for managing the change
- Progress: Are we on track with how we envisioned the change unfolding
- Problems: Setbacks that have occurred and lessons that have been learned (Champ, 1997; Hammer & Stanton, 1995)

BOX 8-9　COMMUNICATING ABOUT CHANGE

- Segment the audience; address different groups of stakeholders differently in terms of timing, media, and emphasis.
- Use multiple channels of communication; supplement verbal communication with nonverbal messages in the form of memos, posters, and so forth.
- Use multiple voices; different messengers will present different viewpoints (this helps to ensure that every listener will find someone with whom they can identify).
- Communicate clearly; keep in mind the essential core of the change message: Purpose, process, progress, and problems.
- Honesty is the only policy—"I don't know" is better than a lie.
- Use emotions, not just logic; convey passion and enthusiasm about the change.
- Use communication to heal, console, encourage, and express appreciation.
- Communicate tangibly. Back up words with actions and evidence.
- Communicate, communicate, communicate.
- Listen, listen, listen.

Source: Hammer, M., & Stanton, S. (1995). *The reengineering revolution: A handbook.* New York: Harper-Business.

This core message needs to be repeated and communicated clearly, honestly, and in tangible terms. Talking through the change process is more effective when a nurse consultant communicates with passion and enthusiasm as well as logic. A nurse consultant also needs to use communication skills to encourage, console, and express appreciation. Finally, talking through the change process requires two-way communication. Nurse consultants need to both listen and respond to what consultees have to say. Box 8-9 summarizes the skills a nurse consultant needs to communicate effectively about change.

CHAPTER SUMMARY

Because consultation is fundamentally a problem-solving process, change is inherent in all nursing consultation relationships. A request for nursing consultation is, in effect, a request for help to make a change. To be effective as problem solvers and changemakers, nurse consultants need an understanding of both the mechanics of change and the emotional responses change precipitates. To function effectively in the change-maker roles of strategist and implementor, the nurse consultant needs to be able to assess a consultee's perspective of change, as well as actualize and communicate about change.

APPLYING CHAPTER CONTENT

1. Reflect on two change situations in which you have recently been involved, one of which was successful and the other unsuccessful. What factors can you identify that contributed to these different change outcomes?
2. Consider the change scenarios of (a) adding a nurse practitioner to a clinic that is staffed only by physicians and (b) transforming a wing of a rural acute care hospital into a long-term intermediate care facility.
   - Conduct a force-field analysis on each of these change scenarios. How could you use this information to facilitate the proposed change? Specifically, how could you use this information to sell and talk through the proposed change?
   - What specific sources of resistance would you anticipate in each of these scenarios? How would you attempt to address these?
   - What types of losses would occur with each of these scenarios? How could consultees be compensated for these losses?
   - How could the application of change-actualizing strategies such as building coalitions and implementing a "pilot" change be used in each of these scenarios?

References

Anderson, E., & McFarlane, J. (2000). *Community as client: Theory and application in nursing* (3rd ed.). Philadelphia: Lippincott.

Bolman, L., & Deal, T. (1991). *Reframing organizations: Artistry, choice, and leadership*. San Francisco: Jossey-Bass.

Brack, G., Jones, E., Smith, R., White, J., & Brack, C. (1993). A primer on consultation theory: Building a flexible worldview. *Journal of Counseling and Development, 71*, 619–628.

Bridges, W. (1991). *Managing transitions: Making the most of change*. Reading, MA: Addison-Wesley.

Champ, J. (1997). Preparing for organizational change. In F. Hesselbein, M. Goldsmith, & R. Beckhard (Eds.), *The organization of the future* (pp. 9–16). San Francisco: Jossey-Bass.

Cohen, W., & Murri, M. (1995). Managing the change process. *Journal of AHIMA, 66*(6), 40–47.

Fuqua, D., & Kurpius, D. (1993). Conceptual models in organizational consultation. *Journal of Counseling and Development, 71,* 607–618.

Haffer, A. (1986). Facilitating change: Choosing the appropriate strategy. *Journal of Nursing Administration, 16*(4), 18–22.

Hammer, M., & Stanton, S. (1995*). The reengineering revolution: A handbook.* New York: HarperBusiness.

Hansen, H. (1995). The advanced practice nurse as a change agent. In M. Snyder & M. Mirr (Eds.), *Advanced practice nursing: A guide to professional development* (pp. 197–213). New York: Springer.

Helvie, C. (1998). *Advanced practice nursing in the community.* Thousand Oaks, CA: Sage.

Kanter, R., Stein, B., & Jicks, T. (1992). *The challenge of organizational change.* New York: Free Press.

Lewin, K. (1947). Frontiers in group dynamics. *Human Relations, 1,* 5–41.

Lewin, K. (1951). *Field theory in social sciences.* New York: Harper & Row.

Lippitt, G., & Lippitt, R. (1986). *The consulting process in action* (2nd ed.). San Diego: University Associates.

McDougall, G. (1987). The role of the clinical nurse specialist consultant in organizational development. *Clinical Nurse Specialist, 1*(3), 133–138.

Perlman, D., & Takacs, G. (1990). The 10 stages of change. *Nursing Management, 21*(4), 33–38.

Price, J., & Reiss-Brennan, B. (1989). Consulting telesis: A systems approach. *Nursing Management, 20*(11), 80A–80E.

Robbins, H., & Finley, M. (1996). *Why change doesn't work.* Princeton, NJ: Peterson's.

Schein, E. (1987). *Process consultation, volume II: Lessons for managers and consultants.* Reading, MA: Addison-Wesley.

Schoolfield, M., & Orduna, A. (1994). Understanding staff nurses responses to change: Utilization of a grief-change framework to facilitate innovation. *Clinical Nurse Specialist, 8*(1), 57–62.

Smith, D. (1996). *Taking charge of change.* Reading, MA: Addison-Wesley.

Tiffany, C., & Lutjens, L. (1998). *Planned change theories: Review, analysis, and implications.* Thousand Oaks, CA: Sage.

Ulschak, F., & SnowAntle, S. (1990). *Consultation skills for health care professionals.* San Francisco: Jossey-Bass.

THE NURSING
CONSULTATION PROCESS

Gaining Entry
in Community Consultation

Starting a relationship with a new client has always been the real challenge for me. (Metzger, 1993)

 KEY CONCEPTS:

scanning, contracting, physical entry, psychological entry, hidden agenda

---

 KEY TERMS FOR YOUR SEARCH ENGINE:

community (or organization) and entry, community and scanning

INTRODUCTION

How many times have you found yourself in a working relationship that you felt was just not a "good fit"? The situation may have involved working with a patient, a student, or another nurse. As in many other helping relationships, in traditional nurse–patient relationships, nurses often have no choice about with whom they work or for whom they provide care. In most cases, nurses simply receive a patient assignment and carry out a plan of care.

The working relationship is different in nursing consultation. Nurse consultants have the opportunity and the responsibility to determine their "fit" with a consultee and client system before becoming involved in a problem-solving relationship. Nurse consultants also

have the opportunity to get acquainted and begin to establish trust and credibility with a consultee before the actual work of a consultation relationship begins. These "fit-determining" and getting acquainted activities and opportunities occur during the gaining entry phase of the nursing consultation process.

The focus of the gaining entry phase of the nursing consultation process is building and defining the consultation relationship. The specific tasks that need to be accomplished during this phase are environmental scanning, contracting, gaining physical entry into the problem setting (i.e., community), and initiating psychological entry with both consultees and the community as a whole. Taken together, these tasks serve a twofold purpose.

First, environmental scanning provides a nurse consultant with information needed to make a decision regarding whether to continue the consultation relationship. More specifically, completing the activities of the gaining entry phase enables a nurse consultant to obtain a more accurate definition of a comunity's expectations for the consultation relationship; this helps a nurse consultant to avoid entering a relationship that will become an excercise in frustration for all parties involved. Second, the tasks of contracting, gaining physical entry, and initiating psychological entry establish the tone and set the stage for the subsequent working phases of the nursing consultation process (Figure 9-1). Thus, the work of the gaining entry phase prepares a

pathway for effective consultation (Monicken, 1995).

The gaining entry phase of the nursing consultation process begins at the time of a community's request for help and culminates with an agreement to formalize a problem-solving relationship. Although accomplishing each task in the gaining entry phase is essential to a successful nursing consultation relationship, the way in which each task is carried out will differ according to the unique features of each consultation situation. The tasks of the gaining entry phase may vary in their timing, degree of formality, level of complexity, and relative emphasis, depending both on the interaction pattern being used to guide the problem-solving activities and on whether

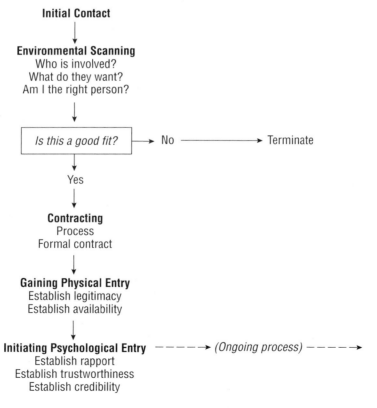

Figure 9-1   The Gaining Entry Phase of the Nursing Consultation Process.
The activities of the gaining entry phase set the tone for the subsequent working phases of the nursing consultation relationship.

the nurse is acting as an internal or external consultant.

This chapter discusses each of the tasks that comprise the gaining entry phase of the nursing consultation process. The specific purpose of each task, strategies for carrying out each task, and potential dilemmas associated with each task are considered. Variations in how the tasks of the gaining entry phase might be carried out are illustrated by scenarios that appear in a series of boxes throughout the chapter. As you read this chapter, consider the following questions:

- What different sets of dilemmas might internal and external nurse consultants face during the gaining entry phase of the nursing consultation process?
- How does the gaining entry phase differ when the consultee is an individual or group?
- How does gaining entry fit into the change process?
- What can be done during the gaining entry phase to facilitate the change process?
- What are some problems that might arise later in the nursing consultation process that could indicate incomplete, unsuccessful, or careless completion of the tasks of the gaining entry phase?

ENVIRONMENTAL SCANNING

Environmental scanning is the informal assessment or scouting that a nurse consultant begins at the time of initial contact with a potential consultee or a community's contact person. During environmental scanning, a nurse consultant gathers information and forms impressions that support a decision about whether or not to enter into a working relationship with the community and its representatives (i.e., the consultees). To reach this decision, a nurse consultant compares how well his or her skills, interests, resources, and work style match those needed or desired by the consultees and the community as a whole.

Strategies for Environmental Scanning

One of the challenges of environmental scanning is getting enough information to make the decision to continue or not continue a nursing consultation relationship. Since, at this point, a nurse consultant does not have a formal contract that enables and facilitates access to information needed for an in-depth

assessment of the community, information sources may be limited to those that are more or less "public property." Informal scouting and exploratory meetings are the information-gathering strategies used most frequently during the environmental scanning process of the gaining entry phase.

Scouting

"Scouting" means investigating a problem and a community by performing informal research (Metzger, 1993). Scouting can include searching out news reports about a community, reading a community's written materials about itself (such as brochures), and conducting informal interviews with persons who know something about the problem issue or problem setting. Scouting also entails unobtrusive observation of interactions in order to get a feel for the interpersonal processes, culture, and power relationships in a community. Most consultants find it helpful to spend some time simply "hanging around" a community, its members, and their interactions as this provides valuable information about the community's culture, availability of resources, and possible barriers to problem solving. For example, in a neighborhood, observation of residents' interactions can provide clues as to their openness and cultural characteristics such as formality versus informality and tolerance of diversity. Likewise, observations about the general state of repair of public areas and private homes can provide information about financial resources and constraints, as well as a sense of community pride. Even these informal observations can give the nurse consultant some idea about the degree of fit with the client system and the likelihood of successful problem solving.

Exploratory Meetings

An exploratory meeting with the contact person (who may or may not be a consultee) can provide information about a community's openness, commitment, and compatibility issues, as well as their perceptions of a problem. Questions that a nurse consultant might ask during an exploratory meeting include:

- How can I be helpful?
- How did you happen to call me?
- What is problematic about your situation?
- How do you know this is a problem?
- How would you like things to be different once the problem is resolved?

In addition to involving the contact person and the nurse consultant, it is helpful if an exploratory meeting includes someone who will be a member of the consultee group or is a well-respected member of the community. This person may be able to convince other consultees and members of the community of the value in engaging in the proposed consultation relationship.

It is usually helpful to hold an exploratory meeting in the community (such as a school or health care agency) or sector of the community that will be the focus of problem-solving efforts. Holding an exploratory meeting "on-site" facilitates observation of the problem setting and reinforces the work-related (rather than social) nature of a nursing con-

sultation relationship. Sometimes, however, holding an exploratory meeting at a neutral location may give contact persons or consultees a greater sense of control because they are away from the problem setting; an off-site meeting may also decrease any perceived pressure to agree to an immediate contract (Dougherty, 1995).

An external nurse consultant needs to decide whether to charge for an exploratory meeting. (Strategies for determining charges for nursing consultation services are discussed in Chapter 17.) While nurse consultants often consider exploratory meetings a cost of doing business, charging for these meetings can provide a test of a community's motivation and commitment to get help (Schein, 1987, 1988). Charging for an exploratory meeting also acknowledges that the consultee or contact person often gains useful information and insight from the conversation that has taken place during the meeting. Sometimes, this insight makes continuing the consultation relationship unnecessary.

Realistically, an internal nurse consultant may not be able to charge for an exploratory meeting. This is because an internal nursing consultation project is usually considered to be within the nurse consultant's "usual" scope of responsibilities in the community. An internal nurse consultant should try, however, to schedule any exploratory meetings during regularly scheduled (and paid) work hours.

Dimensions of Environmental Scanning

Environmental scanning is like going on a first date and making a decision about whether to go out again. As suggested by the preceding discussion of strategies for environmental scanning, the primary roles a nurse consultant assumes during environmental scanning are those of observer, questioner, and listener (Lippitt & Lippitt, 1986). The specific questions a nurse consultant seeks to answer during environmental scanning are: (1) "Who is involved?" (2) "What do they want?" and (3) "Am I the right person?"

Who Is Involved?

The process of identifying who is involved in the consultation relationship has two dimensions. The first involves identifying the persons who comprise the client system, their specific roles within the community, and how they are related to one another. The second involves identifying qualities or attitudes held by these persons that might facilitate or hinder a problem-solving relationship.

Identifying Roles and Relationships. First, a nurse consultant needs to identify all of the parties involved in the problem situation (i.e., who comprises the client system). This is important because there are no surer obstacles to implementing a plan of action than those presented by parties who have been left out—or feel they have been left out—of the process (Monicken, 1995). Second, a nurse consultant needs to identify the roles of the persons in the client system as well as determine how these persons and their roles are related to one another.

It is important to pinpoint the identity of the client. (Recall from Chapter 1 that clients are the targets or intended beneficiaries of the nursing consultation relationship but are not typically involved in the problem-solving process.) The client in a community nursing consultation situation can be the entire community or a sector within the community. In other nursing consultation relationships, the client may be an individual patient, a group of patients, students, a community, a work unit, or an entire organization. Determining the client's identity can be especially difficult in community and organizational consultation situations because there may be a number of parties that directly benefit from the consultation process. For example, who is the client in a nursing consultation project that

focuses on work redesign or nursing staff cross-training in a community clinic? Is the client the group of patients who are served by the clinic (benefit = better, more cost-effective care) or the clinic itself (benefit = more efficient use of resources and a better organizational financial picture)? Identifying the client is important since the client's needs and welfare must be the primary concern when the consultant and consultees develop problem-solving interventions.

Sorting out relationships within the client system is another important task for the nurse consultant. The first relationship to sort out is that between the contact person and the consultees since it is the consultees with whom the nurse consultant will be directly working to solve the consultation problem. A person who is serving only as the contact person will not be involved directly in problem-solving activities and may have only a limited vested interest in the problem situation and its resolution. Questions that should be asked about the contact person and the consultees include:

- Is the contact person a consultee, a representative of the consultee group, or a representative of the client?
- If the contact person is not a consultee, do the consultees know that help is being sought? (Resistance tends to be lower when consultees have a role in identifying both a problem and a need for help.)
- Is the contact person in a supervisory relationship over the consultees? (If so, the consultees may feel coerced to participate in the consultation process and the nurse consultant may encounter a higher degree of resistance.)

It is also important to determine the relationship between the contact person and the fee payer for the nursing consultation relationship. Ideally, this is the same person since it is the fee payer who has control over the financial resources available to the nurse consultant for problem-solving activities. Moreover, the fee payer's sanctioning of proposed consultation interventions (as well as sanctioning by others in positions of authority) sends a powerful message to consultees, the community as a whole, and the nurse consultant about the legitimacy of the nursing consultation relationship. If the contact person is not the fee payer, the nurse consultant needs to make every effort to include the fee payer in any exploratory meetings that take place.

Assessing Personal Qualities and Attitudes. After a nurse consultant identifies all the parties involved in the consultation relationship and the relationship between these parties, the next step is to identify any personal qualities or attitudes within these parties that may help or hinder the problem-solving process. During this part of environmental scanning, a nurse consultant focuses on the following two questions:

- Is the consultee (and the client system as a whole) someone with whom I want to work?
- Does this situation offer the opportunity for a compatible and mutually beneficial relationship?

To answer these questions, a nurse consultant needs to examine the openness, readiness to change, and level of commitment to change of both the consultee and other members of the client system.

Openness. Openness corresponds to a willingness to assume ownership for both the consultation problem and the outcomes of the consultation process. Openness has two dimensions. First, openness means a community is willing to share information about the perceived problem. This is necessary if the nurse consultant is to diagnose the problem accurately and formulate appropriate problem-solving interventions. Second, openness means consultees and other members of the

community are willing to explore a variety of problem-solving interventions. Openness in regard to problem-solving interventions helps to ensure that the interventions chosen are both appropriate and feasible. Because the consultees are usually the members of the community who are most directly affected by the consultation process, their openness is critical to the success of the nursing consultation relationship. After all, they are the persons who are most intimately involved in the consultation process and who are being asked to change their behavior or persuade the community as a whole to do so. The following consultee behaviors may indicate a lack of openness:

- Consultees seem too certain about a problem and its cause.
- Consultees press the nurse consultant for a quick fix to a superficial problem.
- Consultees only want reassurance for a course of action that is already underway.
- Consultees miscast the nurse consultant as an expert who will cure all of the community's problems for them.

A nurse consultant who encounters one or more of these behaviors during environmental scanning needs to confront the consultee about the discrepancy between their behavior and their professed desire for change. (Confrontational interventions are discussed in Chapter 11.) A nurse consultant who continues a consultation relationship when there is a lack of openness needs to accept the possibility of being held responsible if the consultation problem remains unresolved or recurs.

Readiness to Change. Readiness to change refers to a willingness to devote the time, money, energy, personnel, and other resources needed to solve a problem. Readiness to change generally corresponds to a community's degree of "pain" or dissatisfaction with the status quo. In general, a community that is experiencing a higher degree of pain is more likely to devote time, energy, and resources to problem solving.

Readiness to change can be explored by asking consultees to develop a list of reasons for not pursuing a problem solution and a parallel list of reasons in favor of problem solving (Lippitt & Lippitt, 1986). Readiness to change is suggested when consultees are able to both come up with more reasons than not for proceeding with problem solving and counter the reasons given for not pursuing a problem solution.

Exploring readiness to change can give a nurse consultant some idea about how a formal problem-solving relationship with the consultee group and the larger community might unfold (Kurpius, Rozecki, & Fuqua, 1993). Think, for example, about how readiness to change might be indicated in a situation in which a school district superintendent (the contact person) asks a nurse consultant to help implement an abstinence program within the district's junior high and high schools. The ideal scenario would be that the reasons in favor of this change (such as decreasing pregnancies and sexually transmitted diseases among students) outweigh the reasons opposing it. If, however, the consultee group comes up with an equal list of reasons for and against the abstinence program, implementation of the program would progress more slowly. If the consultees identify more reasons for not implementing the program, implementation efforts would most likely trigger conflict. When this latter situation occurs, a consultant needs to convince consultees of the benefits of the proposed change. A nurse consultant can also attempt to change norms and values in the consultee group and community that are inhibiting readiness to change. (These nurse consultant actions are examples of empirical–rational and normative–reeducative problem-solving approaches, respectively. Both of these approaches to problem solving are discussed in Chapter 11.)

Commitment to Change. Consultees' level of commitment to a proposed change is another attribute that determines the likely success of a consultation relationship. A high level of commitment is associated with a willingness to see the consultation process through rather than rush through or skip steps. Consultees usually display a higher level of commitment when they identify the consultation problem themselves rather than when someone else (such as a contact person) tells them that a problem exists. Initially, at least, consultees should display more commitment to and enthusiasm for the consultation relationship than the nurse consultant (Ulschak & SnowAntle, 1990). Commitment is suggested by behaviors such as attentiveness and active participation at meetings. If commitment to change is low, a nurse consultant may have difficulty maintaining the relationship and may encounter efforts to undermine the consultation process. In addition, if a nurse consultant's commitment to the project is greater than the consultees', problem solutions may be formulated without consultee input and may fail to resolve the problem situation. The nurse consultant can respond to a low level of commitment with strategies similar to those used to address a lack of readiness to change.

What Do They Want?

The second question that drives environmental scanning focuses on the consultees' and community's expectations for the nursing consultation relationship. In particular, a nurse consultant needs to be on the lookout for hidden agendas. Hidden agendas are unspoken reasons for seeking consultation or unspoken expectations about the consultation relationship. For instance, in the previous example of a consultation request to implement an abstinence program, is the real purpose to improve students' health and well-being, or is the real purpose of the project to impose certain religious values? Common hidden agendas in nursing consultation situations include the following:

- Trying to use the nurse consultant to evaluate consultees' work performance
- Using the consultation process to make decisions about terminating a consultee's employment
- Using the consultation process to support a decision that has already been made
- Using the nurse consultant as a "go-between" in a community in which parties are unwilling to communicate with each other directly

Identifying where a community is in its "life cycle" can help uncover unvoiced needs or desires (Kurpius et al., 1993) (see Table 9-1). Consider a community in an early stage of development such as a newly established nurse practitioner clinic. This client system, while it may not voice these concerns directly, may need help setting boundaries (how many patients to see, with which preferred provider plans to affiliate), establishing priorities (what equipment to buy), and resolving time management issues. Alternately, a community in a state of decline or crisis may be looking for a "rescuer" on whom they can become dependent or for a scapegoat on whom they can blame their problems.

A nurse consultant needs to verify any suspected hidden agenda. Once verified, a hidden agenda should be put "on the table" and the nurse consultant should negotiate responsibilities regarding the unspoken issues and expectations. A decision about whether to continue a consultation relationship when a hidden agenda is uncovered depends on the nurse consultant's personal value system as well as an assessment of whether more good than harm (for all parties involved) will result from continuing the relationship.

Am I the Right Person?

One of the most important predictors of a mutually productive nursing consultation relationship is compatibility between the nurse consultant and consultee group. While these two parties don't necessarily need to like each other, they do need to level with each other about their respective needs and values. In order to answer this final question that underlies environmental scanning, then, a nurse consultant must decide whether his or her values, preferred working style, skills, and interests are a good match for the problem situation. A nurse consultant's decisions about each of these factors further helps to determine his or her "rightness" for the problem situation.

Values. Being the right person for any job is largely based on the compatibility of a nurse consultant's and a community's values. Shared values that are particularly predictive of a productive working relationship are openness, participation, and mutual accountability. When these values are held by one party (for example, the nurse consultant) but not the other (in particular, the consultee), the problem situation will most likely be characterized by frustration and resentment.

Preferred Working Style. A match between a nurse consultant's and consultees' working styles also influences a nurse consultant's rightness for a particular problem situation. Working style encompasses both the interaction pattern that is driving the nursing consultation relationship and the consultant's and client system's needs for inclusion and control. To get a sense of the importance of these issues, consider how difficult it would be to implement a process consultation interaction pattern if the consultees only want to purchase content or skill expertise. Consider, also, the problems that could arise if a nurse consultant is someone who likes to have control over the situation and the consultees have this same tendency.

Skills. Being the right person for a nursing consultation situation also means a nurse consultant's skills and those needed for solving a specific consultation problem match.

TABLE 9-1. INDICATORS OF A COMMUNITY'S LIFE CYCLE STAGE

A community's life cycle stage is more than a function of its chronological age. Life cycle stage is also reflected by the community's energy level, creativity, tolerance of uncertainty, stability, and productivity

Life Cycle Stage	Energy Level	Creativity	Tolerance	Stability	Productivity	Concerns
Early	High—sometimes chaos seems to reign	High—lots of openness to ideas	High—willingness to take risks	Low—rapid change with little recovery time	Initially low, but increasing	Setting boundaries and limits; harnessing energy so that it is productive
Mid	Steady—adequate to maintain productivity	Tends to come in waves	Lower—emphasis is on homeostasis	High—both a major value and a concern	Stable, peaks during this stage	Maintaining productivity while avoiding complacency
Aging	A tendency toward slowing down	Generally low, satisfied with status quo	Low—not willing to take risks	Initially high, but can decline if threatened by decreased demands for services	High, but can decline if not responsive to changes in the environment	Continuing to maintain productivity by responding to environment; avoiding decline

Not only will a mismatch result in a problem remaining unresolved, a nurse consultant can be held liable for an unsatisfactory consultation outcome. Thus nurse consultants have a legal and ethical responsibility to avoid involvement in nursing consultation relationships for which they lack the appropriate skills. (Additional factors related to liability issues in nursing consultation are discussed in Chapter 15. Ethical considerations in nursing consultation are presented in Chapter 16.)

Interests. The final consideration in determining whether a nurse consultant is the right person for a particular problem situation is that of interests. "Interests" includes a desire to be involved in a problem situation for reasons such as a problem's being perceived as interesting or worthwhile, as well as more practical interests such as compatibility of the community's timeline for the project with a nurse consultant's other commitments. Another practical reason or interest for deciding whether a consultation opportunity is right for a consultant is the political implications of involvement in the problem situation. An opportunity to make contact with persons who can help with career development or provide a letter of reference can be a political reason for accepting a consultation opportunity. On the other hand, some consultation opportunities might adversely affect one's reputation or current position. Think, for example, of the possible risks involved in helping a family planning clinic implement abortion services.

BOX 9-1   DETERMINING GOODNESS OF FIT

The presence of the following conditions suggests goodness of fit between a nurse consultant and a consultation opportunity:

- Clarity of roles and interrelationships among members of the client system
- If the contact person is not a consultee, consultee awareness that help is being sought
- Involvement of the fee payer in early discussions about the consultation relationship and process
- Openness of the consultees and client system
- Both consultee and the community show signs of readiness to change
- Both consultees and the community show signs of commitment to the consultation process
- Absence of hidden agendas or ability to satisfactorily negotiate responsibilities regarding hidden agendas
- Compatibility of values
- Compatibility of work styles
- Compatibility of nurse consultant's skills with those needed to solve the consultation problem
- Nurse consultant is interested in the problem situation
- Compatibility of the community's timeline for the project and the nurse consultant's availability
- Political reasons or acceptance of the political implications of involvement in the consultation relationship

Summarizing Environmental Scanning: Is this a Good Fit?

As mentioned earlier (and illustrated in Figure 9-1), environmental scanning provides a nurse consultant with information needed to reach a decision about continuing a proposed consultation relationship. If a nurse consultant interprets the information obtained from environmental scanning to indicate a "goodness of fit," the second task of the gaining entry phase—contracting—gets under way. If, however, a nurse consultant determines there is not goodness of fit, the relationship should be terminated. Box 9-1 summarizes factors that are associated with goodness of fit between a nurse consultant and a problem situation.

It is important that a nurse consultant learn to say no to consultation requests that appear, for one reason or another, to not be a good fit. Learning to turn down a consultation request is a means of self-care for nurse consultants. Proceeding with a consultation relationship in a "poor fit" situation can result in frustration for both the nurse consultant and the consultees and, as mentioned earlier, can expose a nurse consultant to liability problems. In addition, nurse consultants who say yes to every consultation request can find themselves expected to solve every problem that comes along and therefore become overburdened. Overextending oneself as a nurse consultant can ultimately lead to burnout and ineffectiveness.

The two scenarios presented in Box 9-2 illustrate how the task of environmental scanning can vary in different consultation situations.

CONTRACTING

If, as a result of environmental scanning, a nurse consultant decides to engage in a formal problem-solving relationship with a community, the gaining entry phase progresses to the task of contracting. In nursing consulta-tion, this task has two dimensions: the contracting process itself and the product, a formal contract. The purpose of the contracting process is for the nurse consultant and consultees (or other representative of the client system) to come to an agreement about how to meet mutual "wants" related to the consultation relationship. The contracting process culminates in the development of a formal contract, which delineates and protects the wants of the parties involved in the consultation relationship. Some nurse consultants choose to develop a series of contracts throughout a consultation relationship. For example, a nurse consultant might carry out separate contracting processes and develop distinct formal contracts for (a) the problem identification and action planning phases of a nursing consultation relationship and (b) any involvement in the actual implementation of the problem solution.

At this point, contracting is discussed as a process and tool for gaining entry to a client system so that the problem-solving phases of the nursing consultation process can get under way. (A more in-depth discussion of consultation contracts can be found in Chapter 17. Examples of contracts and a checklist of contract components are also included in that chapter.)

The Contracting Process

The contracting process is a discussion between the nurse consultant, contact person, and consultees, and possibly other members of the community, that focuses on both defining how the nursing consultation process will evolve and exploring expectations about one another's roles and responsibilities during the consultation relationship. The purpose of the contracting process is to come to agreement about how the consultant's, consultees', and community's needs and desires will be met during the nursing consultation process.

BOX 9-2   VARIATIONS IN ENVIRONMENTAL SCANNING

Scenario 1: External Consultation, Purchase of Expertise Interaction Pattern

In this consultation scenario, initial contact consists of a telephone request from the director of a retirement community to a nurse educator with a special interest in gerontology. The director is asking the nurse educator to develop a survey for use at the retirement community. Analysis of the survey data is also requested. The stated goal is to develop a "report card" of the community's health so that the retirement community can plan relevant wellness programs for its residents.

Environmental scanning is conducted by means of informal observations and interview at the retirement community. The following roles and interrelationships among members of the client system are identified:

Contact person: Director of the retirement community
Fee payer: Chief financial officer for the retirement community
Consultees: Staff members who will be administering the surveys; they are aware that consultation is being sought
Client: Residents of the retirement community
Stakeholders: Retirement community, residents' families

Other Key Issues Explored During Environmental Scanning

Possible hidden agendas: Is there an expectation that the wellness programs will generate income for the retirement community?
Compatibility of timeline for project with the nurse consultant's other commitments
Extent of on-site support such as financial resources, copying, computer resources and expertise

Scenario 2: Internal Consultation, Process Consultation Interaction Pattern

In this scenario, the school nurse for a grade school is approached by the school's principal to help teachers and staff develop skills for handling behavior problems in children who have attention deficit hyperactivity disorder (ADHD).

Environmental scanning takes place during an off-site exploratory meeting with the principal. The following roles and interrelationships among members of the client system are identified:

Contact person: Principal
Fee payer: School district superintendent, through the principal
Consultees: Teachers and staff; they are not aware of the consultation request
Clients: Children with ADHD
Stakeholders: Other children attending the school, parents, the school, the school district

Other Key Issues Explored During Environmental Scanning

Is teacher and staff participation voluntary or mandatory?
Do teachers and staff perceive that this problem exists?
Possible hidden agendas: Is there an expectation to evaluate teacher and staff performance in any way?
What type of organizational support is there for this project (money, staff time)?
Will the school nurse be paid extra for this project or is it considered "part of the job"?

The contracting process may begin at the time of initial contact or during the exploratory meeting between the nurse consultant and consultees or contact person. Whether the contracting process can be completed in one meeting or requires a series of meetings depends on the complexity of the problem situation as well as on the initial compatibility and extent of agreement among the parties involved in the contracting process. In complex problem situations such as long-standing or community-wide problems, the contracting process typically requires more time and involves multiple discussions, in part because a greater number of stakeholders may be affected by the consultation process. Complex problems are also more likely to require a more extensive problem identification phase and the development of a more detailed action plan. All of these factors increase the number of roles, the number of wants, and the extent of responsibilities that will need to be negotiated during the contracting process.

Members of the client system who should be included in the contracting process are the contact person, the fee payer, and a representative or two of the consultee group. The contact person should be present to clarify the consultation request and goals. The fee payer needs to be present so that resources available to support the consultation process are taken into consideration. Consultees need to be present since they are the individuals who will be expected to carry out the tasks to address the consultation problem. Which of these parties actually accepts or signs the contract will vary. However, it is important that whoever signs the contract assumes the responsibility for seeing that the terms of the contract are upheld.

Box 9-3 lists questions that can be used to guide the contracting process. The parties

BOX 9-3   QUESTIONS TO GUIDE THE CONTRACTING PROCESS

Questions for Members of the Client System (Community)

What do I want to have happen as a result of this consultation relationship?
What am I willing to do to accomplish these goals?
How much help do I want accomplishing these goals?
How much time can I devote to this project? When can I give this time?
What resources (including skills) can I bring to this project?
What constraints and limitations of resources am I aware of that could affect my involvement in this project?

Questions for the Nurse Consultant

What do I want from this consultation relationship—fee expectations, other less tangible payoffs?
What am I willing to do to accomplish the goals of this consultation? Am I willing to be involved in the implementation of any recommended problem solution or do I see implementation as solely the responsibility of the consultees?
How much time am I willing to devote to this project? When do I have this time?
What resources and support from the client system do I need? How much participation from the consultees do I expect?

involved in contracting can respond to these questions either verbally or in writing. Responses can then be compared and differences negotiated and resolved. At the conclusion of this process, the formal contract is drawn up by either the nurse consultant or a representative of the client system.

It is important to recognize that both a nurse consultant and consultees (as well as other members of the community) enter the contracting process with a set of unspoken expectations about the consultation relationship (Dougherty, 1995). From the consultees' perspective, this "psychological contract" reflects expectations about what will be gained from the nursing consultation relationship and what obligations such as tasks and resource commitment will be accepted. For the nurse consultant's part, the psychological contract includes expectations about what will be given (e.g., time) in the problem-solving relationship and what responsibilities or specific tasks will be taken on. It also includes expectations about what (e.g., fees) is to be gained. For a formal consultation contract to be successful, these implicit wants must be made explicit during the contracting process. When the contracting process overlooks the issues of the psychological contract, the nursing consultation process can be disrupted by the resentment that builds because the involved parties' needs are not being met.

The Formal Contract

A formal contract developed as a result of the contracting process serves as a tool for protecting the interests of the parties involved in the consultation process. It does this by delineating the roles and responsibilities (including specific tasks and timelines) of the nurse consultant and consultees and by clarifying accountability issues such as evaluation, feedback, and fees. The contract further protects the interests of those who will be involved in

the consultation process by making explicit the ground rules that will be followed for confidentiality and terminating the consultation relationship. Chapter 17 includes a checklist of the specific components that should be included in a formal consultation contract.

The actual format of a contract will vary according to the nursing consultation situation. A brief memo may be adequate as a contract for many internal nursing consultation situations. In other situations, a consultation contract might take the form of either a written letter of understanding that is signed by one or both parties or a formal document with legal language. The format that is used for the contract generally mirrors the culture of the client system (e.g., its degree of formality), the degree of familiarity between the consultant and the consultee or representative of the client system, and the working style of the person who actually develops the formal contract. The format should, however, be acceptable to both signing parties.

Box 9-4 illustrates how contracting might be accomplished in two different nursing consultation scenarios.

GAINING PHYSICAL ENTRY

The third task of the gaining entry phase in the nursing consultation process is to gain physical entry into the problem setting/community. Gaining physical entry has a twofold purpose: to establish the legitimacy of the nursing consultation relationship and to establish the parameters of the nurse consultant's involvement with the consultees and other members of the community. Successfully gaining physical entry means that a nurse consultant is accepted as a temporary member of the community. Consultees (or the contact person) as well as the nurse consultant have responsibilities in terms of facilitating physical entry into the problem setting.

BOX 9-4   VARIATIONS IN CONTRACTING

Scenario 1: External Consultation, Purchase of Expertise Interaction Pattern

In this scenario, the contracting process takes place over the telephone at the time of initial contact. The only parties involved are the contact person (the director of the retirement community) and the nurse consultant (a nurse-educator in another state). The formal contract takes the form of a written letter of understanding that is developed by the nurse consultant. Two signed copies of this letter are sent to the contact person—one for the retirement community's files and one that is to be returned to the nurse consultant after it is signed by the director.

Scenario 2: Internal Consultation, Process Consultation Interaction Pattern

In this scenario, the contracting process takes place in a meeting at the school. The principal (who will also be a consultee), the superintendent, and two teachers are present. The formal contract is developed by the principal. It is a formal document with "legalese." The contract is reviewed by the teachers and signed by the principal, superintendent, and nurse consultant. Both the principal and the nurse consultant retain a copy of the signed contract.

Consultee Roles in Facilitating Physical Entry

A consultee or the contact person typically initiates the process of gaining physical entry by formally introducing the nurse consultant and announcing her or his purpose and specific activities to the consultee group and key members of the community. Ideally, these introductions occur in person. However, memos and e-mail messages are other strategies that can be used to introduce the nurse consultant to the consultee and other members of the client system. It is especially helpful to a nursing consultation relationship when the nurse consultant and the consultant's mission are introduced by someone who is in a position of influence within the client system. For instance, this person could be the director of a community service agency or key governmental figure in a geographically defined community. In organizational and community settings, administrative-level sanctioning of a nursing consultation relationship is associated with increased cooperation with problem-solving efforts (Dougherty, 1995).

Another way in which the contact person or consultee can facilitate the nurse consultant's physical entry into the community is by making available some sort of physical working space within the community. Assigning work space further demonstrates a sanctioning of the nurse consultant's activities. It also sends a message about willingness on the part of the community to allocate the resources needed to support the nursing consultation process.

Nurse Consultant Roles in Gaining Physical Entry

A nurse consultant gains physical entry into the problem setting/community by being

BOX 9-5   VARIATIONS IN GAINING PHYSICAL ENTRY

Scenario 1: External Consultation, Purchase of Expertise Interaction Pattern

In this consultation scenario, the nurse consultant gains physical entry when she is taken on a tour of the retirement community and introduced to staff and residents. In addition, flyers are posted in the community dining and recreational areas and a letter of introduction is sent to each resident. The nurse consultant is also given an office in a central location.

Scenario 2: Internal Consultation, Process Consultation Interaction Pattern

In this scenario, the principal facilitates gaining physical entry by introducing the consultation project to all teachers and staff at a monthly meeting. Even though the nurse consultant is a part-time employee in the school, it is important not to assume that all staff have had previous contact with the nurse consultant.

The nurse consultant's strategy for gaining physical entry is to distribute a memo that includes information about office location and hours of availability.

---

available to the consultees and other community members. A nurse consultant demonstrates commitment to the consultation relationship by being at an assigned work space on a predictable basis. At the same time, however, a nurse consultant should mingle and meet with consultees and key stakeholders in their own areas. This demonstrates interest in the consultees and their experiences of both the problem and the problem-solving process. It also facilitates both psychological entry into the client system and gathering information about the problem situation. A nurse consultant who is working with hospital staff, for example, should make an effort to spend time with and be available to the staff on all shifts.

A nurse consultant can also facilitate physical entry and being accepted as a temporary member of the community by minimizing interruptions and disruptions in the consultees' and community's normal activities. This can be done by making every possible effort to adapt problem-solving activities to the problem setting's usual schedule.

Box 9-5 illustrates how gaining physical entry might occur in the two consultation scenarios previously described.

INITIATING PSYCHOLOGICAL ENTRY

The final task of the gaining entry phase is to initiate psychological entry into the client system. As mentioned in Chapter 2, efforts to gain psychological entry occur throughout the entire nursing consultation process. The outcome of gaining psychological entry is "engaging" the consultees. Successful psychological entry decreases the chance that consultees will resist involvement in problem-solving efforts. Psychological entry occurs by creating "buy-in" for the problem-solving process and by fostering consultees' willingness to participate in problem-solving activities and accept the implications of the problem-solving process. Effective psychological entry occurs to the extent that a nurse consultant establishes rapport with the consultees, and the consultees perceive the nurse consultant as trustworthy and credible.

Establishing Rapport

A nurse consultant and consultees have established rapport when their working relationship is characterized by harmony, synergy, and mutual respect. Following a community's rules, regulations, and communication channels and patterns demonstrates respect for the community and is one set of strategies that can be used to establish rapport. Paying attention to cultural norms in highly visible areas such as language and dress helps a nurse consultant look less like an outsider; this, too, helps the nurse consultant establish rapport. For example, an external nurse consultant who is working with clinic staff might look less conspicuous wearing a lab coat over street clothes. This simple action can facilitate staff openness and acceptance of the nurse consultant and, therefore, help establish rapport.

Establishing Trust

A nurse consultant is perceived as trustworthy when consultees feel safe and validated or accepted in their interactions with the nurse consultant. A nurse consultant can build a reputation of trustworthiness by being empathetic and demonstrating understanding of consultees' fears and concerns about being involved in problem-solving activities. In the present health care climate, it is realistic for consultees to be worried about how community-wide problem-solving outcomes might affect their health, their access to health care, the costs incurred in seeking health care, and so forth. A nurse consultant who acknowledges these concerns conveys empathy, which helps establish a perception of trustworthiness. A nurse

consultant also builds a reputation of trustworthiness by respecting confidences, refusing to take sides, following through on commitments, and avoiding involvement in issues that are not a part of the consultation contract.

Establishing Credibility

A nurse consultant who has established credibility is perceived by consultees and a community as believable. One strategy a nurse consultant can use to establish credibility is sharing relevant experiences and stories from community problem situations similar to that being experienced by the client community. A nurse consultant can also establish credibility by planning problem-solving activities that will demonstrate an immediate beneficial effect. (Chapter 11 discusses this strategy further.)

Box 9-6 illustrates how psychological entry could be initiated in the two consultation scenarios discussed previously in this chapter.

CHALLENGES IN GAINING ENTRY

As straightforward and commonsense as the process of gaining entry in nursing consultation seems, this phase is not without potential difficulties and challenges. A nurse consultant who is aware of these potential dilemmas can monitor for their occurrence and address them before they compromise the entire nursing consultation process. The difficulties that arise most frequently during the gaining entry phase are resistance and inattention to details.

Resistance

As discussed in Chapter 8, resistance is a common reaction to any situation that involves

BOX 9-6   VARIATIONS IN INITIATING PSYCHOLOGICAL ENTRY

Scenario 1: External Consultation, Purchase of Expertise Interaction Pattern

In this consultation scenario, the director's perception of the nurse consultant's trustworthiness and credibility actually precipitated the initial contact. This reputation facilitated the development of psychological entry. The nurse consultant also uses the following strategies in an effort to gain psychological entry:

- To establish rapport, the nurse consultant is careful to use language that was not too "ivory tower." Research and data analysis principles are explained in a simple and straightforward manner.
- To establish trustworthiness, the nurse consultant conveys empathy for the contact person's fears that both the project will be too complex and "the Board of Directors won't do anything with this information." The nurse consultant also suggests that a goal of the project might be to develop meaningful ways of presenting the survey findings to different possible audiences.
- To establish credibility, the nurse consultant shares survey techniques and data presentation strategies that have been successful with another client system.

Scenario 2: Internal Consultation, Process Consultation Interaction Pattern

The nurse consultant in this scenario had previously established rapport, trustworthiness, and credibility with the consultees as a school nurse. However, psychological entry still needs to be gained so that the school nurse will be accepted in the new role as nurse consultant.

- To establish rapport, the nurse consultant pays attention to the cultural norm of "no shoptalk during lunch."
- To establish trustworthiness, the nurse consultant conveys empathy for the teachers' feelings of frustration when a child with ADHD disrupts the entire classroom.
- Teachers and staff are also assured that observations of their interactions will not be reported to the principal.
- To establish credibility, the nurse consultant shares a couple of simple techniques that can be put to immediate use and will yield immediate positive results.

---

change. The nurse consultant needs to recognize that resistance is a survival mechanism that protects a consultee or a community from perceived threats. Resistance that occurs during the gaining entry phase is often an emotional response consultees are having regarding the proposed problem-solving process and change.

Consultees might be resistant to the nursing consultation relationship for several reasons. They may have an aversion to the foreseen outcome of the consultation relationship (e.g., an abstinence program in schools). Consultees might also be resistant because they perceive that the costs of the proposed problem solution will outweigh its benefits. Will the hoped-for benefits of the program—fewer teen pregnancies and sexually transmitted diseases—outweigh potential risks such as taking time away from teaching other content, not informing students of safe sex practices, and perhaps advocating a value system that is not universal? Consultees could also be resistant to the abstinence program because they believe the nursing consultation outcome will divert resources from other areas of need in the schools. Finally, consultees' resistance can represent a desire to maintain things as they are in order to protect "turf" and vested interests.

When resistance is encountered during the gaining entry phase, a nurse consultant should respond by first acknowledging it as a natural part of change. A nurse consultant should also encourage consultees to express or "vent" the concerns that are causing the resistance. Finally, a nurse consultant needs to avoid taking the resistance personally. A defensive reaction can be viewed as insecurity and can threaten the nurse consultant's credibility as a problem solver.

Inattention to Details

Both a nurse consultant and consultees can jeopardize the entire nursing consultation relationship if they fail to pay attention to the details of the gaining entry phase. A nurse consultant can jeopardize the consultation relationship by failing to clarify consultees' concerns during environmental scanning activities. This failure can result in a contract that is meaningless. Ignoring the limitations of one's competence in relation to a problem issue will result in a contract that cannot be fulfilled. Promising too much and failing to be specific about what roles will be taken on are examples of nurse consultant oversights during contracting that can jeopardize a consultation relationship. Finally, failing to adapt to a community's culture, concerns, and work processes may make it impossible for a nurse consultant to gain psychological entry into the client system. This will increase consultees' resistance to change and set up the nursing consultation relationship for failure.

Contact persons and consultees also have responsibilities during the gaining entry phase. Overlooking these responsibilities can put the entire nursing consultation process in jeopardy. Failure to clearly explain the consultation problem or verify a nurse consultant's skills can result in developing a contract that will fail to solve the problem issue. A contact person or the consultee group also needs to clarify specific expectations about the nurse consultant's roles and behaviors during the problem-solving process. Finally, consultees have the responsibility to be clear about any limitation of resources so that this is taken into consideration during development of a formal consultation contract.

DOCUMENTING ACTIVITIES OF THE GAINING ENTRY PHASE

Just as nurses are accustomed to documenting their direct care interactions with individual patients, nurse consultants need to become accustomed to documenting their implementation of the nursing consultation process. A written record of a consultation relationship not only reminds the nurse consultant about what is occurring in a given consultation situation, it also serves as a learning device or record of what works and what doesn't work. A written record of a consultation relationship also serves as a means of demonstrating both fulfillment of the terms of the consultation contract and adherence to professional standards of practice. Documentation, therefore, can provide legal protection to a nurse consultant. Box 9-7 provides a documentation checklist for the gaining entry phase of the nursing consultation process. Similar checklists will also be found in the next five chapters for the subsequent phases of the nursing consultation process.

BOX 9-7 DOCUMENTATION CHECKLIST: THE GAINING ENTRY PHASE

Documenting Initial Contact

- ☐ Date and time of contact
- ☐ Manner of contact—telephone call, letter, in person
- ☐ Contact person—name, title, position in the client system
- ☐ Referral source
- ☐ Stated consultation problem
- ☐ Stated desired consultation outcome
- ☐ Action taken and rationale

Documenting Environmental Scanning

- ☐ Date and time of scanning activity
- ☐ Activity undertaken—meeting, interview, reading, and so forth
- ☐ Information source (be exact)
- ☐ Information gained
- ☐ Implications of information for a consultation relationship
- ☐ Conclusions drawn
- ☐ Action taken and rationale

Documenting Contracting

- ☐ Preliminary discussions—date, persons present and their roles in the client system, content of discussion, decisions made
- ☐ Decisions about formal contract—format, who will develop, who will review, who will sign
- ☐ Keep a copy of signed contract

Documenting Efforts to Gain Physical Entry

- ☐ Actions taken—date and time, by whom, members of the client system who were involved
- ☐ Follow-up—comments on effectiveness of actions
- ☐ Notes about what might have been more effective; possible next steps

Documenting Efforts to Initiate Psychological Entry

- ☐ Actions taken—date and time, rationale, parties involved and their response, personal feelings about the action's effectiveness
- ☐ Notes about possible next steps

CHAPTER SUMMARY

The activities of the gaining entry phase of the nursing consultation process lay the foundation for the actual working phases of the consultation relationship. Environmental scanning is used to determine the fit between the nature of the nursing consultation request and a nurse consultant's interests and abilities. Activities undertaken in the process of gaining physical and initiating psychological entry into a community establish the legitimacy of the nurse consultant's involvement and foster the nurse consultant's acceptance. Problems that occur during later phases of a nursing consultation relationship can often be traced to an unsuccessful or careless gaining entry phase. Specifically, failure to identify the real consultation issue, promising too much (especially with too few resources), failure to adequately specify roles and responsibilities, failure to recognize the limits of one's competence with respect to the identified problem, failure to acknowledge a "poor fit" with the problem situation, and failure to adapt to a community's particular concerns and ways of working all reflect a lack of attention to the details of the gaining entry phase. This inattention can undermine the entire nursing consultation process.

APPLYING CHAPTER CONTENT

1. Reflect on both a successful and an unsuccessful consultation situation in which you have been involved. How did the entry phase seem to differ in these two situations? What would you have done differently in the unsuccessful scenario?

2. What criteria would need to be met for you to consider a consultation opportunity a personal "good fit"? Consider your skills, values, and needs as you speculate on these criteria.

References

Dougherty, A. (1995). *Consultation: Practice and perspectives in school and community settings* (2nd ed.). Pacific Grove, CA: Brooks-Cole.

Kurpius, D., Fuqua, D., & Rozecki, T. (1993). The consulting process: A multidimensional approach. *Journal of Counseling & Development, 71,* 601–606.

Lippitt, G., & Lippitt, R. (1986). *The consulting process in action* (2nd ed.). San Diego: University Associates.

Metzger, R. (1993). *Developing a consulting practice.* Newbury Park, CA: Sage.

Monicken, D. (1995). Consultation in advanced practice nursing. In M. Snyder & M. Mirr (Eds.), *Advanced practice nursing: A guide to professional development* (pp. 183–195). New York: Springer.

Schein, E. (1987). *Process consultation, volume II: Lessons for managers and consultants* (2nd ed.) Reading, MA: Addison-Wesley.

Schein, E. (1988). *Process consultation, volume I: Its role in organization development* (2nd ed.). Reading, MA: Addison-Wesley.

Ulschak, F., & SnowAntle, S. (1990). *Consultation skills for health care professionals.* San Francisco: Jossey-Bass.

10

Problem Identification in Community Consultation

. . . (T)here are two reasons for (conducting) community health assessments: information is needed for change, and it is needed for empowerment. (Hancock & Minkler, 1997)

 KEY CONCEPTS:

iterative, key informant, triangulation, framework

 KEY TERMS FOR YOUR SEARCH ENGINE:

community and health data, community (or organization) and assessment

INTRODUCTION

The problem identification phase of the nursing consultation process marks the beginning of the working relationship between a nurse consultant and a community. In fact, in many ways, the activities that take place during the problem identification phase function as an intervention in that they interrupt routines, may affect community members' expectations regarding change, and may influence how they think about themselves and their community. The goal of the problem identification phase, however, is to determine and then communicate the cause of the problems that have prompted the request for nursing consultation.

The problem identification phase consists of three tasks: assessment, diagnosis, and communication of assessment findings. The importance of each task to a successful nursing consultation outcome cannot be emphasized enough. A nurse consultant may solve the wrong problem—or solve the actual problem in an ineffective way—if incomplete or inaccurate information is collected or if conclusions about a problem's cause are inaccurate. A nursing consultation relationship is also likely to be unsuccessful if assessment findings and problem explanations are not effectively communicated to the client system or are not accepted by the client system. Box 10-1 reviews the purpose and focus of each task in

BOX 10-1   TASKS OF THE PROBLEM IDENTIFICATION PHASE IN NURSING CONSULTATION

Task 1: Assessment

Purpose: To identify factors in the nursing consultation problem situation that cause or contribute to the consultation problem
Focus: Information-gathering activities

Task 2: Diagnosis

Purpose: To make a decision and reach a conclusion about the cause of the nursing consultation problem
Focus: Analysis and interpretation of assessment findings

Task 3: Communication of Findings

Purpose: To legitimize and create ownership of the problem's cause
Focus: Packaging and delivering information to different members of the client system

---

the problem identification phase of the nursing consultation process.

The tasks of the problem identification phase are iterative in nature; that is, completing one task may require backtracking and refining what was done earlier (see Figure 10-1). For example, if a community does not accept the nurse consultant's assessment findings and conclusions about the cause of the consultation problem, the nurse consultant will need to backtrack to the diagnosis process. Likewise, the need to refine a problem diagnosis may require more information gathering. Being willing to repeat the tasks of the problem identification phase is important since findings and conclusions from this phase lay the foundation for subsequent development of the nursing consultation action plan.

This chapter explores each task of the problem identification phase: assessment, diagnosis, and communication of assessment findings. The chapter begins by describing different purposes of assessment and different information-gathering strategies. Next, theoretical perspectives through which a nurse consultant can approach assessment and diagnosis activities are illustrated. Finally, the chapter addresses some of the dilemmas that can arise during the problem identification phase of the nursing consultation process. As you read this chapter, think about the following questions:

- How does the purpose of a specific nursing consultation assessment affect information collection strategies, explanations about a problem's cause, and the problem solutions that will most likely be proposed?
- How might a nurse consultant need to carry out the tasks of the problem identification phase differently for an individual versus group or community client?

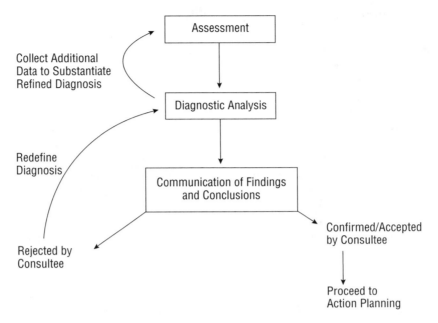

Figure 10-1   The Iterative Nature of the Problem Identification Phase.
Performing one task may necessitate repeating what has already been done in a previous task.

- What specific skills does a nurse consultant need to effectively carry out this phase of the nursing consultation process? What nurse consultant roles predominate during this phase?

- What would be some advantages and disadvantages of carrying out problem identification activities as an internal and external nurse consultant?

ASSESSMENT: GATHERING INFORMATION ABOUT THE NURSING CONSULTATION PROBLEM

The first task in the problem identification phase of the nursing consultation process is assessment. The purpose of assessment is to determine the relationship between characteristics of a community and the nursing consultation problem. In a sense, assessment activities aim to identify and explain the gaps between "what is" and "what ought to be" within the community. Thus, the focus of assessment is information gathering. The

information that the nurse consultant gathers provides data on which to base conclusions about a problem's cause and enables a nurse consultant to develop an action plan that will attack causes of a consultation problem rather than just symptoms (Harrison, 1994). Because assessment uncovers strengths as well as weaknesses, it also provides a foundation on which to build specific problem-solving strategies.

The assessment activities that take place during the nursing consultation process are, in many ways, more complex than those that take place during traditional nurse–patient relationships. The increased complexity is due to the nature of the nursing consultation relationship: Although a nurse consultant is interacting with a consultee (e.g., group of community members), the ultimate goal of a nursing consultation relationship is enhanced client (i.e., total community) well-being. Because of this, assessment in nursing consultation must consider: (a) the community's pattern of health responses or its response to a specific health care or health care delivery issue, (b) factors (including strengths) that contribute to the community's response, (c) the consultees' responses to the community problem, (d) factors that contribute to the consultees' responses, and (e) the interaction between the consultees and the larger community. These interactions and responses are possible causes of the nursing consultation problem and are also potential intervention points for nursing consultation problem solutions. To detect these interactions and responses, a nurse consultant must clearly identify the purpose of the assessment (or answer the question, "What am I trying to find out?") and must select appropriate information-gathering strategies.

Identifying Assessment Purposes

Every nursing consultation assessment has one or more of the following purposes: description, problem clarification, need assessment, or desire analysis. Each assessment purpose reflects different community health issues and one or more key questions a nurse consultant must answer before a problem solution can be proposed. Identification of the purpose of an assessment is important because it influences the selection of information sources and information-gathering strategies. Clarity about the purpose of an assessment also helps a nurse consultant bring into focus details in the problem situation that might otherwise be overlooked or disregarded (Ridley & Mendoza, 1993). Finally, identifying the specific purpose of

assessment activities and anticipating how the purpose is best addressed also increases the efficiency with which the assessment can be carried out.

Description

The purpose of a descriptive assessment is to describe both factors in a community that might be contributing to the consultation problem and resources that can be mobilized to solve the problem. A descriptive assessment, therefore, focuses on answering the question, "What is the history and context of this problem?" The information collected by a nurse consultant who is doing a descriptive assessment is primarily observational in nature. Put simply, a nurse consultant who is doing a descriptive assessment just "gets out and looks around" the community. Because a descriptive assessment is primarily observational in nature, it is sometimes referred to as a "windshield" or "shoe-leather" assessment. Occasionally, information gained by observation is supplemented by information from records and public documents. Community characteristics that are typically observed during a descriptive assessment include the following (Helvie, 1998):

- Quality of housing—age, single or multiple family, vacancies, general upkeep
- Neighborhood hangouts—location, who they are frequented by, whether they are open or closed to strangers
- Schools—location, general upkeep
- Vacant lots—number, location, condition
- Neighborhood decay—abandoned cars, trash, and so on
- Geographic boundaries and their effect (e.g., segregation of ethnic groups and social classes)
- Racial and social class composition, location, and evidence of interaction
- Transportation system
- Presence of shops, food stores, malls, and eating establishments

- Open spaces and their use
- Churches—denominations represented, location
- Health care facilities—services offered, location, accessibility
- Protective services (e.g., fire, police) and their visibility

A descriptive assessment is most useful for forming preliminary ideas about possible causes of a community's problem, as well as resources and constraints that will affect addressing the problem (Helvie, 1998). These preliminary ideas can then be used to formulate more comprehensive assessment activities. The following example illustrates this point: A nurse consultant is asked by representatives of a small rural community to help them determine reasons for their community's high incidence of cardiovascular disease so that preventive programs can be developed. The nurse consultant carries out a descriptive assessment and notes the following: the presence of a large number of fast-food restaurants within the community, a lack of open spaces and recreational opportunities, a seemingly disproportionate number of obese individuals in the community, and evidence that it is only within the last five years that the community's rate of cardiovascular disease has exceeded that of demographically similar communities. Based on this information, the nurse consultant's preliminary idea is that the consultation problem is linked in some way to residents' diet and exercise habits.

The fact that a descriptive assessment provides only preliminary and not conclusive evidence about a problem's cause should be apparent from this example. Cardiovascular disease is a multifactorial problem and can have causes other than diet and exercise habits: genetics and smoking are just two other possible explanations for this community problem. The descriptive assessment in this example merely provides the nurse con-

sultant with some direction for a more focused assessment that considers, among other factors, whether or not residents actually eat at the fast-food restaurants and how their diet and exercise habits have changed over the past five years.

Problem Clarification

When the purpose of a nursing consultation assessment is problem clarification, data-gathering activities are designed to clarify the nature and magnitude of an identified problem and to identify factors that are associated with the problem. The key question in a problem clarification assessment is, "What factors are associated with this problem?"

A problem clarification assessment differs from a descriptive assessment in terms of the scope of information-gathering activities it entails. For example, when the purpose of an assessment is problem clarification, written surveys and interviews are often used to supplement observations. In addition, problem clarification may include comparing characteristics of members of the community who are affected by the consultation problem with those who are not affected by the consultation problem.

A nursing consultation assessment can begin with the purpose of problem clarification. In some cases, though, a problem clarification assessment is used to follow up on preliminary ideas about a problem's cause that have been developed as a result of a descriptive assessment. Consider how a problem clarification assessment could be used as a "phase two consultation assessment" in the preceding scenario: The nurse consultant suspects (because of findings from a descriptive assessment) that there is a link between the dietary habits of a community's residents and the community's high incidence of cardiovascular disease. To follow up on this preliminary idea about the problem's cause, the nurse consultant conducts a problem clarification assessment. Community residents are surveyed about their weight history and eating habits, particularly about eating fast food. Weight histories and eating habits are compared for residents with and without a known history of cardiovascular disease. To further clarify this problem, the relationship between residents' cardiovascular risk status (based on serum lipid levels and family history), weight, and eating habits is explored. As this example illustrates, the scope and depth of a problem clarification assessment allow more confidence to be placed in a statement about a problem's cause.

Need Assessment

A need assessment is the systematic and objective appraisal of the health-related service needs of a client system (Cook, 1989). The purposes of a need assessment are to assess a community's need for change, determine the community's capacity for change, discern ways to enhance this capacity, and identify ways in which a community can accomplish the desired change (Helvie, 1998). A need assessment seeks to answer the question, "What is needed to have a healthier community?" In order to answer this question, a nurse consultant may conduct interviews, administer surveys, review documents, and make observations.

In nursing consultation, a need assessment is indicated when a community needs help identifying and developing specific strategies to enhance its general well-being or well-being in relationship to a specific health indicator. A need assessment is similar to a doctor–patient nursing consultation interaction pattern in that consultees are asking for a diagnosis of what is wrong and a prescription for how to fix it. A need assessment would be an appropriate assessment purpose if a group of nurse practitioners (the consultees) asked a nurse consultant to develop strategies in order to help a free clinic (the client/com-

munity) improve its financial well-being. Information collected during the need assessment might include supply use, staffing patterns, appointment scheduling, and donation patterns and sources. If assessment findings revealed that developing donation patterns and sources could solve the clinic's problem, the nurse consultant could work with the consultee to develop a fund-raising program.

Desire Analysis

When the purpose of nursing consultation assessment activities is desire analysis, a nurse consultant focuses on identifying factors that will facilitate or hinder implementation of a change or problem solution that has been specified by consultees to achieve a specific goal. Thus, the question that informs a desire analysis is "What do we need to address in order to accomplish this change (or implement this specific activity)?" A desire analysis differs from a need assessment in that the consultees have already identified the specific problem to be addressed, as well as how they want to address it, before seeking consultation. Nurse consultants gather information to answer this question by means of observations, interviews, surveys, and selected document review.

Desire analysis would be the appropriate assessment purpose if, in the previous example, the consultee group of nurse practitioners had approached the nurse consultant with a request to develop and implement a fund-raising event to solve the clinic's financial problems. The nurse consultant's assessment would focus on identifying factors that could help or hinder implementation of this request. The outcome of a desire analysis is a delineation of factors that need to be addressed before preceding with a planned problem solution or change.

Box 10-2 summarizes the different purposes of assessment activities in the nursing consultation process.

BOX 10-2   PURPOSES OF NURSING CONSULTATION ASSESSMENT

Purpose	Key Question	Focus
Description	What is the history and context of this problem?	To discover factors that might contribute to a problem
Problem clarification	What is causing this situation?	To clarify the nature and magnitude of an identified problem and to identify associated factors
Need assessment	What is needed to have a healthier community?	To appraise the health-related needs of a community
Desire analysis	What do we need to address in order to implement this change?	To identify factors that will facilitate or hinder desire fulfillment

Selecting Information-Gathering Strategies

In addition to identifying the specific purpose of a nursing consultation assessment, a nurse consultant must determine the best way of collecting the needed information. While a nurse consultant's choice of information-gathering strategies should be based primarily on the purpose of the assessment, information-gathering decisions need to also take into account feasibility issues such as time, resources, and consultant and consultee abilities. A nurse consultant's goal should be to select strategies that will yield reliable, valid, and believable information as efficiently as possible.

A variety of information sources and information-gathering strategies were mentioned in the preceding section about assessment purposes. This section highlights the strengths, limitations, and usefulness of the information-gathering strategies used most frequently by nurse consultants. In-depth discussions of these strategies can be found in any research methods textbook.

Surveys

Surveys are a cost-effective means of collecting information about knowledge, perceptions, concerns, and attitudes from large groups. Surveys offer flexibility in terms of format (for example, they can use forced-choice as well as open-ended questions) and distribution options (such as mail or group administration). A major advantage of surveys is that they are unobtrusive and allow anonymous responses. As a result, individuals may be more likely to give accurate responses to somewhat intrusive questions such as use of illegal drugs. The data generated by surveys tend to be quantitative in nature and lend themselves to high impact presentations such as tables, charts, and graphs.

A major disadvantage of surveys is the time required for their preparation. The format of a survey (such as Likert scale or checklist) needs to take into consideration both the types of information desired and the characteristics (such as reading level) of the survey's intended respondents. Careful wording to avoid cultural or gender bias, logical sequencing of questions, and attention to appearance are other details that a nurse consultant should attend to during the survey construction process. Another disadvantage of surveys is that they do not allow respondents to seek clarification to questions or elaborate on their responses. A final drawback is that the return rate for surveys tends to be fairly low. A low return rate can leave a nurse consultant wondering if the attitudes and perceptions of individuals who returned the surveys are different in any way from those who did not.

In nursing consultation assessments, surveys are useful for collecting information about personal characteristics that could be related to a problem's occurrence. Surveys are also useful for determining satisfaction with community resources and reasons why resources are not being used, and for gathering opinions about how consultees and community residents would prefer to solve a specific problem.

Interviews

Interviews allow a nurse consultant to collect more in-depth and detailed information than is generally possible with a survey. Interviews also allow a nurse consultant to probe and clarify responses.

A drawback of interviews is that they tend to be more costly to administer than are surveys, in terms of both time and human resources. As a result, interviews tend to be used selectively, that is, with carefully chosen key informants rather than large groups. Interviews also require respondents to sacrifice anonymity; this may limit the content that some individuals are willing to discuss in an interview. An additional drawback of interviews is that the data they yield tend to be more time consuming to analyze than do survey data. In addition, because interview data tend to be narrative or qualitative in nature, the conclusions generated from interviews can be harder to sell to consultees who are accustomed to diagnosing problems and justi-

fying change efforts with numbers (such as dollar amounts).

Nurse consultants often use key informant interviews as a strategy for accessing expert or "insider" opinions and insights about a problem situation. Key informants can provide insight into how to decrease resistance to a proposed change and help identify potential allies and other problem-solving resources. Typical key informants in community consultation are public officials, school personnel, religious leaders, business leaders, agency directors, and unofficial community spokespersons. In a desire analysis assessment, key informant interviews might be a productive way of gathering information about factors in the community that could facilitate or hinder a proposed problem solution.

Nurse consultants also use focus group interviews and community forums as ways of gathering information. A group format can be more efficient than multiple individual interviews and has the added advantage of enabling a nurse consultant to observe a group's communication and interpersonal processes. Thus, a group interview or forum can help a nurse consultant identify behaviors and group processes within a community that could be contributing to the nursing consultation problem.

Observation

Observation can be a relatively simple way of gathering information about a problem setting and how its members function on a day-to-day basis. A nurse consultant can use information obtained from observation to identify and clarify issues during subsequent surveys and interviews. Observations can also confirm information gained from other strategies.

A decision a nurse consultant must make before using observation as an information-gathering strategy is that of how much to tell consultees (or other community members) about what is being observed. Observations that are made without awareness (i.e., "participant observations") are more likely to capture "natural" behavior but raise ethical issues about informed consent and full disclosure. Also, a nurse consultant must carefully plan what to observe so that important details and behaviors aren't missed and that observations are consistent and objective.

Reports and Records

Nurse consultants can take advantage of a variety of existing reports and records that allow unobtrusive and relatively inexpensive information gathering. A number of reports about a community's health status and health resources are available on the World Wide Web. Three particularly useful Web sites are listed below:

- Bureau of Primary Health Care, *http:// www.bphc.hrsa.dhhs.gov/*. This Web site provides county-level health status data for every county in the United States.
- Bureau of Primary Health Care Programs, Initiatives, and Offices, *http://www.bphc. hrsa.dhhs.gov/bphc/index_1.htm*. This Web site lists the programs sponsored by the Bureau of Primary Health Care.
- Health Resources and Services Administration State Profiles, *http://stateprofiles.hrsa. gov/*. This Web site provides state-level profiles of health resources and health status.

Other reports and records that may be useful in the problem identification phase of the nursing consultation process will need to be obtained directly from a community or various agencies and subsystems within it. For example, records available from public health departments might help determine the severity of a nursing consultation problem (e.g., child abuse or teen pregnancy). A community's financial records may help a nurse consultant identify the resources or lack of resources available for solving a consultation problem. In the free clinic scenario, review of the appointment schedule over time (e.g., patterns of "no shows") and changes in clinic visits in response to events such as adding a new provider or changing hours or operation could help a nurse consultant detect possible causes of the clinic's financial problems. Finally, a nurse consultant can use reports and records to generate content for surveys and interviews as well as to confirm information obtained by other means.

Like other information-gathering options, reports and records are not without their limitations. The quality of information recorded can vary in terms of both content value and legibility. In addition, data from reports and records can be biased because of problems with selective recording, storage, and retrieval. That is, reports may provide information on only favorable or extreme (and not typical) situations, or records may be saved or retrieved for review only if they portray a community favorably. Finally, some data available in records and reports (even those obtained over the internet) may be out of date because of the usual time lag between data collection, publication, and public availability of information.

Box 10-3 summarizes the advantages and disadvantages of these different information-gathering options. Box 10-4 identifies data collection strategies for information about different community characteristics.

Triangulation

Nurse consultants should incorporate triangulation into an assessment plan whenever possible. Triangulation refers to using multiple data sources and/or multiple data collection strategies to generate information. The purpose of triangulation is to "converge on the truth" about a community's problem. Since each information-gathering option has its own limitations and each data source may have some inherent bias, it stands to reason that if a nurse consultant collects more than one type of data about a problem, the conclu-

BOX 10-3 INFORMATION-GATHERING OPTIONS FOR NURSING CONSULTATION

Option	Advantages	Disadvantages
Surveys	Cost-effective Can collect a variety of information Probably best option for collecting information from large groups Yield numerical data Offer anonymity	Require time to construct Low response rates
Interviews	Allow collection of in-depth and detailed information	Costly to administer Take more time to analyze No anonymity Narrative data may be less convincing than numbers to some groups
Observation	Can detect process and communication problems Inexpensive	May raise issues regarding disclosure and informed consent
Reports, records	Inexpensive Generally easy to access	Problems with selective recording, storage, and retrieval Problems with currency of data

BOX 10-4 DATA SOURCES FOR SELECTED COMMUNITY INFORMATION

Information Needed	Importance	Data Sources
Population data (vital statistics, characteristics)	Impacts health trends and and resource needs	Census data Chamber of Commerce Public health records Internet
Geography (topography climate)	Influences types of health problems seen in a community and access care	Almanac Chamber of Commerce Observation Internet
History of community	Identifies trends in health and health problems, community responses to problems, resources, politics	Library Chamber of Commerce Interviews

BOX 10-4   DATA SOURCES FOR SELECTED COMMUNITY INFORMATION (CONTINUED)

Information Needed	Importance	Data Sources
Economy (employment level, types of work, income, agency/government expenditures)	Influences nature of health problems, access to care, need for community resources	Almanac Chamber of Commerce Census data Interviews Internet
Education (level of education in community, schools and their location and condition)	Influences illness patterns, access to care, understanding of health information	Census data Observation Telephone directory Chamber of Commerce Interviews Internet
Communication (radio, TV, newspapers, billboards: content and coverage of health issues)	Influences types and quality of health information, resources for action, awareness of community concerns	Observation Interviews Telephone directory Library Chamber of Commerce
Politics (parties and leaders, issues and responses)	Reflects community values, involvement, resources barriers to action	Interviews Newspaper Television
Recreational opportunities (types and numbers, access, age use, sponsorship)	Impact health, may serve as a resource for action	Observation Interviews Chamber of Commerce Telephone directory Newspaper Internet
Religion (location, leaders' strength of presence)	Reflects community values, may serve as a resource for action	Observation Interviews Telephone directory
Health resources (services, location, hours)	Indicates resources	Observation Telephone directory Internet
Protective services (visibility, responsiveness)	Indicates resources	Observation Interviews

sions developed about a problem's cause are more likely to be accurate. The value of triangulation was illustrated earlier in this chapter: Conclusions about the causes of cardiovascular disease in a community were more believable when they were based on both surveys and group comparison data rather than only observational data.

DIAGNOSIS: LABELING A PROBLEM'S CAUSE

The second task of the problem identification phase of the nursing consultation process is making a diagnosis. *Diagnosis* is the process of attaching meaning to the information obtained from the nursing consultation assessment. The purpose of diagnosis is to draw conclusions about the cause of a nursing consultation problem. In other words, diagnosis means naming a community's problem as well as identifying its cause. Diagnosis also entails confirming or redefining the scope of a problem, that is, how much of the client system is affected by the problem and how many different factors in the client system contribute to the problem. An accurate diagnosis is important for the success of the subsequent phases of the nursing consultation process.

Before conclusions can be made about the cause of a nursing consultation problem, the raw data from the assessment process need to be analyzed. While it is beyond the scope of this text to discuss specific data analysis procedures in detail, this section provides some simple and general guidelines.

When the assessment data that have been gathered are quantitative or numerical in nature, simple descriptive statistics are usually adequate for summarizing findings (i.e., a tally of responses and calculation of the mean, median, and standard deviation). Sometimes it is meaningful to compare this information for different subgroups, such as community residents who live in different areas or residents who receive specific health care services and those who do not.

Interviews and observations usually yield narrative data that can be analyzed for the presence of recurring themes. The frequency with which the different themes occur can then be counted and compared for different subgroups or periods of time.

To a large extent, the success of a nursing consultation relationship is dependent on the ability of a nurse consultant to draw inferences from assessment data and formulate causal statements with which the consultees agree. Therefore, part of the diagnostic process is getting consultees to both "buy into" a problem's cause and agree to assume their share of responsibility for its solution. One strategy a nurse consultant can use to create consultee buy-in to diagnostic statements is to involve consultees in the actual analysis of the assessment data. For example, consultees can help tally numerical data and can also read narrative data to help identify relevant themes.

In addition to involving consultees in the diagnostic process, it sometimes makes sense to also involve other members of the community. For example, including public officials makes sense because they control the community resources that will need to be accessed to solve the consultation problem. Involving other members of the client system in the diagnostic activities can also function as a form of "interpretive triangulation" and increase the accuracy of a diagnostic or causal statement because different perspectives are being brought into the interpretive process. This is important because a nurse consultant's unintentional misrepresentation of assessment findings and biased interpretation of information can be powerful barriers to the ultimate success of a consultation project.

A final strategy that a nurse consultant can use during the diagnostic process is that of proposing several alternative causes for a consultation problem. This strategy is particularly useful for creating buy-in when consultees or other members of a community have not been involved in data analysis activities. A nurse consultant can share these alternative causes with consultees and other community members and allow them to choose the most likely problem cause, which will be addressed during the subsequent phases of the nursing consultation process (Tiffany & Lutjens, 1998). Consultees may choose a problem cause on the basis of: (a) its reasonability or logic, (b) the feasibility of the problem solutions it implies, (c) perceived "speed" with which it implies the problem can be resolved, or (d) consultees' motivation to respond to a particular causal issue (Dougherty, 1995; Harrison, 1994). Maslow's hierarchy of needs can also be used to help consultees prioritize and choose problem causes (Morgan, Burbank, & Godfrey, 1993). This framework might lead a client system to address basic community needs such as safety before tackling higher-order needs such as community identity.

USING A FRAMEWORK TO GUIDE ASSESSMENT AND DIAGNOSIS ACTIVITIES

Frameworks identify linkages or relationships among the variables in a situation. For the purpose of community assessment and diagnosis activities, the framework a nurse consultant uses reflects a philosophy about linkages that are present among the various characteristics of a problem situation. More specifically, a framework also reflects assumptions about the specific nature of the linkages among the variables in a community and their impact on health.

The advantage of using a theoretical framework to guide assessment and diagnostic analysis is that it helps to focus and bring order to what can otherwise seem like overwhelming tasks (Helvie, 1998). In the problem identification process, a nurse consultant's theoretical perspective guides what kind of information is gathered during the course of assessment. A nurse consultant's theoretical perspective also influences how assessment findings are categorized and interpreted and the label or definition that is given to the problem cause (Anderson & McFarlane, 2000). The definition of a problem's cause, in turn, influences its acceptability to consultees and their community. As mentioned earlier, if

the problem is to be acted on, consultees' acceptance of a problem cause is essential. These points—and the impact of a specific theoretical framework on possible problem solutions—are illustrated by the scenarios that occur throughout this section.

The frameworks discussed in this section are just a sampling of those that can be used to guide assessment and diagnosis activities during the nursing consultation process. The first three (Neuman's System Theory, the Health Belief Model, and Milio's "Upstream" Framework) are described in more detail because they contrast sharply with one another and clearly illustrate how the choice of a theoretical framework influences both data gathering and diagnosis. Nurse consultants can use other nursing frameworks as well as frameworks from the social/behavioral sciences, business, management, and education as appropriate for both the consultation problem and the characteristics of the community/client system.

Neuman's Systems Theory

Betty Neuman, a nursing theorist, maintains that every system (individuals and their subsystems as well as groups and communities) is comprised of an inner core, a normal line of defense, a flexible line of defense, and lines of resistance. Applying these concepts to a community, a community's inner core is its population and their characteristics, as well as community features such as geography, climate, economy, and so forth. A community's normal line of defense is its usual responses to its environment and the level of health that has resulted from these day-to-day coping mechanisms. An intact normal line of defense is associated with health or stability of a community's inner core. Flexible lines of defense reflect temporary community coping mechanisms that are activated when unusual environmental stressors occur and a system's health or stability is threatened. Examples of flexible lines of defense include Red Cross responses to a natural disaster such as floods and development of a hepatitis prevention program in response to a hepatitis A outbreak. Lines of resistance are preventive mechanisms or community strengths that are in place to defend against potential stressors. A community's early response system or policy addressing school closure in the event of bad weather are examples of lines of resistance (Anderson & McFarlane, 2000). Neuman maintains that a system becomes dysfunctional when stressors overwhelm and penetrate the various lines of defense and resistance.

A nurse consultant using Neuman's Systems Theory to guide a community assessment would focus on identifying: (a) stressors, (b) whether present coping strategies represent flexible lines of defense or lines of resistance, and (c) the effectiveness of the coping strategies being used. What the nurse consultant wants to determine is which lines of resistance and defense are intact and which have been threatened or penetrated; these findings form the basis for a statement about the cause of the consultation problem. With this theoretical perspective, problems tend to be attributed to excess stressors and/or ineffective coping. Consultation interventions then, focus on removing stressors or bolstering coping strategies. Box 10-5 illustrates how a nurse consultant could use Neuman's Systems Theory to guide assessment of the problem of increased youth violence in a community.

The Health Belief Model

The Health Belief Model (HBM) is frequently used to explain participation in disease-avoidance activities such as individual compliance with a treatment regimen; the model is

---

BOX 10-5   ASSESSING YOUTH VIOLENCE USING NEUMAN'S SYSTEMS THEORY

A nurse consultant is asked to help a community develop strategies to address the problem of a recent and marked increase in incidents of youth violence. A problem clarification assessment, guided by Neuman's Systems Theory, is carried out. Neuman's Systems Theory is chosen as the theoretical framework for the assessment because the nurse consultant believes that violence occurs when stressors exceed a community's coping capacity. Thus to decrease youth violence, stressors need to be reduced or community coping strategies need to be improved. The consultees agree with this perspective.

Assessment Questions

- What is the "usual" level of youth violence (normal line of defense) in the community? How has this changed?
- What stressors are being experienced by youth in the community? Have these changed? (Possibilities include job layoffs, closure of usual hangouts, increased substance abuse, arrival of new gangs)
- What are the usual coping mechanisms (flexible lines of defense) the community uses to address this problem? Are they being used now? To what extent are they effective?
- What new or emergency coping mechanisms (lines of resistance) are being used? To what extent are they effective?

BOX 10-5   ASSESSING YOUTH VIOLENCE USING NEUMAN'S SYSTEMS THEORY *(CONTINUED)*

Information-Gathering Strategies

- Survey youth and larger community perceptions of stressors and changes in violence, as well as identify community responses to this problem and their perceived effectiveness.
- Interview school personnel to gather more in-depth information about perceptions of the problem and its possible causes.
- Observe mood and interpersonal interactions of youth for evidence of "simmering" violence, anger, frustration.

Findings

- There is community consensus that violence is more frequent and severe than it was 12 months ago.
- Arrival of a new gang in the community and closure of after-hours recreational opportunities are seen as contributing factors.
- The usual coping mechanisms of recreational and job-training programs have been disrupted by economic factors and changes in community leadership priorities.
- "Emergency" community coping mechanism such as more police presence and a curfew have been ineffective.

Diagnosis

Increased youth violence secondary to stressors that exceed effectiveness of coping strategies

Intervention Options

- Remove stressors (probably not feasible).
- Enhance coping strategies—emphasize restoring flexible lines of defense or usual coping mechanisms so that lines of resistance don't need to be activated.

---

equally useful for addressing selected community problems. The HBM maintains that individuals' (or a community's) actions reflect their world view (Butterfield, 1993). More specifically, behavior is determined by: (a) perceptions of susceptibility to a problem, (b) perceived seriousness of the problem if it occurs, (c) perceived benefits of engaging in a problem-avoidance activity, and (d) perceived barriers to participating in the problem-avoidance activity. These perceptions are modified by "cues to action"—environmental variables or events that encourage or discourage action. According to the HBM, a problem exists because of "errors" in perceptions; problems are solved, then, by correcting these perceptual errors or patterns of thinking.

A nurse consultant using the HBM to guide community assessment and diagnosis activities would focus on identifying community attitudes, beliefs, and perceptions that could be the cause of the nursing consultation problem. The diagnosis would identify an "error" in perception as the cause of the problem. Problem-solving interventions would consist of correcting the error in perception by reframing the meaning of the problem situation (e.g., making it seem more serious) and increasing the community's knowledge or understanding of the situation. Box 10-6 illustrates how a community problem of increased youth violence would be assessed if the nurse consultant used the HBM as the theoretical framework for assess-

ment. Note that, in contrast to Neuman's Systems Theory, the HBM downplays environmental influences on problems and views the community itself as solely responsible for the problem situation.

Milio's Upstream Perspective

Nancy Milio's "upstream" perspective is presented as a third contrasting framework that a nurse consultant could use to guide assessment and diagnosis activities in a community. Again,

---

BOX 10-6　ASSESSING YOUTH VIOLENCE USING THE HEALTH BELIEF MODEL

A nurse consultant is asked to help a community address the problem of a recent increase in incidents of youth violence. The violence is present despite opportunities for the community's youth to be involved in weekend and evening job-training and recreational programs. The nurse consultant carries out a problem clarification assessment that is guided by the Health Belief Model. This theoretical framework is chosen because the consultation contact person believes that increased community awareness of the seriousness of this problem will result in the allocation of more resources to address contributing factors.

Assessment Questions

- How susceptible do community residents perceive themselves to be to adverse effects of youth violence? Do they perceive themselves to be at high or low risk?
- How serious do community members perceive the incidents of violence to be? For example, are they viewed only as "normal teenage acting out"?
- What benefits do residents perceive in funding and participating in violence prevention programs?
- What barriers do community residents perceive to increasing funding for and participating in violence prevention programs?
- What cues to action are there regarding the increase in youth violence? In other words, how visible is the problem to community residents?

Information-Gathering Strategies

- Survey community residents about their perceptions of personal susceptibility and the general seriousness of the violence, as well as the perceived benefits and barriers to devoting more resources to addressing the problem.
- Observe for cues to action regarding of violence (e.g., damaged public property).
- Review news reports about the increase in youth violence.

BOX 10-6   ASSESSING YOUTH VIOLENCE USING THE HEALTH BELIEF MODEL *(CONTINUED)*

Findings

- Community residents perceive themselves to be at "low risk" for being personally affected by the violence.
- In general, community residents perceive the acts of violence as "teenage pranks."
- There are few perceived benefits to devoting more resources to addressing the problem.
- Barriers to resource allocation include perceptions of community problems (e.g., street repair) that are of higher priority.
- News reports of incidents of violence (i.e., cues to action) tend to be hidden inside the newspaper rather than appear on the front page.

Diagnosis

Increased youth violence secondary to community complacency about the problem

Intervention Options

- Provide reliable information about the nature and effects of the incidents of violence; make sure these are highly publicized.
- "Advertise" the benefits of addressing this problem as a community.
- Emphasize residents' moral responsibility to contribute to a problem solution; emphasize the cost-effectiveness of prevention programs.

the intent is to illustrate the implications of a nurse consultant's choice of framework for the tasks of the problem identification phase.

Milio's framework focuses on "upstream" or environmental factors that are precursors to poor health or dysfunction (Butterfield, 1990, 1993; Milio, 1976). Milio asserts that individuals (and communities) will make healthy behavioral choices whenever such choices are the easiest ones to make. Milio maintains that poor health (or a nursing consultation problem) occurs when there is an imbalance between the conditions needed for health and the health-promoting conditions (choices) that are realistically available. Health is promoted, then, by making healthy choices or conditions easily available. Milio's framework, therefore, emphasizes society's

responsibility for the health of individuals and communities. This contrasts with the HBM, which maintains that attitudes and perceptions cause health problems.

A nurse consultant using Milio's framework would focus assessment activities on identifying factors in the community's internal and external environments that are contributing to the consultation problem. Of particular interest would be community policies and resources, residents' awareness of these resources, and resource accessibility. Box 10-7 illustrates how the community problem of youth violence could be assessed using Milio's framework. Note that this framework assumes that health-promoting resources will be used if they are available. The "Upstream" Framework overlooks individual resident/commu-

BOX 10-7   ASSESSING YOUTH VIOLENCE USING MILIO'S UPSTREAM FRAMEWORK

A nurse consultant is asked by a community to help them address the problem of a recent escalation of the frequency and seriousness of incidents of youth violence. The community wants to address the problems by increasing recreational opportunities and job training programs that are available to its young people. The nurse consultant decides to use Milio's "Upstream" Framework to guide a desire analysis assessment. The nurse consultant chooses this framework because it holds the community responsible for making the changes needed to solve the problem. The nurse consultant is able to convince the consultee group that this is an appropriate perspective for this problem situation.

Assessment Questions

- Are youth aware of existing recreational and job-training opportunities?
- Are youth participating in these opportunities? If not, why not?

Information-Gathering Strategies

- Survey teens to gather information about awareness and accessibility of recreation and job-training programs.
- Interview selected teens and community leaders in a focus interview format; the intent of the interview is to discover their points of agreement and disagreement about the opportunities the community is making available to its youth.
- Review notices and communication about youth activities in order to determine what messages are given about accessibility (group meeting times, etc.).

Findings

- Most youth are unaware of existing opportunities.
- The programs are available only at two high schools in the community—both of which are in wealthier sectors of the community.
- The programs operate only Monday through Thursday.

Diagnosis

Increased youth violence secondary to lack of awareness and *real* access to community youth-oriented programs

Intervention Options

- Increase publicity about job-training and recreational programs.
- Make programs available on weekends.
- Consider changing or expanding location of program.

nity factors such as values and perceptions that also influence behavior.

Other Frameworks for Consulting with Communities

Neuman's Systems Theory, the Health Belief Model, and Milio's "Upstream" Framework are just three of the many frameworks a nurse consultant can use to guide assessment and diagnosis activities with a community. Open systems theory (described in Chapter 6), the Epidemiological Framework, Gordon's Func-tional Health Patterns, and Orem's Self-Care Theory are four other frameworks that are familiar to many nurses and are useful for nursing consultation. These latter three frameworks, as they apply to community assessment and diagnosis activities, are sum-marized briefly in Box 10-8.

Choosing a Theoretical Framework

Because a single theoretical framework is not equally suitable for all nursing consultation

---

BOX 10-8   ADDITIONAL FRAMEWORKS FOR PROBLEM IDENTIFICATION ACTIVITIES

Epidemiological Framework

Focus: Identification of human and environmental factors that differentiate community mem-bers or the community sector that is affected by the consultation problems from members/sector that is not affected

Assessment Categories

- Host—"who" is affected by the problem and their characteristics (demographics, attitudes, economics, and so forth)
- Environment—"where and when" variables related to the consultation problem; factors such as geography, climate, timing

Diagnosis: The "agent" or the "how and why" of a problem situation. This is usually a combi-nation of host and environment factors.

Gordon's Functional Health Patterns

Focus: Level of functioning in regard to various belief and behavior patterns that are associ-ated with community health

Assessment Categories

- Health perception/health management—adequacy of health and safety efforts
- Nutrition/metabolic patterns—adequacy of nutritional efforts (such as food banks and education)
- Elimination—waste management within the community
- Activity/exercise—transportation and recreational opportunities within the community
- Sleep/rest—community rhythms and cycles
- Cognitive/perceptual patterns—community decision-making processes

(Continued)

BOX 10-8   ADDITIONAL FRAMEWORKS FOR PROBLEM IDENTIFICATION ACTIVITIES *(CONTINUED)*

- Role/relationship patterns—definition of formal and informal roles; interactions within and external to the community
- Sexuality/reproductive patterns—birth rates and patterns; resources for reproductive and family concerns
- Coping/stress behavior—support services available within the community
- Values/beliefs—culture and its impact

Diagnosis: Identification of patterns that are not responsive to community needs

Orem's Self-Care Theory

Focus: The ability of community to perform the functions necessary to maintain its current level of well-being or to improve its level of well-being

Assessment Categories:

- Universal self-care requisites—living space, goods and services, communication, rules and standards of behavior, safety and order, enculturation, opportunities for interaction
- Developmental self-care requisites—needs created by growth and change
- Health self-care requisites—needs that evolve when a community is dysfunctional or its health is threatened
- Therapeutic self-care demands—actions a community must take to meet self-care requisites
- Self-care agency—current level of community well-being

Diagnosis: Identification of self-care deficits

Source: Helvie, C. (1998). *Advanced practice nursing in the community.* Thousand Oaks, CA: Sage.

---

problems, nurse consultants need to be familiar with a variety of frameworks from nursing as well as from other disciplines. Ideally, the framework a nurse consultant selects to guide assessment activities will "fit" the nature of the consultation problem and will lead to meaningful, relevant, and acceptable problem solutions.

With experience, most nurse consultants come to favor certain theoretical frameworks over others. A nurse consultant needs to keep in mind, however, that consultees will become involved in problem solving only if they "buy into" explanations about the problem's cause. Because of this, a nurse consultant needs to make certain that the theoretical framework chosen in a given situation will explain problems in a way that is acceptable to the community. Milio's "Upstream" Framework, for example, would be effective only if the community accepted community (rather than individual) responsibility for problems and problem solving.

INVOLVING CONSULTEES IN ASSESSMENT AND DIAGNOSIS ACTIVITIES

Assessment and diagnosis activities can be carried out by the nurse consultant alone or in a collaborative manner with consultees. Both approaches have advantages and disadvantages. The approach that is used depends on the nature of the consultation problem (e.g., its urgency) as well as the abilities and preferences of the consultees.

When consultees are involved directly in information-gathering and interpretation activities, they will often view conclusions about a problem's cause as more credible. This happens because consultees tend to see the information on a firsthand basis so they know it is valid. This can facilitate ownership of the problem and encourage buy-in or assuming responsibility for problem solutions.

Consultee involvement in information gathering has other benefits and can be especially helpful to external nurse consultants. Because consultees are "insiders" to the community and problem situation, they can help an external nurse consultant locate and access needed information. They may also be more successful than a nurse consultant at retrieving certain types of data such as agency or community financial reports.

While a collaborative approach to assessment and diagnostic analysis has advantages, it also has disadvantages. Sometimes consultee involvement in information gathering and interpretation can cause other members of the community to question the objectivity of the conclusions that are reached. For example, consultees could be accused of interpreting data so that problem solutions will result in personal gain such as additional resources for only a selected segment of the community. A collaborative approach to assessment and diagnostic analysis also takes more time than does a more consultant-directed approach. This is because consultees often need to be taught data collection, analysis, and interpretation skills. Consequently, a collaborative approach is usually not feasible in urgent situations, such as a budget crisis or an infectious disease outbreak.

COMMUNICATING ASSESSMENT FINDINGS

The third and final task of the problem identification phase of the nursing consultation process is communicating assessment findings and diagnostic conclusions to the consultees and other relevant members of the community. The primary purpose of sharing findings with the consultees is to establish legitimacy and encourage ownership of the cause of the consultation problem. A second purpose of communicating assessment findings is to stimulate the consultees' thinking about how the problem might be solved. The communication process also gives consultees the opportunity to give input and support or challenge the nurse consultant's conclusions about the problem's cause. This is important because, as emphasized earlier in this chapter, consultees' acceptance of the problem cause is essential if the consultation process is to be successful.

The primary challenge for a nurse consultant in regard to communicating assessment findings is packaging the information effectively for different community audiences. Often, nurse consultants need to share findings with such diverse groups as agency administrators, public officials, health care providers, and different groups of community members or health care consumers. In most instances, language and style of presentation need to be altered in order to be responsive to the culture, knowledge level, and point of reference or vested interest of a particular audience. The two most common strategies for sharing consultation findings are written reports and formal presentations.

Written Reports

A written report of assessment findings and diagnostic conclusions should begin with an overview of the problem that triggered the request for nursing consultation. The overview should include the community's perspective of the problem (the symptoms and how they are problematic) as well as a history of the problem. The next section of the report should be a summary of how the assessment process was carried out (purpose, information-gathering strategies, and theoretical framework used), and how the information obtained was analyzed. Copies of any data collection tools (surveys and interview schedules, for instance) should be attached as appendices to the report.

The results section of a written report should be an objective reporting of the assessment findings. It is particularly effective to present information graphically (e.g., with pie charts and bar graphs) and in tables rather than in a strictly narrative format. If narrative data have been collected, it is meaningful to include direct quotes, although care must be taken to protect the privacy of the individuals who are being quoted.

The final section of the report is the nurse consultant's interpretation of the assessment findings. This section is where the nurse consultant identifies the cause of the consultation problem. Implications of the problem cause for possible problem-solving strategies are also addressed in this section.

It is important that a report is written in language that is appropriate for the intended audience. Nurse consultants need to be particularly careful about using technical jargon that may not be understood correctly by non–nurse consultees. Conclusions that are presented should be supported with specific facts and observations. Finally, individuals who provided specific information should not be named without their consent. Box 10-9 presents guidelines for preparing a written consultation report.

Formal Presentations

Many of the "ground rules" for preparing a written report can also be applied to formal presentations. Whenever possible, a nurse consultant should arrange for a personal meeting with consultees or the consultation contact person before any formal group presentation of assessment findings and conclusions. This private meeting gives consultees an opportunity to react to the findings. A private meeting avoids having consultees become

---

BOX 10-9   PREPARING A CONSULTATION REPORT

- Begin with an overview of the consultation problem—its history, the symptoms that prompted the consultation request, a description of the difficulties the problem is creating.
- Summarize the assessment process—purpose, what kind of information was gathered, information-gathering strategies, information sources, who collected the information, and theoretical framework used; state the rationale for these decisions.
- Attach any information-gathering tools that were used.
- Describe how the information was analyzed and who was involved in analysis activities.
- Present results objectively—give specific examples, use quotes and graphs to enhance the discussion.
- Protect the privacy of information sources.
- Be sure that report is written in language that is appropriate for the audience.

angry and defensive about any "negative" findings in a group setting. It also gives consultees an opportunity to take part in planning the formal presentation.

The overall goals of a formal presentation about assessment findings and conclusions are to deliver the facts, facilitate discussion, have consultees and the larger community take responsibility for the problem situation and plan the next steps for the nursing consultation relationship. Groups with whom it is appropriate to share assessment findings and conclusions are those who are being asked to take actions as well as those who might be affected by any action that is taken. A sample agenda that should accomplish these goals is presented in Box 10-10.

Communicating assessment findings and conclusions in a group setting can present a number of challenges to a nurse consultant. A particular concern of consultees is that the nurse consultant may catch them "off-guard" and that the nursing consultation assessment might have uncovered information that reveals problems that have been previously hidden (either intentionally or unintentionally). A nurse consultant needs to avoid becoming defensive and arguing with consultees when these reactions occur. Keeping a presentation objective and supporting con-clusions with facts can often decrease consultee hostility. Another effective presentation strategy is to help the community realize that the problem is in the past and the focus is now on the future. In other words, a problem can be reframed as a goal to reach in the future (Kurpius, Fuqua, & Rozecki, 1993).

POTENTIAL DILEMMAS IN THE PROBLEM IDENTIFICATION PHASE

Both methodological and political dilemmas can complicate the problem identification phase of the nursing consultation process. A nurse consultant who is aware of these possible problems will be more likely to recognize their occurrence and respond so that they are less likely to disrupt the tasks of the problem identification phase.

Methodological Difficulties

A methodological difficulty that can complicate the information-gathering process is reluctance of community members being surveyed or interviewed to share unfavorable perceptions of their community. Related to this difficulty is the issue of needing to sort

---

BOX 10-10   SAMPLE AGENDA FOR A GROUP MEETING ABOUT ASSESSMENT FINDINGS

1. Introduction, review of the problem, and reasons for nursing consultation (The primary consultee or contact person should be encouraged to do this; this reinforces support of the nursing consultation process and the consultation relationship.)
2. Overview of the assessment and diagnostic analysis process
3. Presentation of assessment findings and their interpretation (enhanced by graphics)
4. Questions and comments from the audience
5. Validation of findings and conclusions with the audience
6. Recap—summarize what has been agreed upon as the next step

out the meaning of conflicting ideas about the problem situation from different informants. These two dilemmas often represent opposing interests such as job security and fear of retaliation for revealing unfavorable information. A nurse consultant who encounters these difficulties needs to acknowledge the underlying concerns they represent. Additionally, a nurse consultant needs to reassure informants that the confidentiality of the information they share will be respected.

An additional methodological difficulty is constraints on information sources (people as well as documents) that can be accessed. Sometimes involving consultees in information-gathering activities makes accessing these sources easier. Reassuring consultees

---

BOX 10-11   DOCUMENTATION CHECKLIST: THE PROBLEM IDENTIFICATION PHASE

Documenting Assessment Activities

- ☐ Overall purpose of the assessment
- ☐ Theoretical framework that was used and why
- ☐ Date and time of each assessment activity
- ☐ Regarding each assessment activity—purpose, information-gathering strategy, information source, who collected the information; rationale for these decisions; attach any tools that were used
- ☐ Outcome of each assessment activity—information gathered; be objective and specific
- ☐ Difficulties encountered—how they were addressed, whether or not they were resolved
- ☐ Notes about possible next steps
- ☐ Impressions about the assessment process

Documenting Diagnostic Analysis Activities

- ☐ Date and time of each activity
- ☐ Description and rationale for activity
- ☐ Identification of parties involved
- ☐ Difficulties encountered—how they were addressed, whether or not they were resolved
- ☐ Conclusion reached about the cause of the consultation problem
- ☐ Notes about possible next steps

Documenting the Presentation of Assessment Findings

- ☐ Date and time of presentation
- ☐ Audience—be as specific as possible
- ☐ Format of presentation, rationale (attach copy of presentation or report)
- ☐ Difficulties encountered—how they were addressed, whether or not they were resolved
- ☐ Notes about possible next steps
- ☐ Overall (personal, subjective) impressions about how the presentation went

about the confidentiality of information that is shared can also remove access barriers.

A final methodological difficulty that the nurse consultant may face during the problem identification phase is pressure to use quick and, perhaps, cursory and superficial information-gathering strategies. This pressure usually reflects efforts to save time and money as well as prevent discovery of additional problems within the community. A nurse consultant can respond to this pressure by educating the contact person and consultees about the importance of a properly conducted problem identification phase for the ultimate success of the consultation process.

Political Dilemmas

A political dilemma a nurse consultant may face during the problem identification phase is that of being asked to share information obtained during assessment for purposes other than diagnosing a problem's cause. For example, a nurse consultant might be asked to provide input into personnel evaluations and budget decisions in a community agency. A nurse consultant needs to respond to this pressure by emphasizing the confidentiality and purpose of the information that has been gathered. This dilemma can also be prevented (or at least protected against) by addressing the conditions under which assessment information will be shared in the nursing consultation contract.

DOCUMENTING THE ACTIVITIES OF THE PROBLEM IDENTIFICATION PHASE

Documenting the activities of the problem identification phase provides the nurse consultant with reminders of what has transpired during this phase of the nursing consultation process. Documentation also provides the nurse consultant with a learning tool about

what works and what doesn't as a problem identification strategy. Finally, documentation is important because it provides evidence about appropriate fulfillment of the terms of the consultation contract. Thorough documentation can, therefore, provide a nurse consultant with legal protection against charges of inadequate assessment of the problem situation. Box 10-11 is a checklist that can be used for documenting the activities of the problem identification phase.

CHAPTER SUMMARY

The problem identification phase is one of the most important phases of the nursing consultation process. The information gathered during this phase sets the stage for subsequent development of both problem-solving activities and the nursing consultation action plan. Clarity about the purpose of the assessment and selection of appropriate information-gathering strategies and theoretical framework helps to increase the meaningfulness and credibility of the findings and conclusions. Awareness on the part of a nurse consultant about the difficulties that might be encountered during the problem identification phase helps to ensure that the tasks of the phase are accomplished as intended and achieve their purposes.

APPLYING CHAPTER CONTENT

1. Critique the problem identification activities carried out for the youth violence problem presented in this chapter. Which of the frameworks do you think is most effective for this situation? Formulate an assessment for this same consultation problem using another theoretical perspective.

2. Identify a nursing consultation problem in a health care setting or community with which you are familiar. Use two different theoretical frameworks to develop guidelines for implementing a nursing consultation assessment of this problem. Identify the implications of each assessment approach for possible explanations about the problem's cause as well as subsequent interventions. Which theoretical framework seems most appropriate for this problem? Why?

References

Anderson, E., & McFarlane, J. (2000) *Community as partner: Theory and practice in nursing* (3rd ed.). Philadelphia: Lippincott.

Butterfield, P. (1990). Thinking upstream: Nurturing a conceptual understanding of the societal context of health behavior. *Advances in Nursing Science, 12*(2), 1–8.

Butterfield, P. (1993). Thinking upstream: Conceptualizing health from a population perspective. In J. Swanson & M. Albrecht (Eds.), *Community health nursing: Promoting the health of aggregates* (pp. 80–108). Philadelphia: Saunders.

Cook, D. (1989). Systematic need assessment: A primer. *Journal of Counseling and Development, 67*, 462–464.

Dougherty, M. (1995). *Consultation: Practice and perspectives in school and community settings* (2nd ed.). Pacific Grove, CA: Brooks-Cole.

Hancock, T., & Minkler, M. (1997). Community health assessment or healthy community assessment: Whose community? Whose health? Whose assessment? In M. Minkler (Ed.), *Community organizing and community building for health* (pp. 139–156). New Brunswick, NJ: Rutgers University Press.

Harrison, M. (1994). *Diagnosing organizations: Methods, models, and processes* (2nd ed.). Thousand Oaks, CA: Sage.

Helvie, C. (1998). *Advanced practice nursing in the community.* Thousand Oaks, CA: Sage.

Kurpius, D., Fuqua, D., & Rozecki, T. (1993). The consulting process: A multidimensional approach. *Journal of Counseling and Development, 71*, 601–606.

Milio, N. (1976). A framework for prevention: Changing health-damaging to health-generating life patterns. *American Journal of Public Health, 66*(5), 435–439.

Morgan, B., Burbank, P., & Godfrey, D. (1993). Health planning. In J. Swanson & M. Albrecht (Eds.), *Community health nursing: Promoting the health of aggregates* (pp. 109–127). Philadelphia: Saunders.

Ridley, C., & Mendoza, D. (1993). Putting organizational effectiveness into practice: The preeminent consultation task. *Journal of Counseling & Development, 72*, 168–177.

Tiffany, C., & Lutjens, L. (1998). *Planned change theories: Review, analysis, and implications.* Thousand Oaks, CA: Sage.

11

Action Planning with Communities

Careful planning increases the probability of fruitful outcomes and decreases the likelihood of disaster. (Tiffany & Lutjens, 1998)

 KEY CONCEPTS:

goal, objective, Gantt chart, transition, diffusion

 KEY TERMS FOR YOUR SEARCH ENGINE:

community and action, community and planning

INTRODUCTION

Think of the last time you worked with a patient who was having some sort of pain. How did you decide what to do? Most likely, solving this problem involved setting goals (such as maximum pain relief with minimal side effects) and choosing an intervention on the basis of factors such as the nature of the problem (location and severity of pain) and the patient's characteristics (medication allergies, other health problems). The process of deciding on a problem solution is similar when working as a nurse consultant with a community. In nursing consultation, as in individual patient care situations, any presenting problem holds a variety of possible solutions. It is during the action planning phase of the nursing consultation process that a nurse consultant and consultees work together to decide how to specifically go about solving the consultation problem.

Action planning entails planning change. Planned change is a process of well-thought-out actions to make something happen. Planned changes differs from change in that the actions occur in a definite sequence, with each serving as preparation for the next (Anderson & McFarlane, 2000). In nursing consultation, action planning consists of working with consultees to accomplish the following four tasks: setting goals, choosing a problem solution, developing an action plan, and facilitating implementation of the action plan. These tasks occur in a fairly linear fashion despite differences in the nature of the nursing consultation problem, the problem setting, or the nursing consultation interaction pattern being used. Figure 11-1 depicts the tasks of the action planning phases as well as the various activities that occur as a part of each task.

The action planning and problem identification phases of the nursing consultation process are intricately linked in a couple of ways. First, the theoretical framework that a nurse consultant uses to guide assessment and diagnosis activities identifies possible points of intervention for responding to a problem. The selected framework also governs the range of interventions that are likely to be appropriate. Recall, for example, how problem causes and possible solutions differed in the youth violence scenario presented in Chapter 10 when the problem was approached from the perspective of Neuman's Systems Theory, the Health Belief Model, or Milio's "Upstream" Framework. The action planning phase is also linked to the problem identification phase because the basis for a solid action plan is thorough information gathering and solid data analysis. As noted in Chapter 10, inadequate information can lead a consultant to attribute a problem to the wrong cause, which in turn can lead to the development of inappropriate problem solutions. Furthermore, if information-gathering activities fail to detect barriers to potential problem solutions, a nurse consultant may propose a problem solution that the consultees cannot (or will not) implement.

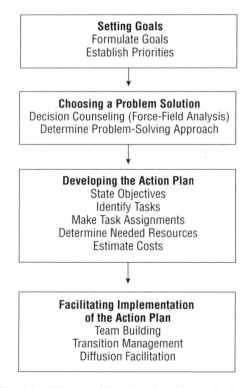

Setting Goals
Formulate Goals
Establish Priorities

Choosing a Problem Solution
Decision Counseling (Force-Field Analysis)
Determine Problem-Solving Approach

Developing the Action Plan
State Objectives
Identify Tasks
Make Task Assignments
Determine Needed Resources
Estimate Costs

**Facilitating Implementation
of the Action Plan**
Team Building
Transition Management
Diffusion Facilitation

Figure 11-1   The Action Planning Phase of the Nursing Consultation Process.
The tasks of the action planning phase occur in a fairly linear fashion despite differences in the nature of the nursing consultation problem, the problem situation, and the nursing consultation interaction pattern that is being used.

The action planning phase of the nursing consultation process is important because it represents the first tangible action to resolve the problem that prompted the request for nursing consultation. The action planning phase is a bridge between the present state and the desired state of a client system; it is the beginning of the "moving" phase of Lewin's description of change (see Chapter 8). It is important to recognize that the stakes are high in this phase for both the nurse consultant and the consultee. The goals that are set and the interventions that are chosen will determine not only whether a community's problem is resolved, but will also determine the side effects associated with solving the problem and whether the solution will produce long-lasting or only temporary results. For example, solving a community's problem of youth violence by developing evening recreational opportunities (as would be consistent with Milio's "Upstream" Framework) could create side effects of safety concerns related to increased traffic or of sports-related injuries.

This chapter discusses each of the four tasks of the action planning phase. In the first section, strategies for working with consultees

to set goals and establish priorities are considered. Next, the process of choosing a problem solution is discussed. The details of developing an action plan and strategies for facilitating implementation of an action plan are presented in the third and fourth sections of the chapter. The chapter concludes with a discussion of some of the difficulties that can arise during the action planning phase. As you read this chapter, consider the following questions:

- How might setting goals and developing problem solutions differ for internal and external nursing consultation situations?
- How might action planning differ with individual and group consultees?
- What skills must a nurse consultant possess to be successful in the activities of the action planning phase? Which of these skills do you possess? Which do you need to acquire or further develop?
- What values and biases would you bring to the action planning phase? How might these affect your success as a nurse consultant?

SETTING GOALS

Goals are statements about how a community wants things to be once the consultation problem has been resolved. Contact persons or consultees often identify goals for a consultation relationship at the time of initial contact with a nurse consultant. These initial goals, however, are often vague ("We want a healthier community") or unrealistic ("We want to eliminate all methamphetamine labs in the city in two months"). In most nursing consultation situations, new and more specific goals are identified once the consultation problem has been clarified and its cause has been determined. Once these new "working goals" have been formulated, the nurse

consultant and consultees work together to prioritize these goals.

The first task of the action planning phase is to help consultees set meaningful and realistic goals. In order to set goals, consultees must have a clear picture about a preferred and feasible future. Developing meaningful and realistic goals is most likely to occur when three conditions are met. First, the tasks of the problem identification phase must be completed satisfactorily; that is, a thorough assessment must lead to an accurate problem diagnosis. Second, consultees must be involved in the two activities of the goal-setting process: formulating goals and establishing priorities. Finally, the goals that are decided on must be clear, understood, and acceptable to the consultees as well as to the larger community (Dyer, 1977).

Formulating Goals

To formulate goals that are meaningful, it is often helpful to have consultees consider exactly how the problem situation is problematic (i.e., what "pains" are being experienced) as well as clarify what is wanted versus what is needed as a consultation outcome. Meaningful goals are value driven because they reflect what consultees would like to see happen in terms of problem resolution. Meaningful goals are also characterized by longevity. That is, not only will they solve the immediate problem, they will also help consultees and a community respond to similar problems in the future.

Goals also need to be acceptable to a community (i.e., in keeping with the community's culture and values) if they are to have longevity. Goal formulation, therefore, needs to consider the personal values of the consultees and the culture of the larger community, as well as how these factors might change in the future.

Organizational development consultants often have consultees explore the anticipated longevity of their goals by engaging in a process called "futurethink" (Chapter 19 discusses this process in greater depth). Consultees are asked to project an image of themselves and their organization five years into the future. In developing this image, consultees are asked to take into account trends in their own organization and work unit, as well as their personal ideas about what constitutes sound organizational practices.

Nurse consultants can engage in a similar activity with both individual and group consultees during the goal-setting process. Community consultees, for example, might be asked to project the following: what their community will look like in five years (size, age distribution, population density, primary businesses), what is going on within the community (demographic changes, health issues, economics), and what is of value to them as a community (safety, connectedness, identity, self-sufficiency). This exercise might help community consultees develop more realistic and acceptable goals for the long-term problem of providing adequate housing and care for low-income elderly persons who need assistance with activities of daily living. By following a similar approach, consultees from a community agency could develop meaningful goals about growth and what services to offer by considering national trends in health care financing, patterns of referrals to the agency, and personal as well as agency values about what services would be both congruent with the agency's mission and profitable.

In addition to being meaningful and acceptable, goals need to be realistic. Realistic goals are hard, but attainable. Goals that are too easy fail to challenge and motivate a community; however, if goals are too hard, consultees will feel overwhelmed before they start working on them (Dyer, 1977). Realistic goals are goals that can be achieved by a community when its resources (e.g., time, workforce, financial resources, skills, and motivation) are taken into account. To formulate achievable or realistic goals, a consultant needs to help consultees determine whether the resources needed to accomplish a goal are available. Reviewing information gathered during the nursing consultation assessment should provide information about resource availability. If not, the nurse consultant will need to backtrack and gather additional information. Appraising resources is important, as failure to identify resource-related barriers to goal accomplishment will leave the nursing consultation problem unresolved. In addition, new problems can be created if scarce resources are depleted or diverted from other needs in the community. Box 11-1 summarizes strategies a nurse consultant can use to help a consultee formulate meaningful, acceptable, and realistic goals.

BOX 11-1   FORMULATING MEANINGFUL, ACCEPTABLE, AND REALISTIC GOALS

To Establish Meaningful Goals

- Clarify what is problematic about the problem situation.
- Clarify what is needed versus what is wanted as a consultation outcome.
- Consider longevity of goals—"Will it still be meaningful in five years?"
- Engage in "futurethink."

To Establish Acceptable Goals

- Consider whether proposed goals are in keeping with personal and the community's culture and values.
- Consider longevity—"Will the goal still fit the community's values and needs in five years?"

To Establish Realistic Goals

- Try to establish goals that are neither too easy nor too hard.
- Identify resources needed for goal accomplishment.
- Review information from the nursing consultation assessment to identify resources available and resource-related barriers that are present.

Establishing Priorities

The creative generation of goals for a nursing consultation relationship with a community needs to be followed by a disciplined process of establishing priorities. A nurse consultant needs to help consultees decide which goal to tackle first. Goals are often given top priority if they address an immediate and overriding problem. Problem scope, severity, and impact are other criteria for setting priorities that make sense (Helvie, 1998). Addressing widespread community concerns creates more buy-in for the nursing consultation process. Addressing "lower order" needs, such as physiological functioning and safety first, is appropriate because, as in individual patient care situations, goals such as self-care and learning new tasks are unrealistic until immediate needs are satisfied (this reflects Maslow's hierarchy of needs). As is the case with individual patients, in nursing consultation situations with communities, consultees' fear and anxiety are often immediate and overriding problems that need to be resolved before the real consultation problem can be addressed.

In other nursing consultation situations, it may make sense to identify some goals as high priority because their accomplishment will provide consultees with knowledge or skills that will facilitate the accomplishment of other goals. For example, in an agency expansion project, it might make sense for initial goals to focus on learning skills such as delegation, time management, and working as a mixed-skill team (e.g., nurses and home health aides), because these skills are foundational to goals that address offering new services and serving a larger population.

Finally, a nurse consultant might advise consultees to give certain goals higher priority because they respond to an immediately solv-

BOX 11-2   ESTABLISHING PRIORITIES: WHICH GOAL TO TACKLE FIRST?

- Goals that address immediate and overriding problems, including safety needs and emotional reactions of consultees
- Goals that address problems that affect a large number of community members or are very serious, even if they affect only limited sectors of the community
- Goals that address widespread community concerns
- Goals that will provide consultees and the larger community with knowledge or skills that will facilitate achievement of other goals
- Goals that are easily attainable and will both increase consultees' (and the community's) perceptions of the credibility of the consultation relationship and build their confidence for proceeding with problem solving
- Goals that address solvable problems—resources are available to attain goals

able problem, are easily attainable, and require no additional resources. Accomplishment of these goals can help demonstrate both a nurse consultant's credibility and the value of the nursing consultation relationship. Accomplishing easily attainable goals can also help consultees build the confidence needed to pursue long-term and more ambitious goals. Box 11-2 provides guidelines for prioritizing goals.

CHOOSING A PROBLEM SOLUTION

Goals and problem solutions are inextricably linked. The desire to achieve a specific goal narrows the range of possible nursing consultation problem solutions. At the same time, because most nursing consultation takes place in an open systems context (see Chapter 6), there are multiple means to any end. Thus, in any nursing consultation situation, a nurse consultant and consultees have a range of possible problem solutions from which to choose. (Reviewing the scenarios presented in Chapter 10 might help to clarify this point.) Selecting the problem solution

that is most likely to be effective involves matching the problem's cause, the goals of the nursing consultation relationship, and the characteristics of consultees (skills) and community (values, culture), as well as resources (time, money, knowledge, skills, infrastructure) to the appropriate problem solution (Tiffany & Lutjens, 1998). Two specific processes involved in the task of choosing a problem solution are decision counseling and selecting an appropriate problem-solving approach.

Decision Counseling

Decision counseling is the process of working with consultees to develop meaningful, acceptable, and realistic problem solutions (Dougherty, 1995). Decision counseling is a give-and-take process between a nurse consultant and consultees and begins with brainstorming about possible ways of attaining goals. Both parties assume responsibility for identifying factors that make a particular problem solution more or less acceptable and appropriate for a problem situation. Of particular interest in decision counseling is exploring both a proposed problem solution's side effects and situational variables that might act as driving or restraining forces to being able to actually implement the problem solution.

Force-Field Analysis

Force-field analysis is a useful exercise for identifying the driving and restraining forces related to a specific problem solution (Anderson & McFarlane, 2000). Driving and restraining forces are characteristics of a problem situation and community that argue for or against a particular problem solution. Force-field analysis can help a nurse consultant and consultees gain perspective about a potential problem solution's possible pitfalls and strong points as they relate to the specific setting and

situation within which the problem solution would take place. Variables that need to be considered as possible driving and restraining forces are identified in Box 11-3.

Once the driving and restraining forces related to a proposed problem solution are identified, the nurse consultant and consultees identify which driving forces can be strengthened and which restraining forces can be decreased. Next, they weight each driving and restraining force (high, medium, and low) in terms of: (a) anticipated degree of impact, and (b) likelihood of occurrence. After the weighting process, driving and restraining forces are tallied separately. Problem solutions with restraining forces that outweigh driving forces are eliminated as viable problem-solving strategies. The force-field analysis process is summarized in Box 11-4.

BOX 11-3   VARIABLES TO CONSIDER AS POSSIBLE DRIVING AND RESTRAINING FORCES

- Potential side effects of the problem-solving strategy in all sectors of a community—desirable side effects should be considered a driving force, whereas undesirable side effects should be considered a restraining force
- Time and timing—how much is needed versus how much is available; if there is a "time crunch," a prescriptive approach to problem solving should be considered
- Teamwork—how much is present versus how much is needed
- Material resources—time, money, equipment
- Human resources—availability, skills, willingness to participate
- Trust—low trust can be a restraining force; try to increase trust with catalytic and confrontational interventions
- Emotions—anxiety and fear are common restraining forces; try to resolve these with acceptant interventions
- Culture and values
- Power—consider who in the community supports and does not support the problem solution
- Historical considerations—Has this problem solution been used before? How did it work?
- Politics—Who will the winners and losers be if this solution is implemented? What impact will this have?

BOX 11-4　THE FORCE-FIELD ANALYSIS PROCESS

Step 1: Identify Support for a Specific Problem Solution

Identify the variables that are present that are supportive of a given problem solution. These are the driving forces for that solution.

Step 2: Identify Barriers to a Solution

Identify the variables that are barriers or restraining forces for a given problem solution. Take into consideration time, human and material resources, emotions, culture, and values.

Step 3: Identify Possible Consequences

Identify the possible consequences of the problem solution. Are side effects desirable, tolerable, or not acceptable? Are these consequences driving or restraining forces?

Step 4: Maximize Supports and Minimize Restraining Forces

Strategize ways in which driving forces can be maximized and restraining forces can be minimized.

Step 5: Weight Factors

Weight each driving and restraining force (high, medium, and low) on the basis of its degree of impact and likelihood of occurring.

Step 6: Tally Weighted Factors

Tally the weighted factors for both driving and restraining forces.

Step 7: Choose or Reject the Problem Solution

If driving forces outweigh restraining forces, consider the solution useable. If restraining forces outweigh driving forces, eliminate the solution from further consideration.

Problem-Solving Approaches

Most problem solutions can be implemented in a number of ways. Once decision counseling has resulted in the identification of a preferred and viable problem solution, a nurse consultant needs to determine the most effective way to implement the problem solution. A "problem-solving approach" is the particular tactic or "manner" (the how) a nurse consultant uses to implement a problem solution (the what).

Whereas decision counseling is a collaborative process between a nurse consultant and consultees, determining the problem-solving approach is generally the prerogative of the nurse consultant. While the decision about which problem-solving approach to use to implement a problem solution generally reflects a nurse consultant's personal philosophy about how problems are best resolved, it is important that it fits the characteristics of the consultees and the larger community.

Empirical–Rational Approaches

Empirical–rational approaches to problem solving are based on the assumption that individuals (consultees) are rational and, therefore, will change their behavior if they believe it is to their benefit to do so (Haffer, 1986). When an empirical–rational approach is used, a nurse consultant focuses on providing consultees with the information they need to lower their resistance to change and alter their patterns of behavior or thinking. Educational strategies (teaching, role modeling, and demonstration) are typical empirical–rational problem-solving strategies (Tiffany & Lutjens, 1998).

Theory–Principles Interventions. Theory–principles interventions (Blake & Mouton, 1990) are a particular type of empirical–rational strategy that focus on helping consultees understand the cause and effect variables in a problem situation. The intended outcome of this type of intervention is that consultees see a problem situation more objectively, are able to think through both immediate and long-term implications of a problem solution, and curb impulsive actions. Theory–principles interventions should increase consultees' problem-solving skills because theories offer explanations for problems and provide problem solutions that can be generalized to similar future situations.

A nurse consultant using a theory–principles intervention would introduce consultees to a relevant theory or framework, help consultees apply this theory to the current problem situation, and compare theory-based outcomes to those that might be attained otherwise. As an example, a nurse consultant might introduce the Health Belief Model (this framework is described in Chapter 10) to the staff of a cardiac rehabilitation program. The staff/consultees could be taught how to apply the model's concepts (perceptions of seriousness, susceptibility, benefits, and barriers) to the nursing consultation problem of helping cardiac rehabilitation patients (the clients) make permanent lifestyle changes. Client outcomes obtained when this model is applied would be compared to those outcomes obtained through other methods. This particular theory–principles application would be considered a success if the consultees were convinced of the value of the model, began assessing and addressing client perceptions of lifestyle change requirements, and experienced a better success rate in achieving the desired outcomes of the rehabilitation program.

A limitation of theory–principles interventions and, in fact, all empirical–rational problem-solving approaches is that they tend to overlook the noncognitive issues in a problem situation. That is, empirical–rational approaches assume that knowledge is enough to inspire behavior change. Other issues that affect a consultee's willingness and ability to engage in problem solving (affective needs, time constraints, resources, etc.) are also not addressed by empirical–rational approaches. As a result, empirical–rational approaches, when used alone, do not usually result in long-term problem solutions.

Referring back to the preceding example, consultees' use of the Health Belief Model to guide their interactions with cardiac rehabilitation patients would most likely be short-term unless the rehabilitation program (client system) also provided the infrastructure and resources needed to incorporate the model into practice, such as rooms for conducting patient interviews and adequate time for patient appointments. Consultees' needs for job satisfaction and the intervention's congruence with consultee, client (e.g., cardiac rehab patients), and societal values would also need to be met for the problem solution to be long term.

Normative–Reeducative Approaches

Normative–reeducative problem-solving approaches presume that people are guided in their actions by social norms, personal meanings, habits, and values. Changes in behavior occur, then, only when consultees' norms or values (or perceptions of these) change (Haffer, 1986). The focus of normative–reeducative approaches to problem solving, thus, is working with consultees to help them clarify and modify their attitudes and values. Teaching is probably the normative–reeducative strategy most frequently used by nurse consultants. Confrontation and catalytic interventions are other normative–reeducative problem-solving strategies.

Confrontation. Confrontation is an appropriate intervention when there is a discrepancy between consultees' professed values and their actual behavior (Blake & Mouton, 1990). A nurse consultant using confrontational tactics with consultees would challenge the consultees to consider how the nursing consultation problem might be resolved if their existing behaviors or attitudes changed. Specific confrontational interventions a nurse consultant might use include asking questions such as "Why are things done this way?," pointing out discrepancies between a consultees' words and actions ("You say this, but your behavior implies . . ."), and playing devil's advocate. Examples of value/behavior discrepancies seen in nursing consultation include articulating a value of client autonomy but encouraging dependency and articulating a value of openness in communication but discouraging consideration of alternative viewpoints. Confrontation would be an appropriate intervention in either of these situations.

The major limitation of using confrontation as a normative–reeducative problem-solving approach is that it tends to trigger consultee defensiveness. Because of this risk, confrontation requires a fairly high level of trust between a nurse consultant and consultees.

Catalytic Interventions. Catalytic interventions are another normative–reeducative approach to problem solving. Catalytic interventions are useful when a nurse consultant needs to both arouse the consultees' interest

in being helped and create a willingness to participate in problem solving (Blake & Mouton, 1990). Catalytic interventions are normative–reeducative in nature because they stimulate a dissatisfaction with the problem situation and sensitize a consultee to how the problem situation might be better if attitudes, norms, and habits are changed. Catalytic interventions that are frequently used by nurse consultants include involving consultees in setting goals, establishing priorities, and choosing problem solutions. Presenting data that clearly demonstrate a problem and the likely effect of a specific solution and persuasive communication skills are additional catalytic interventions (Tiffany & Lutjens, 1998). Role modeling behaviors and values so consultees can see their outcomes is another example of a catalytic intervention.

Prescriptive Approaches

The basic premise of a prescriptive approach to solving nursing consultation problems is that the nurse consultant is the expert and authority and that the problem will be resolved if consultees follow her or his recommendations. Thus, prescriptive approaches involve delegating tasks to consultees and providing specific direction about actions that need to be taken. While this approach may sound counterproductive to the nursing consultation goal of helping consultees learn problem-solving skills, it is useful as an initial intervention when consultees have "reached the end of their rope." It is also useful when consultees have self-doubt and lack the confidence to solve a problem alone (Blake & Mouton, 1990). In these situations, a prescriptive approach can help consultees realize an immediate result, which can help them gain the confidence needed to become a more active participant in problem solving.

A prescriptive approach to problem solving is also indicated in problem situations in which immediate action is needed (e.g., safety concerns or a severe budget crisis) and there is not time for consultee involvement and deliberations about how to solve a problem. In these situations, a prescriptive approach can relieve pressure on the consultees to respond to the immediate crisis. Relieving this pressure helps consultees gain the time and energy needed to be active participants in formulating a long-term solution to the problem.

A third nursing consultation problem situation that may require a prescriptive approach is one in which there is consultee resistance to a mandated change such as change in the eligibility requirements for a clinic's services. A nurse consultant's strategy in this situation is to "force" the change and make sure that those affected see or experience some immediate benefits associated with the change (e.g., being able to provide more comprehensive services to those who are eligible or decrease patient waiting time). Demonstrating these benefits should decrease further resistance and enable the consultant to continue problem solving with more participative approaches.

Acceptant Interventions

Acceptant interventions are approaches to problem solving that are directed toward relieving emotional issues that can act as barriers to participation in problem solving (Blake & Mouton, 1990). Active listening, acknowledgment, and expressing empathy are examples of acceptant interventions. In many nursing consultation situations, acceptant interventions need to be used before the real nursing consultation problem can be addressed; a parallel intervention in nursing would be taking care of a patient's fear or anxiety before trying to teach self-care. A danger with acceptant interventions is that consultees may consider a problem resolved once the emotional issues are relieved. In a clinic merger situation, for example, the danger of using an acceptant intervention would be that consultees might feel better about their work (and even temporarily perform better) once they have had help dealing with their emotional responses to the consultation problem. However, this might not resolve the real problem of staff from two formerly competing clinics who now need to merge different values and procedures to work as a single entity. Acceptant interventions are often followed by empirical–rational and normative–reeducative problem-solving strategies. Table 11-1 summa-

TABLE 11-1. PROBLEM-SOLVING APPROACHES FOR NURSING CONSULTATION PROBLEMS

Problem-Solving Approach	Assumptions	Possible Strategies
Empirical–Rational	Consultees will change their behavior if they think change will benefit them.	Teaching (theory–principles, skills, knowledge) Role modeling Demonstration
Normative–Reeducative	Attitudes, norms, and values must change before behavior will change.	Confrontation Catalytic interventions Teaching (attitudes, values)
Prescriptive	Problems will be resolved if a consultee is told how to change.	Delegation Direction
Acceptant	Emotional issues can act as barriers to problem solving.	Active listening Empathy Acknowledgment

rizes the different problem-solving approaches for nursing consultation problems.

DEVELOPING AN ACTION PLAN

An action plan is a step-by-step blueprint of the work that is required to reach a goal. The action plan details how the problem solution that has been chosen by a nurse consultant and the consultees will unfold. In a sense, an action plan is a contract of the activities that need to be completed in order for a goal to be reached. (The consultation contract is a more comprehensive document than the action plan because it addresses fees, confidentiality issues, and so forth. See Chapter 17 for a checklist of contract components.) In most cases, there are four standard parts to an action plan: objectives, tasks, task assignments, and resources needed, including estimated costs.

A modified Gantt chart (see Figure 11-2) can be constructed to use as the basis from which to compile a narrative action plan, or can be used as the "working" action plan itself. A modified Gantt chart identifies objectives, tasks and their timeline, who is responsible for each task, and resources and costs associated with each task.

Stating Objectives

An action plan begins with a statement of the objective(s) of the nursing consultation relationship. An objective is a translation of the community's goal or desired end state, from a vague and abstract idea, into terms that are more concrete. To put it another way, an objective is the precise behavior or change required to meet a goal. Objectives have four components: (1) the client, (2) the actions needed to meet the goal, (3) the time frame, and (4) the standard to be met. For example, the abstract goal of "Decrease the incidence on pneumonia among the county's elderly

population" might be translated into the more concrete objective of "Achieve 90% immunization rate (action and standard) among persons 65 and older (the clients) within three months (time frame)." Stating objectives in terms of a future condition that can be observed and measured builds in a means of evaluating the success of the consultation project.

Identifying Tasks

The next component of the action plan is a list of the tasks or subobjectives that need to be completed in order to meet the specified objective. To continue with the example of pneumonia immunizations, tasks or subobjectives that might need to be addressed include: obtaining the vaccine, establishing a date for an immunization clinic, arranging a facility for the clinic, advertising the immunizations, and providing transportation in order to facilitate access to the immunization clinic. Particular attention needs to be given to sequencing and prioritizing these tasks. A nurse consultant and the consultees collaborate to identify the tasks that need to be accomplished first in order to lay the foundation for later tasks. It is often helpful to list easier tasks early in the action plan because the successful completion of these tasks can build consultees' confidence for tackling more difficult tasks. Moreover, placing simple tasks at the start of the plan gives the nurse consultant an opportunity to detect any unforeseen problems in the plan (e.g., additional costs) as well as time to assess the consultees' skills and motivation to carry through with the plan. This strategy also gives a nurse consultant the opportunity to revise the plan if needed.

Making Task Assignments

An action plan should also identify who is responsible for each task and specify a

NURSING CONSULTATION PROBLEM: Rural nurse practitioners (the consultation community) need more opportunities to meet continuing educational requirements

OBJECTIVE: Help a nurse practitioner group (the consultees) sponsor a 2-day conference in March that will attract 200 participants and provide 15 contact hours of continuing education

Task	Timeline/Person Responsible								Resources Needed	Estimated Cost
	Sept	Oct	Nov	Dec	Jan	Feb	March	April		
1. Survey members to identify conference topics	NNNN								Mailing list of members, paper, postage	Consultant time (4 hours), paper and postage for 500 surveys
2. Tally survey results		NN								Consultant time (4 hours)
3. Plan conference schedule, set date, identify speakers and location		NNNN CCCC								Consultant time (8 hours)
4. Contact and confirm speakers			CCC							Telephone calls
5. Develop conference brochure			NN CC							Printing costs for 1,000 brochures
6. Mail brochures				CC					Mailing list	Postage for 1,000 brochures
7. Obtain handouts from speakers					CCC					
8. Compile conference materials						NNN CCC				Paper and printing costs for 250 conference notebooks
9. Hold conference							NC		Site, audiovisual equipment	Consultant's time (16 hours), speaker fees, equipment rental fees, site fees, refreshments
10. Evaluate conference								NC		Consultant's time (8 hours)

Responsible party: NNN = Nurse consultant CCC = Consultee

Figure 11-2 Modified Gantt Chart for a Nursing Consultation Problem.
Refer to text discussion for a complete explanation of the components of this chart.

timeline (start and end date) for when each task needs to occur. For a plan to have the best chance of succeeding, the nurse consultant should work with the consultees to identify who needs to be involved; a key to successful action planning is being clear about exactly where responsibility lies for the accomplishment of each task. Failure to specify responsibilities precisely can lead consultees to mistakenly assume that the nurse consultant is responsible for implementing the action plan (Ross, 1993). Should this happen, the nurse consultant could be held wrongly accountable if the nursing consultation problem is not resolved.

Working with a Task Force

In some nursing consultation situations, the consultees will comprise the task force that will assume responsibility for carrying out the action plan. In other situations, a task force may be formed to actually implement the problem solution. Task force members are usually selected on the basis of two considerations: the skills they can contribute and politics or the "clout" their involvement will carry.

When identifying task force members, a nurse consultant must be careful to avoid two common pitfalls. First, it is a mistake to assume that the people who are chosen to work together are willing and able to do so. Thus, consideration needs to be given to the compatibility of task force members and the time needed for team building. (The concept of team building is introduced in a later section of this chapter and discussed in-depth in Chapter 12.) Second, it is easy for a task force to take on a life of its own and become alienated from the larger community and the consultees. An action plan should, therefore, incorporate strategies for regular communication between a task force and the rest of the client system.

Determining Needed Resources and Estimating Costs

Finally, an action plan should identify the human and material resources needed to carry out each task as well as the estimated cost of each task. Resources that need to be considered include personnel, time, office supplies, and information. Costs that need to be estimated include the consultant's fee, costs associated with consultees' involvement in consultation activities (e.g., paid time to attend meetings), travel expenses, and supplies. Identifying needed resources and costs up front can help a community avoid the pitfall of moving ahead with an action plan without having the material and financial resources needed to complete the plan. If a nurse consultant identifies resources that are needed before the action plan can be implemented, the action plan will need to be revised to include acquisition of the needed resources as a necessary subobjective.

Action Planning as Participative Learning

An action plan that is "owned" by the consultee has the greatest chance of being successful (Kurpius, Fuqua, & Rozecki, 1993). Thus, a nurse consultant needs to create opportunities for consultee "buy-in" to the action plan. Buy-in can be facilitated by involving consultees in the action planning process through participative learning strategies (Anderson & McFarlane, 2000).

Participative learning—learning by doing—helps a nurse consultant achieve the tactical goal of developing consultees'—and a community's—own problem-solving skills. Using action planning as a learning opportunity also enhances consultees' capabilities and collaborative skills, encourages commitment and contributions to outcomes, raises consciousness about the dynamics of problem solving, and increases the likelihood of diffusion of the changes needed to address a community's problem (Senge, Kleiner, Roberts, Ross, & Smith, 1994).

FACILITATING IMPLEMENTATION OF AN ACTION PLAN

As discussed in Chapter 1, it is the nature of a nursing consultation relationship that responsibility for implementing the action plan rests with the consultees. Paradoxically, a nurse consultant's success as a consultant is judged, at least in part, by whether consultees implement the action plan and whether the consultation problem is resolved. Nurse consultants, then, have a vested interest in facilitating the implementation of action plans that they help to develop. Consequently, nurse consultants generally incorporate three activities in their relationships with consultees that lay the groundwork for implementing the action plan: team building, transition management, and diffusion facilitation.

Team Building

Team building refers to activities that are specifically designed to develop an effective consultant–consultee team (Dyer, 1977). Adjectives that describe effective teams include "in harmony," supportive, motivated, committed, open, involved, interested, and productive. The goals of team building in terms of the action planning phase include active participation in problem-solving activities and ownership by all team members of the outcomes of the problem-solving process. Team building helps consultees see themselves as beneficiaries rather than as victims of the changes that accompany problem solving (Cohen & Murri, 1995).

Team-building strategies focus on improving the "workings" of groups by enhancing relationships, problem-solving skills, and effectiveness. Thus, team-building strategies

focus on both the social and task-oriented processes (see Chapter 7) that occur within groups. Because team-building strategies decrease resistance and build understanding and support for change, they are an appropriate activity in all nursing consultation relationships.

The specific nature of team-building strategies is limited only by the creativity of the nurse consultant. Typically, team-building strategies incorporate catalytic, confrontational, and acceptant interventions. Team members are asked to engage in self- and group review and analysis by reflecting on the group's image, processes, and values.

Involving group members in problem identification activities and in planning problem solutions are additional team-building strategies. Providing continuous feedback to consultees about the value of their participation in these activities acts as a team-building strategy by maintaining the momentum of a group's problem-solving efforts. These activities enhance team members' capabilities, commitment, contributions, collaborative skills, and hence, the continuity of the problem solution (Senge et al., 1994). Team building and specific team-building strategies are discussed in depth in Chapter 12.

Transition Management

Transition management strategies focus on the psychological processes that people go through as they come to terms with a new situation, such as adjusting to new behaviors that will need to be assumed in order to resolve a nursing consultation problem. These interventions acknowledge that "It isn't the changes that do you in, it's the transitions" (Bridges, 1991). Including transition management strategies in the action planning phase can prevent consultee guilt, self-absorption, resentment, anxiety, and stress from interfering with developing and implementing a problem solution.

Transition consists of three phases: letting go, managing the neutral zone, and launching new beginnings. Nurse consultants can encourage problem solving by facilitating the passage through each phase. To help consultees let go of the past, a nurse consultant can use acceptant interventions such as identifying who is losing what and openly and sympathetically acknowledging the importance of these losses. If possible, losses should be compensated for. A nurse consultant should also clearly define what is over and what is not over and should treat the past with respect. In a merger situation, for example, staff members' loss of identity as members of one of the merging clinics could be compensated for by development of a new logo and name to which staff from both facilities would have to adjust. A nurse consultant should acknowledge past successes of the individual merging clinics while emphasizing the importance of continuing quality care.

The core of the transition process and the focus of transition management interventions is the "neutral zone." The neutral zone is an "emotional wilderness" where old ways are gone but new ways don't yet feel comfortable (Bridges, 1991). The middle of the neutral zone encompasses that period of time during which reorientation and role redefinition are taking place. A nurse consultant can facilitate passage through this transition phase by maintaining clear and consistent open lines of communication and by providing the training and education needed to make the change. Providing consultees with the opportunity to question usual ways of doing things and developing new and creative solutions to difficulties that arise during the transition also facilitate passage through the neutral zone. In a merger situation, for instance, some staff may need to learn to work with new equipment. Peer teaching sessions could be implemented to meet this need (and could simultaneously facilitate the development of teamwork).

Once a change has been implemented, there is an adjustment period during which consultees and community members begin to incorporate the problem solution (new behavior, new attitudes, or new processes) into their usual way of work. A nurse consultant needs to help consultees accept the feelings of incompetence that often arise at this time. Strategies can be built into the action plan to lessen these feelings and let consultees "save face." These strategies will also help ensure that the action plan isn't abandoned because of these feelings. An action plan, for example, might build in temporary lower expectations of quantity (reduced patient load) while still communicating expectations for quality. Box 11-5 summarizes transition management strategies.

Diffusion Facilitation

Diffusion is the process through which a change is communicated to and adopted by a community's members (Helvie, 1998). Diffusion occurs as the result of consciously planning the best way to reach the most people with a planned intervention and to positively influence their health. Diffusion strategies should be a part of all nursing consultation action plans.

To a great extent, diffusion is determined by the inherent characteristics of both a problem situation and the proposed solution. For example, widespread diffusion will occur more rapidly if a proposed change is seen as having a relative advantage or superiority over current processes in terms of unique benefits, economic factors, satisfaction, prestige, time factors, and so forth. Additional characteristics of an intervention that determine the speed and extent of its diffusion through a community are the following (Helvie, 1998):

- Compatibility with the community's norms and values
- Complexity (low)
- Trialability—amenable to being implemented on a small scale to "iron out the

BOX 11-5   TRANSITION MANAGEMENT STRATEGIES

To Help a Community Let Go

- Identify who is losing what.
- Accept the reality and importance of subjective losses.
- Don't be surprised at and overreact to "overreaction."
- Acknowledge losses openly and sympathetically.
- Expect and accept the signs of grieving: anger, bargaining, anxiety, sadness, disorientation, and depression.
- Compensate for losses.
- Give people information—clearly and again and again.
- Mark the endings.
- Treat the past with respect.
- Let people take a piece of the old way with them.
- Show how endings ensure continuity of what really matters.

To Help a Community Manage the Neutral Zone

- "Normalize" the neutral zone.
- Redefine and reframe the neutral zone; use metaphors such as "a bridge to be crossed."
- Create temporary systems.
- Strengthen intragroup connections.
- Use a transition management team.
- Establish checkpoints.
- Use the neutral zone creatively: Allow time for questions and innovation, provide training, and encourage experimentation.

To Help a Community Launch New Beginnings

- Acknowledge ambivalence.
- Consider issues related to timing and allow time: Explain the purpose of the change, paint a picture of how it will look and feel, and give everyone a chance to participate and contribute.
- Reinforce new beginnings: Give consistent messages, ensure quick successes, symbolize the new identity, and celebrate successes.

Source: Bridges, W. (1991). *Managing transitions: Making the most of change.* Reading, MA: Addison-Wesley.

wrinkles" before it is implemented with an entire community

- Modifiability
- Observability—results are visible
- Reversibility
- Risk (low)
- Cost effectiveness

It is equally important that a nurse consultant is aware of factors that can lead to the failure of a change and/or function as barriers to diffusion. Examples of barriers to diffusion include incompatibility of a change with a community's norms and values, high complexity, rigidity or lack of modifiability, and expenses that outweigh perceived benefits. Strategies to prevent these conditions should be built into a nursing consultation action plan. A change and its diffusion can also fail because of innovation failure, communication failure, adoption failure, implementation failure, or maintenance failure.

Innovation failure is the failure of a problem solution to bring about the intended effect. Innovation failure is usually a function of poor design or inadequate pilot-testing and evaluation. Communication failure results in a lack of consultee and community buy-in to the intervention. It can be the result of either ineffective communication skills or neglectful communication. Communication failure can lead to adoption failure. Adoption failure can also occur when an action plan fails to address needed consultee knowledge or skills or needed community resources. Implementation failure occurs when a problem solution is implemented incorrectly or incompletely. Implementation failure can be unintentional (due to an unclear or incomplete action plan) or intentional. Finally, diffusion failure is a result of failing to incorporate transition management or change maintenance strategies into the action plan (change maintenance strategies are discussed in Chapter 14).

POSSIBLE DIFFICULTIES WITH ACTION PLANNING

Conflict, ambivalence, and resistance are the dilemmas that are most likely to complicate the action planning phase of the nursing consultation process.

Conflict

Politics (competing needs and demands) are a frequent source of conflict during the action planning phase. One political conflict that a nurse consultant often faces is that of needing to decide whose needs to satisfy— consultees', the contact person's, the client's/ community's, or his or her own. Sometimes a nurse consultant's own needs may override her or his judgment about what would be appropriate in a given situation. For example, a nurse consultant might want to use a process model of nursing consultation when the consultees have neither the time nor energy to do so.

Conflicts about goals or desired outcomes can also occur during the action planning phase. Consultees, contact persons, and the nurse consultant may disagree on what a desirable or feasible goal might be. As an example, the goal of "becoming healthier" can mean something different to each involved person.

Finally, methods conflicts can arise during action planning. Methods conflicts involve disagreements about both strategies and who should do what. There is a natural tendency for consultees to want a quick and easy problem solution. Consultees have often been living with the problem for some time, and once they decide to ask for help, they want it immediately (Kurpius et al., 1993). Nurse consultants can exacerbate methods conflicts by an inflexible insistence on using their favorite strategies to solve every kind of nursing consultation problem.

A nurse consultant is in a difficult position with all of these conflicts. Negotiation and the use of empirical–rational interventions can help prevent and resolve these conflicts.

Ambivalence

Ambivalence is a mix of positive and negative feelings about a situation. In the action planning phase, ambivalence is a natural reaction and usually reflects realistic concerns about how proposed interventions will affect consultees on a personal level. While ambivalence should be legitimized as normal and expected (acceptant intervention), it also needs to be overcome so that consultees become committed to a problem-solving effort rather than merely compliant with it.

Nurse consultants can respond to ambivalence by using it as a resource (Lippitt & Lippitt, 1986). Listening to and clarifying consultees' concerns often helps a nurse consultant identify important misinformation that needs to be corrected. Ambivalence can also be addressed by demonstrating the validity and feasibility of the action plan through role modeling, rehearsal, and a pilot implementation project. Short-term demonstrable steps toward goal attainment can be developed, progress can be documented, and intermediate accomplishments can be celebrated and rewarded. In short, a nurse consultant can use ambivalence as an opportunity to involve consultees and enrich and revise the action plan so that it has a greater likelihood of success.

Resistance

Resistance to a specific proposed problem solution or to problem solving in general is a third dilemma that nurse consultants often face during the action planning phase. Cues that resistance might be building are highlighted in Box 11-6.

Sometimes, behavior that is labeled as resistance really is normal reality testing. A nurse consultant should respond to consultee comments, such as "I'm not sure we've thought this through" and "I'm not sure this will work" by looking for possible holes in the action plan. When responding to these comments, it is important that a nurse consultant does not become defensive and try to change consultees' attitudes. Rather, a nurse should use this as an opportunity for exploring the completeness and feasibility of the action plan.

Resistance can also reflect a lack of understanding about the reason for a particular problem-solving strategy. When this is the case, a nurse consultant can use empirical–rational interventions to help consultees gain knowledge and, hopefully, understanding about the appropriateness of a particular intervention.

BOX 11-6   IS RESISTANCE BUILDING?

Possible Cues

- The action plan is attacked as impractical.
- Consultees act confused about what the problem is or what the goals of the plan are.
- Consultees intellectualize that the problem is really not a problem.
- The problem is labeled "no longer relevant."
- Consultees moralize about "right" and "wrong" problem-solving strategies.
- More data and details are requested repeatedly.
- "No time" is used as an excuse for not accepting a specific solution or for not participating in the action planning process.
- There is pressure for an easy and quick solution.
- Passive–aggressive behaviors are present, such as arriving late for meetings, leaving early, and acting bored.

DOCUMENTING THE ACTION PLANNING PHASE

Documenting the activities of the action planning phase provides a nurse consultant with a track record of what has transpired during this part of the nursing consultation relationship. Documentation can also serve as a learning tool and legal protection. A nurse consultant needs to document specific activities undertaken, parties involved, rationale for decisions, and outcomes of activities. In addition, many nurse consultants find it helpful to keep anecdotal notes about their impressions of how the consultation relationship is unfolding and ideas for next steps.

Box 11-7 provides a documentation checklist for the action planning phase of the nursing consultation process.

BOX 11-7   DOCUMENTATION CHECKLIST: THE ACTION PLANNING PHASE

Documenting Goal Setting

- ☐ Identification of goal
- ☐ How goal was determined: Parties and process involved, rationale used
- ☐ Conflicts about the goal: Who, what, how it was resolved
- ☐ Prioritization of goals: Criteria used, who was involved in decision, conflicts (who, what, how resolved)

Documenting Intervention Selection

- ☐ Process used to select intervention: Date and time, parties involved
- ☐ Results of force-field analysis: Driving and restraining forces identified, ideas about how to minimize and maximize these forces
- ☐ Problem solution selected: Criteria for decision
- ☐ Conflicts about problem solution: Who, what, how resolved
- ☐ Resistance encountered: Who, what, how resolved

Documenting the Action Plan

- ☐ Objectives and how determined
- ☐ Sequenced list of tasks
- ☐ Task assignments, rationale
- ☐ Resources needed
- ☐ Estimated costs
- ☐ Attach Gantt chart if used

Documenting Implementation Facilitation

- ☐ Date and time of activity, parties involved
- ☐ Description of activity (team building, transition management strategy), rationale
- ☐ Results of activity
- ☐ Ideas about possible next steps

CHAPTER SUMMARY

The activities of the action planning phase represent the first tangible "work" toward responding to the nursing consultation problem. Consequently, the action planning phase is a sensitive and somewhat risky phase of the nursing consulting process for both the nurse consultant and the community. The consultant's reputation as an effective problem solver is on the line. At the same time, the community is beginning to confront the transitions and losses that implementing the action plan (assuming it is accepted) will likely entail. Successful completion of the action planning phase can be determined only after the action plan has been carried out. However, matching goals and problem solutions to fit problem and community characteristics, continually incorporating teamwork and transition management, developing a sufficiently detailed plan of how an intervention should unfold (including its diffusion), and being alert for and attending to possible dilemmas should result in an action plan that is meaningful, acceptable, and feasible and addresses the nursing consultation problem.

APPLYING CHAPTER CONTENT

1. Develop actions plans for a single nursing consultation problem (e.g., the high incidence of pneumonia among a community's elders) using two different theoretical frameworks. State your rationale for the problem solutions and problem-solving approaches that you have chosen. Identify diffusion facilitation strategies you could incorporate into each plan. Speculate as to what dilemmas you might encounter with each plan. Which plan do you think would

have the greatest chance of success and why?

2. Consider the following possible nursing consultation situations: (a) working with an agency that is needing to discontinue a popular health program, and (b) opening a school-based clinic. What types of transition issues would be faced in each of these situations? How would you manage them?

References

Anderson, E., & McFarlane, J. (2000). *Community as partner: Theory and practice in nursing* (3rd ed.). Philadelphia: Lippincott.

Blake, R., & Mouton, J. (1990). *Consultation: A handbook for individual and organization development* (2nd ed.). Reading, MA: Addison-Wesley.

Bridges, W. (1991). *Managing transitions: Making the most of change.* Reading, MA: Addison-Wesley.

Cohen, W., & Murri, M. (1995). Managing the change process. *Journal of AHIMA, 66*(6), 40–47.

Dougherty, A. (1995). *Consultation: Practice and perspectives in school and community settings* (2nd ed.). Pacific Grove, CA: Brooks-Cole.

Dyer, W. (1977). *Team building: Issues and alternatives.* Reading, MA: Addison-Wesley.

Haffer, A. (1986). Facilitating change: Choosing the appropriate strategy. *Journal of Nursing Administration, 16*(4), 18–22.

Helvie, C. (1998). *Advanced practice nursing in the community.* Thousand Oaks, CA: Sage.

Kurpius, D., Fuqua, D., & Rozecki, T. (1993). The consulting process: A multidimensional approach. *Journal of Counseling and Development, 71*, 601–606.

Lippitt, G., & Lippitt, R. (1986). *The consulting process in action* (2nd ed.). San Diego: University Associates.

Ross, G. (1993). Peter Block's Flawless Consulting and the Homunculus Theory: Within each person is a perfect consultant. *Journal of Counseling and Development, 71,* 639–641.

Senge, P., Kleiner, A., Roberts, C., Ross, R., & Smith, B. (1994). *The fifth discipline fieldbook.* New York: Currency-Doubleday.

Tiffany, C., & Lutjens, L. (1998). *Planned change theories for nursing: Review, analysis, and implications.* Thousand Oaks, CA: Sage.

12

Team Building in Nursing Consultation

Partnerships between community members and health care professionals are critical for collaborative decision-making in order to improve health. (Anderson & McFarlane, 2000)

 KEY CONCEPTS:

team building, ice breaker, group energizer, empowerment, participatory research

 KEY TERMS FOR YOUR SEARCH ENGINE:

team building, participatory research

INTRODUCTION

Team building is an activity that is commonly associated with consultation. In fact, some consultants, particularly those who specialize in organization development, make their living providing team-building experiences as their consultation service. These consultants are often referred to as trainers. As introduced in Chapter 11, however, it makes sense to think of team building as a somewhat generic consultation activity. That is, team building, along with transition management and diffusion facilitation, should be incorporated into *all* nursing consultation relationships in order to encourage adoption and implementation of the nursing consultation action plan.

Including team building as an activity in all nursing consultation relationships, especially those with communities, makes good sense for several reasons. First of all, in community consultation relationships, nurse consultants frequently work with a group of consultees. Group members may or may not know one another, and may or may not be willing participants in the consultation relationship. Team-building activities can help members of a consultee group become more comfortable with one another and can help establish the foundation for effective participation in the consultation process. Nursing consultation with communities is also frequently characterized by the use of task forces or work groups

217

to implement an action plan. A task force can include consultees as well as other community representatives. Task force members often need to serve as liaisons to the larger community in the process of carrying out the actual problem-solving activities detailed in the action plan. To be effective in this liaison role, task force members need to be able to team build and create partnerships with and empower sectors of the larger community (the nursing consultation client).

This chapter focuses on team building as a set of strategies for helping members of a group work together effectively. The chapter builds on content presented in Chapter 7 (the differences and dynamics of work groups and teams) and Chapter 11 (an introduction to team building as a generic consultation intervention). The first section of the chapter is an overview of team building, as well as its purpose and rationale. Next, the mechanics of team building, including using games as a team-building strategy, are considered. The final section of the chapter links team building

to the concept of community empowerment. As you read this chapter, think about the following questions:

- Reflect on experiences you have had with team building. What made these experiences positive or negative? What could the consultant/trainer have done differently to make the experience more positive?
- How will a community's culture and values affect the team-building process? What cultural characteristics and values will act as facilitators and barriers to team building?
- How would you implement team building differently as an internal versus external nurse consultant?
- What skills do you bring to team building? What skills do you need to develop? What strategies could you use to develop needed skills?

TEAM BUILDING AS A NURSING CONSULTATION INTERVENTION

Team building refers to activities that are specifically designed to improve the effectiveness of a group that must work together to achieve specified results (Dyer, 1977). While some of the tasks of the nursing consultation process (such as gaining physical entry and initiating psychological entry) and the way in which other tasks are carried out (e.g., involving consultees in the activities of the problem identification phase) will generally help a group of consultees begin to see themselves as a partner in the nursing consultation process, they may not be direct enough or "strong" enough to build a true team culture. Team-building activities are specifically intended to help a group see the value of a team approach and adopt a team approach as their norm for interaction.

In nursing consultation relationships with communities, teamwork and partnerships are important for involvement in political processes, coalition building, community empowerment (discussed later in this chapter), and other community interventions (Helvie 1998). Team-building activities also decrease resistance, help build understanding and support for changes, and help create ownership of the outcome of the problem-solving process. While nurse consultants—and society in general—readily promote the need for teamwork (i.e., cooperation and collaboration), the actual idea of working together as a team tends to imply competition (Ukens, 1997b). Generating a *constructive* competitive spirit, however, motivates group members to maximize their contributions to the group, helps a group develop a "going places" attitude, and makes it more likely that a group will achieve its goals.

BOX 12-1   WHY TEAMS?

- Teams function as coalitions—alliances of individuals working together to gain specific goals or mutual advantage.
- Teams (or coalitions) prevent duplication of effort, pool and therefore maximize resources, and engender greater publicity than might be possible with individuals working alone.
- The complementary skills and perspectives of team members increase the likelihood that a problem solution will fit a community's needs, culture, and resources.
- There is a certain amount of safety in numbers. Teams are not as threatened by taking risks and changing as are individuals who need to fend for themselves.
- Team building fosters the development of long-term problem-solving skills that can be dispersed throughout a community once the nursing consultation relationship has ended.

Team-building strategies are limited only by the creativity of a nurse consultant. Team building is, however, hard work (Katzenbach & Smith, 1993). Because team building is such hard work, takes time, and involves an element of personal risk, many nurse consultants try to avoid incorporating team-building activities into a consultation relationship. The use of teams has, however, emerged as a logical approach to sharpening an organization's competitive edge (Ukens, 1997b), and teams are equally valuable to communities. Whether a group of consultees is a work group or a true team (this difference was discussed in Chapter 7), the point is that when consultees have a "team mentality," the nursing consultation relationship is more likely to be successful. Box 12-1 summarizes the benefits of teams and team building.

THE MECHANICS OF TEAM BUILDING

Chapter 7 presented "team basics"—how to build team performance, how to provide leadership to a team, how to help a "stuck" team. This section goes beyond the basics and discusses specific strategies for building the sense of camaraderie and team spirit that characterizes a team.

"Training Programs" for Teams

When organization development consultants engage with consultees in a team-building program, the process typically occurs as an intense two- or three-day retreat or takes place through a series of workshops or meetings over several weeks (or even months). Nurse consultants working with community clients usually do not have the same luxuries of time and financial resources with which to support intensive team-building activities. They can, however, adapt the principles used by organization training consultants to work with community consultees and clients. While there is no one way to do team building, effective team-building or training programs seem to follow the general process outlined in Dyer's (1977) classic work.

Phase 1 of a team-building program is the preparation phase. The goal of this phase is to get at least minimal commitment from those who are to be involved in the program (this usually is the consultees in a community consultation relationship). Explaining the purpose of team building and decreasing participants' anxiety are two tasks that need to be accomplished during this phase. Sometimes a consultant will conduct individual interviews with the participants in a team-building program so that activities can be tailored to address their concerns and perceived needs for change. A consultant may also use a written survey to gather anonymous perceptions about a community's problems and needed changes. Other consultants might accomplish the goals of the preparation phase by meeting with participants as a group and giving a motivational and/or educational presentation. Sometimes outside speakers are used for these presentations. If consultees haven't worked together before, the consultant may engage them in "icebreaker" activities as a strategy to increase comfort, familiarity, and trust with one another.

Phase 2 of a team-building program is the start-up phase. The goal of this phase is to create a climate for work, get people relaxed, and establish norms regarding openness, confidentiality, and dealing with issues. The consultant may work with group members to help them develop a profile of the group or community as it currently exists and to formulate an agenda for the team-building program. Many consultants use group-energizer or problem-solving games so that a group can be made aware of its positive and negative interaction processes. Other activities that can help a group develop a profile of itself or its community are creating metaphors ("Describe our group as a kind of animal, a combination of animals, a machine, or a type of person") or building collages. The nurse consultant looks for themes that emerge from these activities and shares these themes with the group. These images can be used as the springboard for discussion about changes that need to occur.

Phase 3 of a team-building program focuses on group problem solving. The goals of Phase 3 are to (a) increase a group's awareness of its processes and their impact, and (b) begin to make plans for needed changes in processes. If a group did not engage in group problem-solving games in Phase 2, they generally will do so now. Other groups will attempt to tackle actual problems they are facing. The consultant shares objective data from his or her observations of and interactions with the group about its functioning. The consultant then helps the group establish goals and rules and develop other strategies for improving its interaction processes. Dysfunctional process patterns that are observed fairly frequently in consultees or other groups include domination, lack of participation, defensiveness, avoiding conflict, and the development of cliques and coalitions.

Phase 4, the final phase of a team-building program, is the follow-up phase. Group interactions and processes are observed again to see if they have changed as a result of the feedback and suggestions provided in Phase 3. If consultees' group processes have not improved, Phases 2 through 4 may need to be repeated. Box 12-2 summarizes the phases of a team-building program.

Games as a Team-Building Strategy

Estimates are that only 1 trainer in 50 does *not* use games as a team-building strategy (Sugar, 1998). Games are effective when they are fun and result in learning (Ukens, 1997b). If games are not managed correctly, however, they can leave group members feeling foolish, vulnerable, and betrayed.

How and Why Games Work

Games work because they can simulate the total work environment and provide meaningful experiences that can be translated into

BOX 12-2   PHASES OF A TEAM-BUILDING PROGRAM

Phase 1: Preparation

Goals: Explain purpose of team building; get commitment from team-building participants; decrease participants' anxiety about the program
Strategies: Individual interviews, surveys, motivational or educational presentations, icebreaker games

Phase 2: Start-Up

Goals: Create a climate for work; get participants relaxed; establish norms regarding group processes
Strategies: Metaphors, collages, group energizers or problem-solving games

Phase 3: Group Problem Solving and Analysis

Goals: Increase the group's awareness of its processes; begin to take action on process problems
Strategies: Problem-solving games if not used in Phase 2; feedback to group in regard to observations made of group processes during Phase 2 activities

Phase 4: Follow-Up

Goal: Observe improvement in group interactions and effectiveness as a group
Strategies: Share feedback with group as to its current level of function; repeat Phases 2 through 4 as necessary

---

insights and applications for the work a group needs to do (Sugar, 1998).

The inherent structure of a game is a goal and resistance against achieving the goal. The effort a player makes to overcome the resistance (which can include his or her own anxiety) and achieve the goals is at the heart of the activity and central to making it enjoyable and rewarding. In most games, resistance is supplied by an opponent who is trying to achieve the same goal. The opponent, therefore, even if intrinsic (e.g., anxiety), is a partner in the game (Ukens, 1997b).

Games are also effective because they promote group interaction, require group members to work on the task at hand, and take advantage of each group member's unique abilities. In performing the activity, a group must accept the total situation, including the task to be performed and the strengths and limitations of the group as a whole as well as individual members. Assessment and acceptance are also key tasks when problem solving with communities.

The competitive aspect of a game serves additional purposes. Competitive games help prepare participants for future challenges because the solution to the problem posed by the game can be discovered only with active involvement. Games, thus, show group members that they can and should become effective and contributing group members. Competition also meets needs that individual group members have in terms of social interaction and acceptance, security, self-esteem, and achievement (Ukens, 1997b).

Effective Games

Games are most likely to be effective when they offer active participation, opportunity for diverse inputs, continuous interaction, rapid reinforcement, an integrative review, and immediate application (Sugar, 1998). When group members play games, they want to interact and become personally involved with the content. They do not want trivial or artificial exercises. They want the game to be a thoughtful exercise that evokes meaningful dialogue. Effective games reflect thoughtful game selection and deliberative implementation on the part of the nurse consultant.

Choosing a Game. The first step in choosing a game is to identify the desired learning outcome or what group members are supposed to get out of the game (Sugar, 1998). The game that is chosen should be related to the activity (or theme or goal) of the problem-solving and team-building session. A general rule of thumb to keep in mind when selecting a game for any purpose is that it is better to err on the side of conservative risk taking rather than have participants feel vulnerable or manipulated—especially when issues are sensitive or controversial and trust has not yet been established (Ukens, 1997a).

Icebreakers are organized activities that are used to acquaint group members with one another and to promote openness and sharing (Ukens, 1997a). An example of an icebreaker is having group members form pairs and share the best book they have read. The group then reconvenes as a whole, and partners share each other's responses with the group. Because icebreakers are intended to build a sense of comfort and belonging, they are appropriate in Phase 1 or Phase 2 of a team-building program.

Group energizers are designed to invigorate a group and build team cohesion (Ukens, 1997a). They require whole-group interaction (an example would be solving a puzzle), whereas icebreakers generally require group members to work in groups of two or three and then report back to the entire group. Group energizers are also appropriate for Phase 2 of a team-building program.

Competitive and collaborative (or problem-solving) games are often used during Phase 3 of a team-building program. These games require group members' joint efforts to complete an assigned task. They are designed to be lessons in determination, teamwork, and planning (Ukens, 1997a). Problem-solving games allow group members to practice and assess one another's ability at skills such as creativity, negotiation, strategic thinking, risk taking, and recognizing relationships among variables and events (Sugar, 1998). "Desert Survival" is an example of a popular problem-solving game.

Characteristics of the players should also be considered when choosing a game. There should be as close a match as possible in terms of group members' skills, abilities, interests, and work environment and what the game requires or has to offer. An effective game also offers the right balance between chance and skill. If a game relies on too much chance, players may tend to find it boring and mindless and consider it a waste of time. On the other hand, if there is too much emphasis on knowledge and skills, a game can become an anxiety-provoking test (Sugar, 1998). Finally, a game will be most effective if it is easily explainable and quickly understood—and fun to play. Box 12-3 summarizes factors to consider when choosing a game.

A wide variety of "game books" for consultants/trainers are readily available. These books are most useful if they categorize games in terms of content, number of players, and time requirements, and provide ideas for conducting postgame debriefing. The references by Sugar (1998) and Ukens (1997a, b)

BOX 12-3   CHARACTERISTICS OF EFFECTIVE GAMES

- Relevant to desired team-building or learning outcome
- Require active participation
- Offer opprotunity for diverse inputs
- Engage players in continuous interaction
- Match players' knowledge, skills, abilities, interests, and work environment
- Balance chance and skill
- Easily explainable
- Quickly understood
- Offer opportunity for diverse interpretation and ideas regarding application to the work setting

at the end of this chapter are good examples of useful game books.

Implementing ("Playing") a Game. Selection of the game is just half of the equation for an effective game. For a game to provide its intended experiences, it must be played successfully.

In general, experts recommend limiting playing time for a game to 50 minutes or less. Time also needs to be allowed for game setup (generally half as long as playing time) and debriefing (the same amount of time as allowed for actual play). Using this formula, a 50-minute game would require just over a two-hour block of time (setup, 25 minutes; play, 50 minutes; and debriefing, 50 minutes). Game setup involves arranging the space where the game will be played and organizing the necessary props and equipment. It also involves preliminaries such as forming teams, distributing materials, introducing the game, and reviewing rules and procedures. During the actual play of the game, a nurse consultant needs to keep the atmosphere light and use humor. A nurse consultant must also be ready to intervene if conflict threatens to get out of hand or if the atmosphere becomes too heavy.

Postgame debriefing is an essential ingredient in effective games. The debriefing period can begin by congratulating and rewarding the winners of the game; however, the value of the competition rather than the importance of winning should be emphasized. Next, the nurse consultant should initiate and moderate a discussion that allows venting, encourages sharing of insights, and helps group members link the game to real life by transferring their insights and generalizations to the community problem-solving situation. Debriefing also helps participants develop an awareness of the obligations of each and every member of a group that is confronted with a challenge (Ukens, 1997b). Questions that can be used to guide debriefing include the following (Sugar, 1998):

- *What?* What happened? What did you experience? How did you feel? What did you see and contribute in terms of cooperation, leadership, resourcefulness, decision making, efficiency, and initiative?
- *So what?* What learning happened? What led to these insights? What are things this reminds you of?

BOX 12-4   PLAYING GAMES SUCCESSFULLY

- Check time needed versus time available.
- Pay attention to preliminaries—room setup, equipment, props, game accessories.
- Be sure rules and procedures are understood before the game starts.
- Keep the atmosphere light while the game is being played.
- Be ready to intervene if conflicts get out of hand or the atmosphere becomes too heavy.
- Be prepared to initiate and moderate a guided debriefing to link game experiences to real life.

- *Now what?* What applications can be made to real life? How will you incorporate what you have learned into the work/problem solving we need to do?

Box 12-4 summarizes strategies for playing games effectively.

Nurse Consultant Roles in Team-Building Activities

Too many consultees have had unsatisfactory experiences with team-building programs and activities. Nurse consultants can minimize and counteract the anxiety, misgivings, and skepticism with which many consultees approach team building by remembering some basic nursing consultation and group leadership skills.

First of all, a nurse consultant needs to create a comfortable atmosphere—one that is characterized by honesty, sensitivity, consideration, fairness, and mutual respect (Barczak, 1996). A nurse consultant can set the standard for effective communication within the group by role modeling openness and trust. A nurse consultant should provide an opportunity for all group members to participate (but should not force participation) in discussions by guiding the discussion and guarding

against domination. Finally, the nurse consultant can keep meetings and program sessions meaningful by having an agenda, summarizing discussion, and providing follow-up on the outcomes of previous decisions and meetings.

FROM TEAM BUILDING TO COMMUNITY EMPOWERMENT

Community involvement has been identified as a key element in problem solving with communities (Anderson & McFarlane, 2000). Community participation, in turn, requires mechanisms to mobilize communities to recognize their needs, work as partners with health care providers, and develop a culture of participation. Community empowerment is a mechanism that can help a community develop a culture of participation. Because the consultees in a nursing/community consultation relationship often function as liaisons with a community to implement an action plan, they are in an ideal position to facilitate community empowerment. Team building is inextricably linked to empowerment in that the aim of team building is to develop the same norms of collaboration, cooperation, and trust, as well as the self-confidence and sense of efficacy, that characterize an empowered group or community. Consultees who have participated in successful team-building programs can therefore translate their experiences and learning to their liaison role with a larger community. In a very real way, then, when a nurse consultant empowers consultees by team building, she or he is indirectly empowering a community.

Defining Empowerment

Empowerment is a mechanism by which people, organizations, and communities gain mastery over their affairs (Helvie, 1998). The result of empowerment is community control, improved community quality of life, and social justice. Empowered communities have the knowledge, skills, opportunity, and support to identify, assess, and meet their own needs. Traditionally, health care providers have interacted with communities in a top-down, paternalistic, biomedical model in which health care is viewed as a commodity (Anderson & McFarlane, 2000). Empowered communities, in contrast, are able to view health care as a community lifestyle choice that includes

health promotion, disease prevention, and caring beyond curing. An empowered community, like an effective team, demonstrates four competencies: (1) the ability to identify its needs and problems through effective collaboration, (2) the ability to achieve agreement on goals and priorities, (3) the ability to agree on how to achieve goals, and (4) the ability to collaborate effectively in implementing plans to achieve goals (Helvie, 1998).

Strategies for Empowering Communities

The role of a nurse consultant in regard to community empowerment is helping community members—starting with consultees—to build effective partnerships and develop a sense of efficacy. The first step in community empowerment, similar to team building, is to create a sense of connectedness among community members, others with whom they interact, and their environment. In other words, team attitudes need to be transferred or diffused to a larger, more diverse, and

---

BOX 12-5   THE PARTICIPATORY RESEARCH PROCESS: STRATEGIES FOR SUCCESS

1. Plan for participation—develop effective communication strategies with key stakeholders.
2. Develop the infrastructure for community involvement, such as a steering committee, to maximize community input and articulate diverse points of view.
3. Maximize the number of community members involved in data gathering, data analysis, and the dissemination of findings.
4. Divide the project into small, achievable tasks with target dates for completion; this helps maintain enthusiasm and motivation.
5. Maintain interest in the project by giving continuous feedback on progress and preliminary findings.
6. Acknowledge participants' contributions.
7. When barriers are encountered, let participants help identify alternate strategies.
8. Be sure study findings are shared with the community at the end.

more dispersed group. Education, creating awareness, and open dialogue are keys to creating connectedness. Working with communities to visualize their needs and their preferred future, and involving a broad representation of community members in planning and implementing needed change are additional empowerment strategies.

Participatory research can be a particularly powerful empowerment strategy. Participatory research is problem-focused or context-specific research that is centered on addressing a particular problem and involving all participants (i.e., consultees, implementation task force members, client representatives, and stakeholders) in every step of the research process. The goal of participatory research is social change. Participatory research helps community members gain skills in critical thinking about and analyzing the health concerns of their community. The outcome of participatory research is empowerment in that participants are prepared to help their community identify, understand, determine common goals, and find solutions to resolve community problems. Box 12-5 details the participatory research process.

CHAPTER SUMMARY

Nursing consultation is the process of working with individual or group consultees to resolve a client's actual or potential health concerns. While the consultees in a nursing consultation relationship bear the responsibility for implementing the consultation action plan and resolving the client's problem, the nurse consultant is responsible for ensuring that consultees are motivated and able to implement the plan. Team building should be incorporated into all nursing consultation relationships for the express purpose of "priming" consultees to follow

through with implementation of the problem solutions and activities detailed in the action plan.

Frequently, in the process of implementing the action plan, consultees and/or additional task force members need to interact with community members and engage them as partners in the problem-solving process. Community members become problem-solving partners through the process of empowerment. Translating and diffusing the goals and processes of team building to larger community groups can facilitate empowerment and help create a community that can identify and address its own health concerns.

APPLYING CHAPTER CONTENT

1. Plan and implement a team-building game during a class session or with another small group. How did you select the game you used? How did the audience react to the game? What did you learn about yourself during this process? What would you do differently next time?
2. Think of a community or group with which you are familiar. Would you consider this group to be empowered or not? Explain your answer. What strategies would you use to empower this group?

References

Anderson, E., & McFarlane, J. (2000). *Community as partner: Theory and practice in nursing* (3rd ed.). Philadelphia: Lippincott.

Barczak, N. (1996). How to lead effective teams. *Critical Care Nursing Quarterly, 19*(1), 73–82.

Dyer, W. (1977). *Team-building: Issues and alternatives.* Reading, MA: Addison-Wesley.

Helvie, C. (1998). *Advanced practice nursing in the community*. Thousand Oaks, CA: Sage.

Katzenbach, J., & Smith, D. (1993). *The wisdom of teams*. New York: HarperBusiness.

Sugar, S. (1998). *Games that teach: Experiential activities for reinforcing learning*. San Francisco: Jossey-Bass.

Ukens, L. (1997a). *Getting together: Icebreakers and group energizers*. San Francisco: Pfeiffer and Co.

Ukens, L. (1997b). *Working together: 55 team games*. San Francisco: Pfeiffer and Co.

13

Evaluating Nursing Consultation Efforts

Evaluation is determining the worth (or value) of something.... For community-focused interventions to be timely and relevant, the community database, nursing diagnosis, and health program plans must be evaluated routinely. (Anderson & McFarlane, 2000)

 ## KEY CONCEPTS:

formative evaluation, summative evaluation, effectiveness criteria, performance standard, impact evaluation

---

 ## KEY TERMS FOR YOUR SEARCH ENGINE:

consultation and evaluation

INTRODUCTION

Gaining entry, problem identification, action planning, evaluation, and disengagement—the phases of the nursing consultation process—represent distinct sets of activities that occur in a predictable sequence. Recall from earlier discussion, however, that the activities of adjacent phases may actually overlap (see Figure 2-1), and that there can be a certain amount of back-and-forth movement between phases. Thus, the nursing consultation process is an iterative process: What occurs in one phase provides feedback about previous phases and may necessitate backtracking and repeating tasks. For

example, an inability to agree on goals during the action planning phase may signal a need to revisit the diagnosis that resulted from the problem identification process. Another characteristic of the nursing consultation process is that some activities occur on a more or less continual basis throughout a consultation relationship. To a certain extent, a nurse consultant is *always* assessing, diagnosing, planning interventions, and evaluating (Dougherty, 1995).

In nursing consultation, evaluation involves systematically collecting data and making and communicating judgments about both

229

the activities and outcomes of a nursing consultation relationship. Because a consultee may not actually implement a proposed action plan, evaluation of a nursing consultation relationship does not always focus on determining the success of a particular problem solution or intervention. Instead, the "intervention" that the nurse consultant evaluates is the entire nursing consultation relationship. The evaluation process in nursing consultation consists of the following tasks: (a) planning evaluation activities, (b) conducting the evaluation, and (c) giving evaluation feedback.

Much of the first task—planning—takes place during the action planning phase of the nursing consultation process. The second and third tasks—conducting the evaluation and giving evaluation feedback—occur on two levels. First, these tasks occur as distinct phases of the consultation process and are carried out in order to draw conclusions about the nursing consultation relationship (summative evaluation). Second, these tasks occur on a more or less continual basis and provide the nurse consultant with information for revising the nursing consultation process while it is still under way (formative evaluation). Thus, evaluation in nursing consultation can be thought of as a feedback mechanism that provides ongoing as well as endpoint information to both a nurse consultant and consultees about their success in meeting the goals of the nursing consultation relationship.

This chapter begins with a discussion of how evaluation fits into the nursing consultation process. Next, the specific tasks associated with evaluation—planning an evaluation, conducting the evaluation, and giving evaluation feedback—are discussed. The chapter concludes by considering some of the difficulties associated with implementing evaluation activities in a nursing consultation relationship. While the content in this chapter focuses primarily on summative evaluation as a distinct phase of the nursing consultation process, much of the content applies equally to the ongoing or formative evaluation activities that take place throughout the entire consultation relationship. As you read this chapter, think about the following questions:

- How are assessment and evaluation activities, which both occur continuously throughout the nursing consultation process, distinct from one another?
- How might the evaluation phase of the nursing consultation process be different when the consultee is an individual and when the consultee is a group?
- How might the evaluation phase vary with purchase-of-expertise, doctor–patient, and process consultation interaction patterns?
- What different types of difficulties might internal and external nurse consultants encounter during the evaluation phase?

EVALUATION AND THE NURSING CONSULTATION PROCESS

Evaluation is one of the more complex sets of activities undertaken by a nurse consultant because, in addition to being a distinct phase in the nursing consultation process, evaluation occurs on a more or less continual basis. Evaluation is more likely to be carried out effectively if both the nurse consultant and consultees understand the difference be-

tween formative and summative evaluation, appreciate the purposes of evaluation, and understand how evaluation links to and affects other phases of the nursing consultation process.

Formative and Summative Evaluation

As indicated, evaluation is both an ongoing activity and a distinct phase in the nursing consultation process. Formative evaluation is the evaluation activities that occur on an ongoing basis throughout the nursing consultation process. The purpose of formative evaluation is to provide a nurse consultant and consultees with a steady stream of information about how the nursing consultation relationship is progressing. Formative evaluation provides a nurse consultant with an answer to the question, "Are we on the right track?" Formative evaluation is a decision-making tool that helps a nurse consultant determine whether (a) the consultation relationship is progressing effectively and should be continued as planned, or (b) the consultation relationship is not progressing effectively and earlier phases of the nursing consultation process need to be revisited.

Formative evaluation is often conducted in an informal manner. That is, formative evaluation can be accomplished by simply questioning consultees about how they think the consultation relationship is progressing. Formative evaluation should also entail checking the progress of the nursing consultation relationship against the proposed project timeline and anticipated costs.

Summative evaluation is the evaluation activities that comprise the fourth phase of the nursing consultation process. Summative evaluation activities predominate as the nursing consultation relationship is winding down. The purpose of summative evaluation is to provide a nurse consultant and consultees with answers to the questions, "Have we been successful?" and "Did we do what we planned to do in an efficient and effective manner?"

Like formative evaluation, summative evaluation is a decision-making tool. Information obtained from summative evaluation helps a nurse consultant decide whether (a) the consultation relationship has been successful and can be terminated, (b) the relationship has been partially successful but additional problem-solving efforts are needed and ear-

lier phases of the nursing consultation process need to be revisited, or (c) the relationship has not been a success but should go no further and an "autopsy" should be done (Ulschak & SnowAntle, 1990). Box 13-1 compares the specific questions addressed by formative and summative evaluation of a nursing consultation relationship.

Other Purposes of Evaluation

Evaluation has other purposes in the nursing consultation process besides that of being a decision-making tool. Evaluation can serve as a quality control and accountability device, legal protection, a learning device, and a marketing tool. Evaluation, therefore, is beneficial in a number of ways for a nurse consultant as well as for consultees and an entire community.

As a quality control device, evaluation provides a nurse consultant and consultees with information about the validity of the problem definition that was generated from earlier problem identification and diagnosis activities. In other words, if problem-solving efforts are unsuccessful, it might be because the wrong problem cause was identified. Evaluation also provides information about the quality of decision making that went into goal setting and action planning. For example, were community culture and feasibility issues related to proposed problem solutions considered?

Evaluation promotes accountability in both a nurse consultant and consultees by verifying whether and to what extent they have met the terms of the nursing consultation contract. In this way, evaluation also offers both the nurse consultant and consultees legal protection because it helps to identify whether failing to meet agreed upon and contracted responsibilities are to blame if the nursing consultation relationship is unsuccessful.

BOX 13-1   QUESTIONS ADDRESSED BY FORMATIVE AND SUMMATIVE EVALUATION OF A NURSING CONSULTATION RELATIONSHIP

Formative Evaluation

- What are the objectives at this point in time, and have we accomplished these objectives?
- Are we proceeding on our timeline?
- What stumbling blocks are we encountering? How are we dealing with these?
- Are any new problems arising?
- Do we need to make any changes in the way this project is being carried out?
- What about the clients' openness versus resistance to consultation? Is this changing? If so, in what direction?
- Are needs and issues being met or unmet?

Summative Evaluation

- Was the action plan carried out? If not, why not?
- Were revisions in the plan needed? Why?
- Have the interventions achieved their desired purpose?
- Were there any unanticipated effects?
- What factors facilitated success?
- What factors subtracted from success?
- What factors contributed to effectiveness and efficiency?
- What factors subtracted from effectiveness and efficiency?
- Were the terms of the contract met?
- Did investments of time, money, and effort pay off?
- Was the consultant helpful?
- Did we "pass" or not?
- Would we be recommended or contacted again?

Information obtained from evaluating a nursing consultation relationship can also serve as a learning device. Evaluation can help consultees recognize additional needs or areas and skills that need more work if a problem solution is to be long lasting. Evaluation can also help consultees identify problem-solving skills and interventions that could be useful in similar problem situations that might occur in the future.

Evaluation information may also serve as a learning tool for a nurse consultant. Evalua-

tion feedback such as consultee satisfaction or perceptions of effectiveness can help a nurse consultant identify a need for improvement in particular skills or services. In addition, feedback from many consultation relationships, over time, can help a nurse consultant understand how different consultation approaches and problem-solving strategies are more or less effective for different consultation situations (Kurpius, Fuqua, & Rozecki, 1993). With permission from consultees and the client system, evaluation information can form the basis of research projects, journal articles, books, or other "how to" resources and thus serve as a learning tool for other nurse consultants and communities who are confronting similar problem situations.

A final purpose or benefit of evaluation is that both a nurse consultant and consultees can use information obtained from evaluation as a marketing tool. Consultees (or other community members) can use evidence of improved performance (i.e., community well-being) as a tool for attracting future resources. Favorable satisfaction and effectiveness ratings can promote positive public relations for both internal and external nurse consultants. Since as much as 75 percent of a consultant's activity is from consultee referrals and repeat business (Cosier & Dalton, 1993), this benefit or side effect of evaluation cannot be overlooked.

Linkages Between Evaluation and Other Phases of the Nursing Consultation Process

Formative evaluation, evaluating the nursing consultation relationship as it is unfolding, is one way in which evaluation-related activities permeate the entire nursing consultation process. Evaluation is linked to other phases of the nursing consultation process in another way as well: Activities that take place during earlier phases of the consultation process lay the foundation for the summative evaluation activities that comprise the fourth phase of the nursing consultation process.

During the gaining entry phase, a nurse consultant needs to communicate to consultees and/or the contact person that evaluation is both an expectation of the nursing consultation relationship as well as crucial to its success. To reinforce this expectation, it is important that the nursing consultation contract includes an explicit agreement that evaluation will occur. The contract should also specify any limitations (such as time, budget,

or access to information) that may restrict how evaluation activities are implemented in the consultation relationship.

Throughout the problem identification phase of the nursing consultation process, a nurse consultant should attempt to identify possible sources of evaluation data. A nurse consultant should also be alert for information that might be meaningful to compare on a before-and-after basis as a way of determining the effectiveness of the consultation relationship. Take, for example, a consultation project that is focused on the problem of helping nurses in a home health care agency meet the psychosocial needs of persons with HIV/AIDS. During the problem identification phase of the consultation process, a nurse consultant might collect information on nursing staff attitudes toward caring for persons with HIV/AIDS. As this information is being collected, a nurse consultant should make at least a mental note to reassess these attitudes as a way of determining the effectiveness of the consultation relationship.

During the action planning phase, a nurse consultant and consultees lay an additional foundation for summative evaluation by collaborating to determine how to evaluate specific problem solutions and interventions. To do this, the nurse consultant and consultees develop effectiveness criteria and performance standards for each intervention. In addition, they outline in advance the specific strategies for measuring the objectives of the action plan in order to ensure that the objectives are realistic. If the objectives of the nursing consultation relationship cannot be measured, the nurse consultant and consultees cannot know whether they have attained the objectives or if the objectives are even attainable. Table 13-1 summarizes the evaluation-related activities that occur during each phase of the nursing consultation process.

Because assessment and evaluation both involve data gathering and interpretation and both occur on an ongoing basis throughout

TABLE 13-1. EVALUATION AND THE NURSING CONSULTATION PROCESS

Phase of Nursing Consultation Process	Evaluation-Related Activity	
Gaining Entry	Communicate evaluation and feedback as important components of the nursing consultation relationship Establish expectations that evaluation will occur	Formative Evaluation
Contracting	Agree to evaluation Identify limits to evaluation activities	
Problem Identification	Plan to evaluate the nursing consultation relationship: Identify data sources for postconsultation comparison	
Action Planning	Plan to evaluate specific interventions and problem solutions: Establish effectiveness criteria Identify performance standards Determine data sources and data collection strategies	
Evaluation	Conduct the evaluation: Gather evaluation information Determine whether standards have been met Share evaluation feedback Utilize evaluation findings 1. Goals met → disengage 2. Goals not met → disengage, do autopsy 3. Problem still exists → recycle to earlier phase 4. Unanticipated results → implement secondary interventions	Summative Evaluation

the nursing consultation process, the two sets of activities are sometimes confused with each other. Assessment and evaluation differ, however, in terms of their orientation and utilization, as well as in the relative emphasis assumed during the course of the nursing consultation process (see Figure 13-1). Assessment activities predominate during the initial phases of the nursing consultation process and taper off as the consultation relationship progresses; the opposite progression occurs with evaluation activities. Assessment activities focus on discovering new information about the problem situation and using this information for shaping problem solutions. In contrast, the focus of evaluation is gathering information for determining whether the nursing consultation relationship is on track or needs midcourse correction.

PLANNING EVALUATION ACTIVITIES

Even though evaluation is not emphasized until the fourth phase of the nursing consultation process, as the preceding discussion implies, much of the groundwork for evaluation takes place prior to the evaluation phase itself. In fact, plans for summative evaluation activities should be incorporated into the nursing consultation action plan. The evalua-

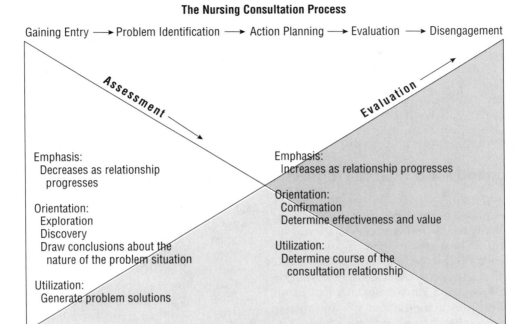

Figure 13-1   Assessment and Evaluation in the Nursing Consultation Process.
Assessment and evaluation both occur continuously throughout the nursing consultation process. Assessment activities predominate in the earlier phases of the process and decrease as the consultation relationship progresses; the opposite occurs with evaluation activities. Assessment and evaluation also have different foci and their findings are used for different purposes.

tion plan reflects decisions about the content of evaluation (what to evaluate), effectiveness criteria, performance standards, appropriate data sources, and data collection strategies. A carefully constructed evaluation plan helps prevent evaluation from being burdensome to implement and yielding data that are meaningless or ignored.

Identifying Evaluation Content

The first step in planning evaluation is identifying evaluation content. Because nursing consultation consists of a product (the problem solution) as well as a process, evaluation activities need to consider both the services provided by the nurse consultant and perceptions

of how well the nurse consultant provided the services. More specifically, evaluation should focus on (a) consultee progress toward goal attainment, (b) specific events in the nursing consultation relationship, and (c) the working relationship between the nurse consultant and the consultees (Lippitt & Lippitt, 1986).

Each evaluation issue or area that is evaluated needs to be considered in terms of three potential levels of impact. Nursing consultation relationships can affect individuals, groups, and the total client system or community, including its extra-community relations in regard to health issues (Helvie, 1998). At the individual level, nursing consultation affects the consultees with whom the nurse consultant is interacting, as well as the clients on whose behalf consultation was sought. Groups that can be affected by a nursing consultation relationship include work units, families, and aggregates of patients. Nursing consultation can also have far-reaching effects on a community as a whole. The content that needs to be considered in the evaluation of a nursing consultation relationship, then, can be pictured as an "Evaluation Area by Impact Level Matrix." This matrix and examples of issues it might address are illustrated in Box 13-2.

Evaluation Area 1: Goal Progress

This evaluation area centers around progress toward or accomplishment of the agreed-upon goals of the nursing consultation relationship. If an action plan is sufficiently detailed and has clearly stated objectives and a timeline, goal progress evaluation should be straightforward. A nurse consultant can simply collect information about whether or not tasks are being carried out and whether or not this is occurring as planned.

Individual-level impacts of goal progress that might be considered include changes in consultee knowledge, attitudes, or behavior (Helvie, 1998). Group-level impacts of goal progress include changes in work group productivity. At the total client system level, effects of goal progress on community health status, policy changes, or community values might be evaluated.

Goal evaluation provides a nurse consultant with valuable information about the quality of the problem identification and action planning phases of the nursing consultation process. For example, goal evaluation can provide feedback to a nurse consultant about the feasibility of both goals and the timeline of the action plan.

Evaluation Area 2: Event Evaluation

Event evaluation considers specific events that have occurred during the course of the nursing consultation relationship. Examples of specific events a nurse consultant might want to evaluate are education or team-building sessions, feedback meetings, and specific data-gathering events such as interviews and surveys. Event evaluation considers reactions to and perceived value of a specific event.

At the individual level, evaluation of a team-building session could include participants' comments about the strategies used and the usefulness of the session. Group-level impacts of the same team-building session that could be evaluated include how much the session disrupted the client system's productivity. A total client system impact of a team-building session to consider would be the cost–benefit ratio; that is, did expenses for the session pay off?

Event evaluation provides a nurse consultant with information that can be used to improve similar future events that are scheduled to occur during the consultation relationship. It also provides information that a nurse consultant can use when designing future consultation projects with other client systems and other problem situations.

Evaluation Area 3: Relationship Evaluation

One of the most significant predictors of successful consulting is the relationship a nurse consultant is able to establish with consultees and other members of a client system (Ross, 1993). For this reason, a nurse consultant needs to be continuously gathering information and informally monitoring how individuals, consultee groups, and the total client system (e.g., community) are reacting to him or her as a consultant. In many ways, relationship evaluation assesses the extent to which a nurse consultant has been able to gain psychological entry into the client system. Thus, relationship evaluation considers a nurse consultant's abilities to establish rapport and credibility and communicate effectively. These abilities reflect an awareness of the culture of a community

BOX 13-2 EVALUATION AREA BY IMPACT LEVEL MATRIX FOR EVALUATION: EXAMPLE QUESTIONS

Evaluation Area	Individual Impact	Group-Level Impact	Total Client System Impact
Goal Progress	Have there been changes in consultee behavior, attitudes, or knowledge? What side effects have been experienced because of goal accomplishment?	How has health status changed for the client group? How has goal accomplishment affected morale and productivity?	What has been the cost–benefit ratio of goal accomplishment?
Specific Events	What was the perceived effectiveness of team-the event?	How did the event affect work flow of the unit? Were all groups able to participate in the event?	How much time and productivity was lost because of participation in the event?
Nursing Consultation Relationship	Have there been any changes in consultee insight and skill?	How did the relationship affect teamwork and collaborative skills?	Has the relationship had an impact on community self-esteem and sense of efficacy?

and the ability to accommodate interactions and interventions to the community's culture. Relationship evaluation also focuses on consultees' perceptions of the nurse consultant's fulfillment of the consultation contract and her or his technical skills as a consultant.

Individual-level impacts of a nursing consultation relationship that could be considered include individual consultees' satisfaction with the nursing consultation relationship. Group-level relationship impacts could include increased teamwork, collaborative skills, and sense of efficacy. A possible community-level relationship impact could be an enhanced public image or community self-esteem secondary to engaging in the consultation relationship. Feedback about perceptions of the nurse consultant–consultee relationship can help a nurse consultant identify areas for personal and professional development.

Selecting Effectiveness Criteria

The second decision made when developing an evaluation plan is selecting the criteria that will be used to determine the effectiveness or success of the nursing consultation relationship. Selecting effectiveness criteria can be one of the more difficult tasks in developing an evaluation plan. It is also one of the most important tasks, because if effectiveness criteria fail to pass the tests of meaningfulness and relevance, it may prove difficult to persuade the consultees that undertaking an evaluation is worthwhile. Even if an evaluation is undertaken, if effectiveness criteria are perceived by consultees as being irrelevant or meaningless, it is unlikely that evaluation results will be used.

Effectiveness criteria should be selected by both the nurse consultant and consultees. Occasionally, other members of the client system (e.g., community representatives, the consultation contact person) may also be involved in developing criteria. For example, an agency administrator (who is paying the nurse consultant's fee) may want to have

some say about what constitutes effectiveness in a consultation project in which the entire agency is the client. Questions that can be used to help select meaningful and relevant effectiveness criteria are "What needs to happen for this relationship to be considered a success?" and "What would success look like in this situation?" Effectiveness criteria that should be considered for evaluating any nursing consultation relationship are cost–benefit ratio, behavior or performance change, cognitive or knowledge change, affective or attitude change, and "reactions."

Cost–benefit ratio considers the net "payoff" of the nursing consultation relationship. Of specific interest is whether what was gained from the relationship outweighs costs (time, money, stress, etc.). The effectiveness criterion of *behavior or performance change* considers whether behavior changes among consultees and community members occurred as planned and contributed to the problem solution. Considering *cognitive or knowledge change* as evidence of effectiveness makes sense when educational strategies are used as a problem solution. If the criterion of *affective or attitude change* is used, a nursing consultation relationship is considered effective if consultees' attitudes changed in such a way as to contribute to the problem solution. Finally, the effectiveness criterion of *"reactions"* considers consultees' satisfaction with the nursing consultation relationship and perceptions of the relationship's effectiveness.

Which of these criteria are most meaningful and relevant will depend on the nature of the nursing consultation problem, the goals of the consultation relationship, and the identity of the client. Not all criteria are appropriate in every nursing consultation situation. Also, different effectiveness criteria might be appropriate for different impact levels of a nursing consultation relationship. For example, a change in knowledge might indicate effectiveness of the nursing consultation relationship at the individual consultee impact level, while work group efficiency might be a more valid effectiveness criterion at the group impact level. At the total client system impact level, cost–benefit information might be considered the most meaningful and relevant indicator of effectiveness. The scenario presented in Box 13-3 illustrates determining effectiveness criteria.

It is important to recognize that effectiveness evaluation is different from impact evaluation. Effectiveness evaluation focuses on goal accomplishment. In contrast, impact evaluation considers multiple effects of the nursing consultation relationship, and effectiveness is only one possible effect (Anderson & McFarlane, 2000; Helvie, 1998). Referring to the scenario in Box 13-3, note that effectiveness evaluation is concerned with determining the extent to which outcomes and reactions asso-

ciated with the nursing consultation process resulted in achieving a community clinic's goal of an increased caseload of pediatric patients in order to receive more grant funds from the state. Impact evaluation would look for other possible effects of the nursing consultation relationship and its outcomes, for example, healthier children, better access to care, increased waiting time for an appointment, increase in clinic revenue, increased expenses incurred by the clinic group as a result of seeing more pediatric patients, changes in provider job satisfaction, and so forth. In summary, while there can be many favorable outcomes at different impact levels for any nursing consultation relationship, effectiveness evaluation focuses only on goal accomplishment and, therefore, the effect of the relationship on client/community well-

BOX 13-3   DETERMINING EFFECTIVENESS CRITERIA: A NURSING CONSULTATION SCENARIO

The Consultation Problem

A community clinic asks a nurse consultant to help them increase their caseload of pediatric clients so that they will be eligible for more state grant monies.

Parties Involved

Consultees: Clinic personnel
Clients: Community clinic
Stakeholders: Children and their parents, other health care providers, taxpayers

Possible Effectiveness Criteria

Cognitive or knowledge change: Have the consultees' knowledge changed in such a way that they know how to attract pediatric clients?
Behavior change: Have behaviors changed in such a way that more parents want to bring their children to the clinic?
Goal accomplishment: Has the clinic secured more grant funding?
Reactions: How did the consultees rate their satisfaction with the consultant and the consultation relationship?

being. In our working scenario, this would translate into the receipt of increased grant monies for the clinic.

Specifying Performance Standards

The third decision that a nurse consultant needs to make in developing a nursing consultation evaluation plan is that of performance standards. A performance standard is a reference point against which specific consultation outcomes are compared in order to make a judgment of success or failure. A nursing consultation relationship is successful when its outcomes match or exceed predetermined performance standards. Common performance standards include the following: operating more effectively than before the nursing consultation relationship, meeting minimal accepted standards such as those established by an accrediting agency, and meeting ideal standards established by oneself or some group (Harrison, 1994).

What constitutes an appropriate performance standard is determined by the nature of the nursing consultation problem and the consultees' goals. For example, in the scenario about the nurse consultant working with the community clinic, performance standards that could be used to determine the success of the nursing consultation relationship include the following: (a) The clinic's caseload of pediatric patients doubles in volume as compared to its preconsultation level, (b) the clinic's pediatric caseload accounts for 50 percent of daily office visits, and (c) the clinic qualifies for and receives additional state funding.

Identifying Data Sources

The fourth decision that needs to be made when formulating an evaluation plan for a nursing consultation relationship involves identifying appropriate sources of evaluation data. Data sources that should be considered include consultees, other members of the community/client system (e.g., the consultation contact person, fee payers, or family of a target patient group), and other stakeholders. Recall that one of the distinguishing characteristics of nursing consultation is that health care consumers or community members always stand to be affected by the consultation relationship, either directly as clients or indirectly as stakeholders. With this in mind, a nurse consultant should always make an effort to gather evaluation information from community members, regardless of their role in the nursing consultation relationship.

Evaluation data from clients and stakeholders who are health care consumers can target current "performance" (e.g., incidence rate of a condition, perceptions of well-being) and reactions to the consultation relationship as well as expectations about future performance. Again, using the scenario of the nurse consultant working with the community clinic, current evaluation data from the parents of pediatric patients might focus on satisfaction with the care provided on a single occasion. Future-oriented evaluation data might focus on the likelihood that parents will use the clinic again for their child's health care needs. Future-oriented evaluation data can provide a nurse consultant and consultees with information about both the likely longevity of their problem solution and the need to conduct additional problem-solving interventions on an ongoing basis.

An additional source of evaluation information in a consultation relationship is oneself as the consultant. One's own perceptions about how things went and what worked (as well as what didn't and why) provide valuable information for structuring subsequent consultation relationships and increasing one's effectiveness as a nurse consultant. Essentially, what a nurse consultant needs to ask is, "If I had to do it over, what would I do the same and what would I do differently?" A nurse consultant should also evaluate any personal reactions (such as satisfaction) to the consultation relationship and personal cost–benefit ratio. This self-evaluation can provide a nurse consultant with information about what types of problem situations are a good fit for her or his skills and about how to formulate future consultation contracts.

Determining Data Collection Strategies

The final decision that needs to be made by a nurse consultant and consultees about the consultation evaluation plan is how to collect the evaluation data, including data collection techniques, timing of data collection, and collecting comparison data. Ideally, individuals who are affected by the consultation relationship should be involved in making the decisions about how evaluation data will be collected. In addition, involving consultees in collecting and analyzing evaluation data increases the credibility of the findings and the likelihood that the information will be used.

Data Collection Techniques

Observations, interviews, surveys, and document review can all be used to gather evaluation data about the nursing consultation relationship. The usefulness and limitations of each of these techniques were discussed in Chapter 10. The nature of the information desired, who the data sources are, and feasibility issues all influence decisions about how specific evaluation information would be best obtained.

One specific technique for generating evaluation data involves compiling a case study about the community/client system. A case study is an in-depth narrative report that includes detailed descriptions of observations of changes in consultees, clients, and the community as a whole that occur as a particular consultation relationship unfolds. Case studies have the advantage of generating rich qualitative data on an ongoing basis. These data can contribute to a nurse consultant's own learning and can be shared with consultees to provide positive feedback and increased insight into how consultees' behaviors and values influenced the consultation outcome. Case study data alone, however, may be less convincing than quantitative data to administrators, payers, and other stakeholders in a consultation relationship. Case study data are also inherently subjective and, therefore, prone to consultant bias. A nurse consultant, for example, may "see" hoped-for improvements in a community's health status that cannot be confirmed objectively.

The Timing of Data Collection

Deciding how to best time the collection of data in order to get a reliable indication of effectiveness requires consideration of a different set of issues. Evaluation data from surveys and consultee interviews might produce overly positive results due to a "novelty" effect if collected too soon after a problem has been resolved. That is, the evaluation results might appear positive only because the intervention or change is new and different and its side effects have not had a chance to develop. On the other hand, data collected too soon could reveal largely negative results if consultees are reacting to the discomfort of being in an adjustment period. Finally, if evaluation data are collected too late, changes that occurred may have become accepted as the status quo and thought of as "how things have always been." In these situations, effectiveness or success might be underestimated. Timing dilemmas are often handled best by collecting both immediate and delayed evaluation data.

Collecting Comparison Data

Decisions about data collection strategies also involve consideration about what kinds of comparisons need to be made in order to demonstrate effectiveness of the nursing consultation relationship. Comparisons can be made over time as well as between groups.

Pre- and Postcomparisons. Comparisons of relevant pre- and postconsultation data from any source can provide objective and quantitative data about changes in attitudes or the frequency of undesirable behaviors or events. A pre- and postconsultation review of the number of cases of hepatitis A that can be traced to food service workers, for example, would provide a nurse consultant with one piece of information about the effectiveness of consultation efforts addressing hepatitis A vaccinations and safe food handling with owners of fast-food restaurants. The drawback of pre- and postconsultation data is that they require obtaining the same information from the same source at two points in time. If the data source is records, changes in documentation practices may have occurred between the pre- and post–data collection points. If before and after attitudes are being compared, testing effects (such as recall of previous responses) and attrition or "dropout" of some group members may bias findings and affect their meaningfulness and accuracy.

Longitudinal Comparisons. When the purpose of a nursing consultation relationship is to effect change in a variable that has fluctuating values (such as playground accidents at a school), it is often appropriate to track indicators of effectiveness over a longer period of time. In a longitudinal comparison, it is desirable to see a general trend of improvement that overrides any natural transient or situational variations. A nurse consultant working with a school to improve playground safety might look for a general trend in decreased accidents over time despite occasional and expected increases that could be explained by the weather and the types of activities in which students engage or general school absenteeism. Time and cost factors are the primary barriers to collecting longitudinal data about the effectiveness of nursing consultation interventions. Longitudinal evaluations can also delay bringing closure to a nursing consultation relationship.

Using a Comparison Group. Comparisons between consultees or sectors of a community that were "exposed" to the nursing consultation relationship interventions and those that were not can also be a means of generating effectiveness information. One difficulty of using this type of comparison, however, is the possibility of preexisting differences between the groups. For instance, different styles of leadership on two smoking cessation support groups, only one of which participated in the nursing consultation intervention, might be the real explanation of any postconsultation differences that are detected between the two groups. A second drawback of using comparison groups is the possibility of "contamination effects." Participants in the groups involved in the consultation relationship might share what they learned with members of the comparison group staff and cause changes in their behavior.

Box 13-4 summarizes the advantages and disadvantages of these different strategies for collecting comparison data.

The importance of triangulation was emphasized as a strategy for providing a check against bias during the problem identification phase of the nursing consultation process; it is also a recommended strategy when evaluating nursing consultation efforts. Combining reports of decreased smoking with time-series data about fewer respiratory illnesses, for example, would provide a more convincing picture of the effectiveness of the nursing consultation relationship with the smoking cessation support group than would either piece of information alone.

Box 13-5 summarizes the decisions the nurse consultant needs to make when planning the summative evaluation of a nursing consultation relationship.

CONDUCTING AN EVALUATION

Evaluation can be conducted in either a consultant-directed or a collaborative manner. An

BOX 13-4 STRATEGIES FOR COLLECTING COMPARISON DATA FOR NURSING CONSULTATION EVALUATION

Pre- and Postconsultation Comparisons

What it involves: Collecting the same information from the same sources before and after the nursing consultation relationship

Advantages: Since information is gathered from the same source, changes in performance are easy to see and interpret

Disadvantages:
- Can be cumbersome
- Practices of recording the data to be compared (e.g., in medical records) may have changed between the two data collection periods
- Testing effects—individuals may recall their previous responses and respond in the same way
- Low response rates may bias postconsultation results

Longitudinal Comparisons

What it involves: Collecting outcome data at multiple points in time

Advantages: Probably the best way of identifying the effects of the consultation relationship on variables that have fluctuating values; also the best way to determine long-term effects of a problem solution

Disadvantages:
- Take time
- Are costly to implement
- Delay achieving closure of the nursing consultation relationship

Comparison Groups

What it involves: Collecting information on the same variable from individuals who were participants in the nursing consultation relationship and those who were not

Advantages: No need to worry about testing effects

Disadvantages:
- Need to find a valid comparison group
- Preexisting group differences may explain differences in performance
- "Contamination" of nonparticipants by participants in the consultation relationship

---

evaluation that is carried out solely by the nurse consultant can often be completed in a more timely manner than can a collaborative evaluation. A consultant-directed evaluation allows a nurse consultant to work quickly and not have to rely on consultee cooperation or teach consultees evaluation-related skills. Consultant-directed evaluation is most appropriate when a nurse consultant is under pressure to wrap up the consultation relationship in a

BOX 13-5   PLANNING SUMMATIVE EVALUATION: ESSENTIAL DECISIONS

Decision 1: Evaluation Content

Evaluation areas: Goal progress, specific events, the nurse consultant–consultee relationship
Impact levels: Individual, group, total client system

Decision 2: Effectiveness Criteria

Cost–benefit ratio
Behavior change
Knowledge change
Attitude change
Reactions

Decision 3: Performance Standards

Before and after changes
Compare to other groups
Compare to minimum standards
Compare to an ideal

Decision 4: Data Sources

Consultee
Client
Other members of the client system
Patients
Nurse consultant

Decision 5: Data Collection Strategies

Techniques:
- Surveys
- Interviews
- Observations
- Case study

Timing:
- Immediate
- Delayed

Comparisons:
- Pre- and postconsultation
- Longitudinal
- Comparison group

hurry and when the inability to conduct evaluation in a timely manner might mean that evaluation would not be conducted at all. It is also appropriate when consultees are focused on implementing the action plan and dealing with the psychological transitions that accompany problem solving to the exclusion of actively contributing to the evaluation process. A disadvantage of consultant-directed evaluation is that its findings may be perceived as biased by consultees and other members of the community. For example, a nurse consultant might conclude that the consultation relationship has been successful, but consultees or community members might perceive otherwise since they have not had firsthand experience "seeing" and "hearing" the evaluation data.

Conclusions that are derived from an evaluation that has been conducted in a collaborative manner are often more believable to consultees and other members of a client system. This is because consultees have had an opportunity to see and hear the evaluation data as the data come in. Consultees who are involved in the evaluation process also see how effectiveness and impact evaluation can offer different perspectives on the success of the consultation relationship. Another advantage of involving consultees in evaluation activities is that it gives them the opportunity to develop skills that will enable them to conduct their own evaluations in the future. Finally, consultees who are involved in evaluation have the opportunity to see the importance of evaluation as a feedback mechanism and learning device; this increases the likelihood that they will incorporate evaluation activities into their own work setting.

GIVING EVALUATION FEEDBACK

Evaluation is useless unless the information that has been gathered is acted on and used to either make midcourse corrections in the nursing consultation relationship or reinforce positive changes that have occurred in the problem situation. Sharing evaluation findings with consultees and other members of a community is the first step in using the findings to shape the subsequent course of a nursing consultation relationship.

Feedback helps evaluation accomplish its intended purposes. If consultees are not aware of evaluation findings, they will be unable to use the information as a decision-making, learning, or marketing device. Giving evaluation feedback, then, functions as a catalytic intervention (see Chapter 11) because it increases awareness of how the nursing consultation relationship is progressing. Feedback can also serve as reinforcement for continuing the nursing consultation relationship and problem-solving efforts. Sharing evaluation findings also helps to bring closure to a nursing consultation relationship.

Strategies for Giving Effective Feedback

For evaluation feedback to be effective, a nurse consultant must make decisions about who needs to hear what information and how this information can be "packaged" so that it is accepted and used. In a consultation situation in which a nurse consultant is working with a food bank about how to put together nutritious combinations of foods for distribution, the nurse consultant would want to provide detailed ongoing (i.e., formative) evaluation feedback to the food bank staff and volunteers. Most likely, this feedback would be shared informally and verbally. Depending on the situation, it might also be important to share evaluation information with food donation programs, food recipients, and the agency administrator. The content and format of an evaluation report would most likely vary, however, for each of these audiences.

If evaluation findings are to be shared in a public forum such as an entire community or with the media, it is wise to first present the findings privately to the primary consultees or contact person. This provides an opportunity for a nurse consultant to preview possible reactions to and enlist support for the evaluation findings as well as involve consultees or the contact person in the group presentation. This involvement is perceived by the audience as a sanctioning of the evaluation findings and increases the likelihood that they will be used.

Because evaluation includes a component of judgment, sharing evaluation findings is different from sharing other kinds of information such as problem assessment findings. Before consultees or clients will hear judgmental news, a nurse consultant must be perceived as both credible and trustworthy. There also needs to be "readiness to hear" or agreement that feedback is a legitimate activity to engage in at this point in time.

The difficulty involved in giving needed negative feedback about consultation effectiveness can tempt a nurse consultant to withhold negative information in order to save face and avoid consultee reactions such as defensiveness. However, negative evaluation findings are at least as important as favorable findings in terms of being a learning device. Sometimes negative findings can be neutralized by being paired with positive findings. For example, a nurse consultant might be able to neutralize negative evaluation findings about the cost–benefit ratio of a consultation relationship by pairing them with favorable reports of community satisfaction. Negative findings can also be reframed as opportunities for further growth.

A nurse consultant also needs to be careful about how positive evaluation findings are shared with consultees and a community. If findings are presented too enthusiastically or in terms that are too "glowing," consultees may be tempted to think a problem has been solved once and for all and may ignore the need for change maintenance strategies and ongoing self-monitoring. A nurse consultant who is presenting positive evaluation findings needs to be clear that these are "here and now" findings—and that they will continue only if there is ongoing effort on the part of the consultees and community.

Throughout the feedback process, a nurse consultant needs to be mindful of the feelings that may be triggered by evaluative feedback and alert for possible signals of poor timing or violation of cultural norms. Both defensiveness and a too eager acceptance of feedback can signal recognition as well as denial of the validity of the evaluation findings. Premature closure of a feedback session often indicates confirmation of, but lack of support for, evaluation findings. A nurse consultant can deal with these reactions by acknowledging the validity of the feelings that most likely underlie the reaction (e.g., frustration or embarrassment), making an effort to share favorable findings and strengths, and trying to reframe evaluation findings. For example, it might make sense to reframe an immediate postconsultation finding of ineffectiveness in terms of cost–benefit ratio as a poorly timed evaluation and an indication for additional follow-up. Other strategies for effectively communicating findings from the evaluation of a nursing consultation effort are highlighted in Box 13-6.

Evaluation can be a painful and anxiety-provoking process for all involved. Because evaluating nursing consultation efforts entails gathering data about a nurse consultant's own effectiveness as well as about goal attainment by the community, a nurse consultant, too, can react to evaluation findings with defensiveness and denial. Many of the tips in Box 13-6 for effectively sharing feedback can be reinterpreted and used by a nurse consultant as strategies for interpreting personal evaluation findings. For example, a nurse consultant needs to consider how timing can affect personal receptivity to evaluation findings (bad news is always worse when one is tired!). A

BOX 13-6   GIVING EFFECTIVE EVALUATION FEEDBACK

- Keep the feedback objective and nonjudgmental.
- Keep feedback pertinent to the focal issues (i.e., the nursing consultation experience and its effectiveness); remember relevance and meaningfulness.
- Support conclusions with specific examples; avoid broad generalities.
- Share strengths as well as weaknesses—what was accomplished or effective as well as what was not.
- Consider timing issues.
- Consider cultural norms.
- Recognize the need of all parties to "save face."
- Share formative evaluation findings with clients on an ongoing basis.
- Keep individual evaluation responses confidential.
- Give verbal feedback before written feedback.
- Share findings privately with key players in the problem situation before "going public."
- Try to demystify evaluation and reframe negative findings.
- Consider that sharing evaluation findings can function as both a catalytic and confrontational intervention.

nurse consultant should also look for specific examples to support general statements about personal effectiveness and avoid putting too much stock in broad generalities. Finally, just as consultees and community members are expected to accept only meaningful and relevant evaluation information, a nurse consultant should only attend to evaluation comments that address effectiveness in the present consultant role, not other roles (such as expert clinician or supervisor) in which the nurse consultant may also be familiar to consultees.

POSSIBLE DIFFICULTIES IN EVALUATING NURSING CONSULTATION EFFORTS

Many of the difficulties related to evaluating nursing consultation efforts such as timing, effectiveness issues, and the emotional responses to evaluation have been mentioned in earlier sections of this chapter. In this section, the focus is on three specific sets of

potential difficulties: political dilemmas, hidden agendas, and barriers to implementing evaluation.

Political Dilemmas

A political reality of working with communities is the tension between securing private (individual level) and public (group or community level) benefits. Because repeat business is such a large part of any consultant's "portfolio," there is a myopic temptation to share only good news with a community. While buying into the motto "the customer is always right" and sharing only favorable evidence of effectiveness may help all parties initially save face, it can be disastrous for both the nurse consultant and the community in the long run, especially if interventions produce only short-term change or result in unanticipated side effects or costs. A response to this difficulty is learning to package unfavorable findings so they are more acceptable to consultees and community members.

Hidden Agendas

One of a nurse consultant's tasks during the gaining entry phase of the nursing consultation process is to determine what, if any, hidden agendas might be prompting the consultation request. During the evaluation phase, consultees' or a community's hidden agendas may place limits on what can be evaluated, what data can be accessed, and what findings are appropriate to share with which parties in the client system. Among the hidden agendas that can become apparent during the evaluation phase is the tendency to use findings to either protect an ineffective but popular individual or program or get rid of an effective but unpopular individual or program. For instance, a nurse consultant may be asked to reframe negative findings about a community agency's inability or unwillingness to provide the resources to implement a change in service eligibility as staff inability or unwillingness to meet resultant increased needs within the existing structure of care delivery. The potential difficulty of hidden agendas can be addressed proactively when a nurse consultant and consultees establish parameters for reporting evaluation information in the nursing consultation contract and the evaluation plan.

Nurse consultants can also have hidden agendas that compromise the integrity of the evaluation phase of the nursing consultation process. Because favorable evaluations are effective consultation marketing tools, the temptation exists for evaluation activities to be structured and findings to be used strictly to serve marketing purposes. The danger, of course, with following this agenda is that the nurse consultant's needs, and not those of consultees or clients, are served by the evaluation. For example, a nurse consultant can put together a portfolio that documents consultation activities to promote him- or herself for a position in a community organization. Failing to gather or report data about the impact of interventions, however, might hide the fact that many repeat requests for consultation reflect an inability to help clients solve certain types of problems on the first attempt. A nurse consultant needs to recognize that this shortsighted response to negative evaluation findings is unlikely to protect his or her reputation on a long-term basis. Instead, negative evaluation findings need to be used as guidelines for further professional development.

Barriers to Implementing Evaluation

Because evaluation can be an uncomfortable process, both consultees and consultants tend to come up with excuses for not including it as part of the consultation process. Evaluation is often perceived as an activity that only adds more time and expense to a consultation relationship. Evaluation also is often viewed as self-serving for the nurse consultant but of little value to consultees or the client system. In today's health care environment of cost containment, these arguments are understandable but also somewhat shortsighted. Monitoring, documenting, and ensuring the quality of changes in health care practices that have resulted from consultant recommendations is vital for protecting and promoting the practice of nursing and nursing consultation as well as for ensuring that the health of communities and individual health care is not compromised. Nurse consultants need to actively educate consultees about the purposes and benefits of evaluation.

The barriers that are most difficult to overcome in evaluating nursing consultation efforts are determining what constitutes meaningful, relevant, and feasible effectiveness criteria and valid performance standards. Few effectiveness criteria will suit the interests of all participants and stakeholders in the consultation process equally; this dilemma can result in avoidance of the entire evaluation phase. One response to the effec-

BOX 13-7   DOCUMENTATION CHECKLIST: EVALUATION ACTIVITIES

Documenting Formative Evaluation

- ☐ Consultee and nurse consultant perceptions of task accomplishment
- ☐ Consultee perceptions of key events and cost–benefit ratio
- ☐ Consultee perceptions of nurse consultant effectiveness
- ☐ Nurse consultant's impressions about the effectiveness of the nursing consultation relationship to date
- ☐ Adherence to timeline for tasks (if no, give rationale)
- ☐ Adherence to budget (if no, give rationale)
- ☐ Unanticipated side effects and how they are being responded to
- ☐ Date and time of each evaluation activity
- ☐ Source and method of data collection for each evaluation parameter
- ☐ Parties with whom formative evaluation findings were shared and reactions of these parties
- ☐ Actions taken as a result of evaluation findings

Documenting Summative Evaluation

- ☐ Goal accomplishment (give evidence)
- ☐ Consultee and nurse consultant evaluation of key events
- ☐ Consultee and nurse consultant evaluation of the nurse consultant–consultee relationship
- ☐ Other effects of the consultation relationship—describe, provide specific examples, identify as positive or negative
- ☐ Adherence to timeline (if no, give rationale)
- ☐ Adherence to project budget (if no, give rationale)
- ☐ Consultee satisfaction with the consultation relationship
- ☐ Nurse consultant satisfaction with the consultation relationship
- ☐ Cost–benefit ratio of the consultation relationship
- ☐ Date and time of each evaluation activity
- ☐ Data sources for each evaluation parameter
- ☐ Data collection strategy (timing, method, who implemented) for each evaluation parameter (attach tools)
- ☐ Effectiveness criteria and performance standards used for each evaluation parameter
- ☐ Difficulties encountered during summative evaluation—how they were handled, whether or not they were resolved
- ☐ Parties with whom evaluation findings were shared—format, their reactions
- ☐ Actions taken as a result of summative evaluation findings

tiveness dilemma is developing an evaluation plan that incorporates multiple evaluation areas and impact levels. Also, incorporating the concept of triangulation into data collection strategies can give a more convincing and accurate picture of effectiveness.

DOCUMENTING EVALUATION ACTIVITIES IN NURSING CONSULTATION

Documenting the evaluation activities that occur during a nursing consultation relationship serves many of the same purposes as evaluation itself. More specifically, documenting evaluation activities provides visual feedback and reminders to a nurse consultant about how to proceed with the nursing consultation relationship as well as serves as a learning tool in terms of providing information about interactions and interventions that were more and less successful. Documenting evaluation activities can also provide protection against possible legal charges of not adapting the consultation process to the evolving needs of a particular nurse consultant–consultee relationship. Box 13-7 provides a checklist for documenting the evaluation activities that take place during the nursing consultation process.

CHAPTER SUMMARY

The benefits of evaluating nursing consultation relationships—for nurse consultants, their consultees, and communities/client systems—underscores the importance of ensuring that the difficulties inherent in evaluation don't cause evaluation to be avoided as a part of nursing consultation. Systematically planning and implementing evaluation activities increases the likelihood that evaluation is feasible and yields information that is meaningful and relevant. Evaluation is more likely to be perceived as a worthwhile activity if it is kept simple and evaluation findings are actually used to enhance the effectiveness of the nursing consultation process.

APPLYING CHAPTER CONTENT

For each of the following scenarios, describe how you would evaluate the effectiveness of your consultation efforts. Specifically address the following issues:

- Areas to evaluate (including evaluation areas and impact levels)
- Effectiveness criteria
- Performance standards
- Sources of data
- Methods of data collection (including timing and comparisons)
- Reporting strategies
- Dilemmas or difficulties you might encounter and how you would respond to them

SCENARIO 1

You are a nurse-educator who has been providing consultation to a local community agency as they formulate their self-study report in preparation for an accreditation site visit. Your primary interventions have been meeting with the agency staff and sharing with them your impressions of their program and areas that might be problematic in the report. You also read the final self-study report before it is submitted to the accrediting agency.

SCENARIO 2

You are a nurse practitioner who has been providing consultation to a day care facility.

The issue that prompted consultation was perceptions of "acting out" behaviors by one of the toddlers who attends the day care. Your interventions have included education about toddler developmental issues and appropriate behavior management strategies.

SCENARIO 3

You are a nurse-manager who is working as an internal consultant with a hospital unit that has recently undergone work redesign. The issues that prompted the consultation request were perceptions of low morale on the unit and patient care concerns. Specifically, ratings on patient satisfaction surveys have dropped and there has been an increase in incident reports. Your interventions have included listening to staff complaints, explaining the rationale behind redesign, and providing in-service education on communication and delegation skills.

SCENARIO 4

You are a clinical nurse specialist in a rehabilitation facility. A nurse colleague asks you for help dealing with a patient who seems to be in denial about his poor prognosis and is refusing pain medication. Your interventions with the nurse can be characterized as being acceptant and confrontational in nature. You also make some specific suggestions for intervening with this patient.

References

Anderson, E., & McFarlane, J. (2000). *Community as partner: Theory and practice in nursing* (3rd ed.). Philadelphia: Lippincott.

Cosier, R., & Dalton, D. (1993). Management consulting: Planning, entry, performance. *Journal of Counseling and Development, 72*, 191–196.

Dougherty, A. (1995). *Consultation: Practice and perspectives in school and community settings.* Pacific Grove, CA: Brooks-Cole.

Harrison, M. (1994). *Diagnosing organizations: Methods, models, and processes* (2nd ed.). Thousand Oaks, CA: Sage.

Helvie, C. (1998). *Advanced practice nursing in the community.* Thousand Oaks, CA: Sage.

Kurpius, D., Fuqua, D., & Rozecki, T. (1993). The consulting process: A multidimensional approach. *Journal of Counseling and Development, 71*, 601–606.

Lippitt, G., & Lippitt, R. (1986). *The consulting process in action* (2nd ed.). San Diego: University Associates.

Ross, G. (1993). Peter Block's Flawless Consulting and the Homunculus Theory: Within each person is a perfect consultant. *Journal of Counseling and Development, 71*, 639–641.

Ulschak, F., & SnowAntle, S. (1990). *Consultation skills for health care professionals.* San Francisco: Jossey-Bass.

14

Disengagement from Consultation Relationships

If the entry stage is characterized by the question, "Hello, what can I do for you?" then the disengagement phase is characterized by the question, "What do we need to take care of before I say good-bye?" (Dougherty, 1995)

 KEY CONCEPTS:

readiness, dependency, institutionalization, psychodynamics

 KEY TERMS FOR YOUR SEARCH ENGINE:

consultation and termination

INTRODUCTION

Typically, traditional nurse–patient relationships "just end." In the traditional nursing process, a patient's discharge may be anticipated or even planned, but, as desirable as it may be, there is seldom an opportunity for a systematic and planned relationship closure process. In the nursing consultation process, however, there is a formal disengagement phase. Disengagement is the strategically planned and mutually agreed upon series of activities that ultimately results in the termination of the nurse consultant–consultee relationship. Disengagement, then, is a process rather than a single abrupt event.

This chapter begins with an overview of the disengagement phase—its purposes, its importance, and its relationship to the other phases in the nursing consultation process. Next, a nurse consultant's tasks in the disengagement phase are discussed. The chapter closes by considering some of the difficulties that a nurse consultant may encounter when implementing the disengagement phase. As you read this chapter, think about the following questions:

• How might implementation of the disengagement phase differ for internal and external nurse consultants?

- How might disengagement differ with individual and group consultees? How would it differ with a peer consultee?
- How might a community's culture affect disengagement?

- What facilitates and impedes successful implementation of the disengagement phase?
- How would you approach disengagement if you were "fired" as a nurse consultant?

AN OVERVIEW OF DISENGAGEMENT

The themes of the disengagement phase are "letting go" and "securing the future." The theme of "letting go" applies to both the nurse consultant and consultees. What is "let go," however, is only the problem-solving relationship between a nurse consultant and consultees. Disengagement does not necessarily mean that all personal or professional contact with a consultee ends. For example, in an internal consulting situation, a nurse consultant remains a part of the client system and most likely interacts with consultees (and perhaps clients) after the nursing consultation or problem-solving relationship has ended.

The second theme of the disengagement phase is "securing the future." Disengagement is an opportunity for both a nurse consultant and consultees to link the past with the future. That is, the activities of the disengagement phase provide an opportunity for a nurse consultant and consultees to review what has happened during the nursing consultation process and to ensure a secure future for the problem solution and resultant changes in the consultees and the community or client system.

The Purposes of Disengagement

Although "letting go" and "securing the future" describe the overall focus of the disengagement phase, a more immediate goal of disengagement is to ensure that any problems that have been solved as a result of the nursing consultation relationship remain solved.

Thus, the primary purpose of disengagement is to facilitate "refreezing," that is, to ensure institutionalization of consultees' new points of view and new behaviors into everyday working relationships (Helvie, 1998; Schein, 1987).

A second purpose of disengagement is to encourage consultee self-reliance and prevent dependency on others for problem solving. This purpose supports the overall goal of nursing consultation to provide consultees with problem-solving skills that can be transferred to future problem situations. This purpose of disengagement is also in line with the professional responsibility of nurse consultants to become progressively unnecessary to consultees and a client system (Lippitt & Lippitt, 1986). The disengagement phase in the nursing consultation process helps prevent continuing a consulting relationship when it would only serve to meet the needs of the nurse consultant.

The Importance of Disengagement

How many times have you been involved in a consultation situation, either as a nurse consultant or as a consultee, in which the changes that had resulted from the consultation relationship evaporated as soon as the consulting relationship ended? On occasion, consultation efforts result in only short-term change and consultees regress to old ways of interacting with clients. In other situations, change is so fragile that counterreactions arise and must be dealt with quickly in order to protect the problem solving that has occurred (Lippitt & Lippitt, 1986). A strategically planned disengagement phase is important as a strategy for fostering the continuance of the outcomes of the nursing consultation relationship.

The disengagement phase is an opportunity to acknowledge the relationship that has developed between a nurse consultant and the consultees. Very often, nursing consultation occurs because of a difficult and complex problem situation. As a nurse consultant and consultees work together to solve problems, a valued, trust-based, interpersonal relationship develops. Disengagement is an opportunity for the nurse consultant to recognize and validate the importance of this dimension of the nursing consultation relationship (Barron, 1989). This validation is important for establishing a basis for future personal and professional contact between the nurse consultant, consultees, and with the larger community.

Keep in mind that disengagement culminates in the termination of the nurse consultant–consultee relationship only in regard to a particular problem-solving activity. When disengagement activities have been successful, termination should be accompanied by a mutual sense of satisfaction about both the consultation relationship and what has been accomplished. If the problem-solving relationship between a nurse consultant and consultees has been mutually satisfying, the door is always open for reinvolvement or additional work at the consultees' request.

Linkage to Other Phases in the Nursing Consultation Process

While disengagement is a distinct phase in the nursing consultation process, much of the groundwork for successful disengagement is laid in earlier phases. During the gaining entry phase of the nursing consultation process, a nurse consultant needs to clearly establish the temporary, problem-focused nature of the consultation relationship. A nurse consultant needs to make sure that consultees understand that the focus of the nursing consultation relationship is solving a particular problem and learning problem-solving skills for future use. The nursing consultation contract should clearly identify the criteria that will be used to set the activities of the disengagement phase into motion.

During the action planning phase of the nursing consultation process, a nurse consultant and consultees decide together how the nurse consultant will transfer responsibility for maintaining change to consultees and the time frame for this transfer. In particular, the nature of the supports and resources that will be developed and installed into the community or client system in order to institutionalize the problem solution need to be identified (Lippitt & Lippitt, 1986). The action plan should be clear in terms of who is responsible (the nurse consultant, the consultees, or someone else in the community) for developing and securing these supports.

The disengagement phase is linked most clearly to the evaluation activities that occur during the nursing consultation process. Ongoing formative evaluation may provide a nurse consultant and consultees with feedback that success is unlikely in a particular problem-solving relationship. For example, formative evaluation information may reveal a lack of resources or consultee motivation for continuing the nursing consultation relationship in any kind of an effective manner. If this is the case, the nurse consultant and consultees should proceed with disengagement activities (Kurpius, Fuqua, & Rozecki, 1993).

In many nursing consultation situations, disengagement begins with the onset of summative evaluation activities. Collecting "endpoint" evaluation information (e.g., on satisfaction or perceptions of success) often serves as a "natural" signal to consultees that the nursing consultation relationship is winding down. In other cases, disengagement does not begin until after findings of summative evaluation provide a nurse consultant and consultees with the information needed to decide whether the goals of the nursing consultation relationship have been accomplished. If a nursing consultation problem has been resolved or the consultees have accepted a nurse consultant's recommendations, the nurse consultant and consultees can proceed with the previously planned disengagement activities. If, on the other hand, evaluation findings indicate that the nursing consultation problem remains unresolved, a nurse consultant and consultees have three options available to them: (1) continue with current problem-solving efforts, (2) revisit an earlier phase of the nursing consultation process (such as problem identification or action planning), or (3) proceed to the disengagement phase because success seems unlikely (Ross, 1993). (Recall that in some cases, evaluation findings will indicate a need to implement secondary or supplemental interventions in response to new problems or side effects to problem solving that have occurred.) Figure 14-1 illustrates how the disengagement phase is linked to other phases in the nursing consultation process.

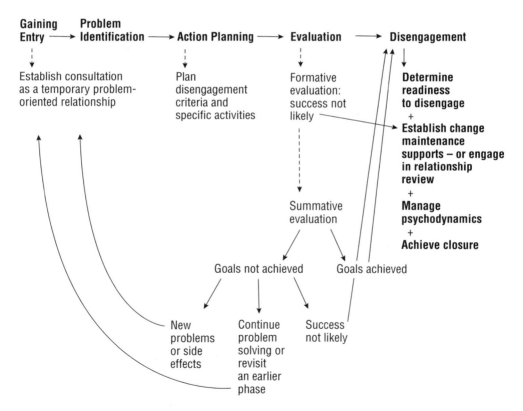

Figure 14-1   Disengagement in Nursing Consultation.
While disengagement is a distinct phase in the nursing consultation process, the foundation for successful disengagement is laid during the gaining entry and action planning phases of the nursing consultation process. Information from both formative and summative evaluation activities helps a nurse consultant and consultees decide whether to proceed with disengagement activities or revisit an earlier phase in the nursing consultation process.

A NURSE CONSULTANT'S TASKS IN DISENGAGEMENT

Nursing consultation is characterized by a peer relationship between a nurse consultant and consultees; that is, the nurse consultant and consultees share responsibility for completing the tasks of each of the phases of the nursing consultation process. The situation is somewhat different in the disengagement phase, in which the nurse consultant assumes primary responsibility for successful task completion. This makes sense because disengagement occurs at a point in the nursing consultation relationship when the consultees need to concentrate on new ways of thinking and new behaviors that will ensure that the nursing consultation problem remains resolved after the nurse consultant leaves the problem setting. To accomplish the goals of the disengagement phase (and thus of the entire nursing consultation process), a nurse consultant must successfully complete four tasks: (1) accurately determine the consultees' readiness to disengage, (2) put supports in place to institutionalize the changes that have occurred as a result of the consultation relationship, (3) manage the psychodynamics that accompany disengagement, and (4) achieve closure or terminate the nursing consultation relationship.

Determining Readiness to Disengage

The activities of the disengagement phase of the nursing consultation process should not begin until both the nurse consultant and consultees agree that the consultation relationship should be terminated. Ideally, this occurs because the goals of the nursing consultation relationship have been achieved and the nurse consultant is no longer of value to the community or client system. However, disengagement is sometimes initiated because it has become clear that a successful outcome

to the nursing consultation relationship is unlikely. In either case, a nurse consultant should be alert for cues or indications that it is time to wind down the consultation relationship.

Information from the summative evaluation of the nursing consultation relationship should provide a nurse consultant with evidence (in terms of consultee behavior and characteristics of the nursing consultation relationship) that it is appropriate to proceed with the tasks of disengagement. Attainment of project goals or acceptance of the nursing consultation action plan is one piece of evidence that suggests it is appropriate to proceed with disengagement. Another cue of readiness to disengage would be consultees' statements about readiness and self-confidence to continue without the nurse consultant (such as, "I think we've got it now"). Evidence that refreezing has occurred and that new behaviors, attitudes, and problem-solving skills have become the norm for consultees and the client system also supports disengagement. The best evidence that it is appropriate to proceed with disengagement is when a nurse consultant hears mutually developed recommendations and conclusions about a problem's cause being verbalized and owned by the consultees (Monicken, 1995). An undesirable but nonetheless important indicator of readiness to begin disengagement is evidence that consultees are growing more dependent on the consultation relationship in spite of new problem-solving abilities and goal achievement. Increased dependence is suggested by consultee passivity and withdrawal from problem-solving activities and by "stall tactics" such as the reappearance of previously resolved resistance to the problem solution and the changes it implies.

As an example of how readiness to disengage might present itself, consider the scenario of a nurse consultant who has been working with a domestic violence program to help it secure mental health services for women in the program. One indicator of readiness to disengage could be letters of agreement from several mental health service providers to accept referrals from the domestic violence program. Another cue would be an actual increase in the number of women in the program who receive mental health services. In contrast, increased or continuing reliance on the nurse consultant for assistance making referrals could indicate dependency and a need to begin disengagement activities as a strategy to promote the program's self-reliance and future problem-solving skills. In this case, however, a lack of provider willingness to see referrals or women's dissatisfaction with the referral network would need to be ruled out as explanations for what appears to be dependency.

Sometimes, the disengagement phase needs to begin because there is evidence that success is unlikely in a particular nursing consultation relationship. This conclusion may result from either formative or summative evaluation findings. Evidence that success is unlikely in a nursing consultation relationship includes consultees' withdrawal from problem-solving activities, unfulfilled promises of community support for problem-solving resources and activities, and verbalization by consultees (or other influential parties in the community) that the nursing consultation problem no longer exists. Continuing a nursing consultation relationship under these circumstances only serves to meet the needs of the nurse consultant.

The preceding point is especially important, for a nurse consultant needs to be alert for indications of becoming too enmeshed with consultees or in the client system. The danger of prolonging the nursing consultation relationship in this situation is that the nurse consultant loses objectivity and, consequently, becomes less helpful in problem solving. When a nurse consultant trades empathy for emotional enmeshment with a consultee, problem solutions that are developed are less likely to take into account the needs of the community or client system and more likely to

be developed to meet needs of the nurse consultant. Nurses who are providing consultation in emotionally charged problem situations that are similar to situations they have lived through (e.g., downsizing and work redesign) are particularly at risk for becoming enmeshed with consultees and losing their objectivity. Again, this is an indication to initiate disengagement activities and, possibly, turn the situation over to another nurse consultant.

Box 14-1 summarizes indicators of readiness to disengage.

Maintaining Change

A nurse consultant's second task in the disengagement phase is to develop strategies that will enable the client system to maintain or institutionalize the changes that have occurred as a result of the nursing consultation relationship. Reduced involvement, intermittent follow-up, and the development of "continuity supports" are typical change maintenance strategies that are used by nurse consultants (Lippitt & Lippitt, 1986).

Reduced Involvement
Reducing involvement with consultees and the community forces the consultees to take on more responsibility for ongoing problem solving. A nurse consultant's contact with the consultees should not abruptly drop to zero, but should decrease gradually and strategically as consultees demonstrate more skill and self-confidence. For example, a nurse who has been providing consultation to a community agency might first decrease full-time involvement and presence in the agency to daily "drop-in" contact. The next step might be to only attend staff meetings rather than have a predictable presence in the agency. A nurse consultant needs to keep in mind that decreasing involvement means reducing regular presence within a client system but not eliminating availability to deal with problems that may arise during the disengagement phase.

BOX 14-1   WHEN TO DISENGAGE

A nurse consultant's sense of timing is a key factor in successful disengagement. A nurse consultant needs to be alert for the following cues that indicate it is appropriate to proceed with the disengagement phase of the nursing consultation process:

- Attainment of the goals of the nursing consultation relationship
- Refreezing has occurred; new behaviors and problem-solving skills have become the norm for the consultees and client system
- Consultee dependency
- Success in the consultation relationship is unlikely even with recycling to an earlier phase
- The nurse consultant is becoming enmeshed with the consultees and client system or community and is losing objectivity

Intermittent Follow-up

While disengagement requires a nurse consultant to reduce contact with consultees and a client system, this phase also involves planned intermittent follow-up or checking back with consultees and other community members. Intermittent follow-up (e.g., by e-mail) that is initiated by the nurse consultant facilitates early discovery of possible difficulties with a problem solution that is being implemented. Intermittent follow-up, therefore, provides a nurse consultant and consultees with opportunities to salvage an action plan that is not as effective as had been anticipated. Follow-up also demonstrates a nurse consultant's continued availability for assistance with problem solving and provides the opportunity to give positive feedback. Finally, follow-up that is initiated by the nurse consultant enables consultees to save face by not needing to ask for help at a time when increased capability at problem solving is supposed to be demonstrated.

Continuity Supports

Continuity supports are situation-specific mechanisms developed and put into place to help ensure that the consultees and other members of the community or client system don't regress to old patterns of thinking and behaving once the nursing consultation relationship has ended. Continuity supports also help prevent the development of counterreactions to the changes in the community that have occurred as a result of the nursing consultation process.

Training a consultee or another influential member of the community to be an internal consultant or "change maintainer" is one continuity support strategy. As an example of this strategy, an external nurse consultant who has been working with the nursing staff of two rival home health care agencies as they merge their services could train one or two of the nurses in group facilitation and mediation skills. This particular type of continuity support might be appropriate because communication problems, value conflicts, and power struggles are most likely to be the issues that will compromise the ability of these two former competitors to work together.

Another strategy that can be used as a continuity support is a "minimum periodic maintenance plan." A minimum periodic maintenance plan is a regular schedule of self-evaluation that is undertaken by consultees to make sure that the performance objectives established during the nursing consultation action plan continue to be met. This continuity support strategy might be promoted by a nurse who has been providing consultation to a school that is developing a school-based clinic. Clinic staff could be assisted to develop an audit process for periodically gathering, analyzing, and responding to data on effectiveness indicators such as utilization of clinic services, types of problems seen, number of referrals made, and student and parent satisfaction with the clinic.

Yet a third continuity support strategy that can be put into place by a nurse consultant is referral of consultees to an informal resource for ongoing support. This strategy is appropriate when change maintenance is likely to require ongoing external support that it is unrealistic for the nurse consultant to provide. This strategy might be used by a nurse consultant who has been providing consultation to a group of public health nurses in regard to adopting critical pathways for their high-risk maternity patients. In this case, the nurse consultant might use referral to a public health department consultee in another community that has successfully implemented critical pathways as a strategy for continuity support.

Finally, nurse consultants can take advantage of technology as a means of providing continuity suppot. A nurse consultant could develop a Web site with hyperlinks to articles and resources of interest, could conduct online chat sessions with consultees, and could use a listserv to distribute automatic updates on topics of interests to consultees.

Managing the Psychodynamics of Disengagement

Disengagement can trigger a variety of emotions in consultees. Most commonly, disengagement triggers feelings of inadequacy and abandonment. These emotions can result in dependency behaviors, withdrawal, passivity, or increased conflict within the group of con-

sultees of the larger community. The emotions triggered by disengagement activities and consultees' reactions to these emotions are referred to as the "psychodynamics of disengagement." A nurse consultant's third task in the disengagement phase is to manage these psychodynamics so that consultees aren't overpowered by them to the extent that there is regression to old habits and former patterns of behavior.

A nurse consultant should inform consultees about the anticipated timeline for disengagement. By doing so, a nurse consultant may prevent or allay some of the consultees' feelings of abandonment. A "weaning period" of gradually reduced frequency and intensity of contact between the nurse consultant and consultees can also ease these feelings. A nurse consultant can also attempt to decrease the stress of disengagement by leaving the door open for future consultation with the consultees and community.

A nurse consultant can respond to the feelings of inadequacy that arise in consultees as the disengagement process gets under way by providing reassurance and evidence to consultees about their readiness to disengage. A nurse consultant can also remind consultees that proceeding with disengagement is actually a vote of confidence about their abilities to maintain the changes that have been put in place during the nursing consultation relationship.

Continuity supports that have been developed as change maintenance strategies can also be used to respond to the psychodynamics of the disengagement phase. Consider how the continuity supports described in the previous nursing consultation scenarios might also be used to help manage the psychodynamics of the disengagement phase:

• In the first scenario, the nurse consultant working with the merging home health care agencies might anticipate increased interstaff conflict once termination of the nursing consultation relationship becomes apparent. With the nurse consultant present less frequently, the competing staffs might each believe that now is their last chance for hanging on to their former ways of doing things. Staff members who have been trained in mediation skills could help the nurses respond to these reactions.

- The second scenario was about a nurse consultant working with a school to develop a school-based clinic. This client system might feel overwhelmed and perceive decreased contact with the nurse consultant as abandonment. Periodic drop-in visits and telephone or e-mail contact on the part of the nurse consultant could help the clinical staff feel more secure and less alone.
- The public health nurses might respond to disengagement with passive resistance and might perceive decreased contact as an opportunity to regress to former ways of delivering care. Periodic self-evaluation and feedback in the form of a chart audit could serve to hold the nurses accountable for the patient care outcomes intended by the critical pathways.

Achieving Closure

A nurse consultant's final task in the disengagement phase is to achieve closure of the nursing consultation relationship. Achieving closure acknowledges both the problem solving that has occurred and the interpersonal relationships that have developed during the course of the consultation process. Closure activities require a degree of intentionality so that both the nurse consultant and the consultees have a sense of satisfaction and pride about what they have accomplished and how it has taken place. Numerous strategies and rituals can be used to facilitate closure, the scope of these activities being limited only by

the creativity of the nurse consultant. Closure activities must also be sensitive to the culture of the community or client system.

A final consultation report is one strategy that can be used to formally signal the transfer of responsibility for maintaining change and ongoing problem solving to the consultees. A final report generally includes an overview of what has occurred and been accomplished during the consultation process, acknowledgment of persons and processes that have contributed to success, and the nurse consultant's thoughts about what the future holds and issues that need ongoing attention. A final "closure report" typically ends with a thank you for the consultation opportunity and an offer to be of future assistance.

Other termination strategies can be more symbolic indicators of the completion of a change process—a celebration, a mock funeral, a ceremonial discarding of old equipment, and so forth. Consider how these types of closure strategies might be incorporated into the disengagement phase of the nursing consultation scenarios used earlier in this chapter:

- In the home health care agency merger scenario, closure could involve an open house of the facility, introduction of a new logo, and new equipment bags for staff, as well as a final report.
- The nurse consultant who has been providing consultation to the school-based clinic could persuade the school district to purchase signage for the clinic and could arrange for a new article or feature on the clinic.
- The nurse consultant who has worked with the public health nurses to implement critical pathways could stage a closure celebration that includes shredding old chart forms and opening packages of new forms.

Strategies for successful disengagement are summarized in Box 14-2.

BOX 14-2   STRATEGIES FOR SUCCESSFUL DISENGAGEMENT

- Know when it is time to leave.
- Provide warning that termination is forthcoming; be specific about when, why, and how it will be done.
- Explain what has happened as a result of the nursing consultation relationship; consider goals that have been met as well as other changes in the culture and climate of the client system that have occurred.
- Recognize members and processes of the community or client system that have been especially helpful; be generous with thank yous.
- Share recommendations for reinforcing the changes that have occurred.
- Celebrate successes.
- Always leave the door open for future contact.

POSSIBLE DIFFICULTIES IN DISENGAGEMENT

As is the case with the other phases of the nursing consultation process, difficulties can arise during disengagement. These difficulties, if not resolved, can undermine successful disengagement. Timing issues and role-related dilemmas are two potential threats to successful disengagement. Another difficulty a nurse consultant may need to face is that of needing to complete the disengagement phase when the nursing consultation relationship has been unsuccessful.

Timing

Even the most carefully planned disengagement phase can end up being ineffective if it is carried out too soon or not soon enough. All too often, disengagement activities are premature. Ending a nursing consultation relationship is sometimes seen by either the nurse consultant or consultees as the best or easiest way out of a consultation relationship or project that is not progressing as anticipated. In other situations, starting disengage-

ment too soon reflects a desire by either the nurse consultant or consultees to "bail out" when the going is getting rough and the consultation relationship is becoming characterized by conflict and confrontation. Nurse consultants who are working with consultees about process issues (communication patterns, power, values, interpersonal dynamics, etc.) are at particular risk for beginning disengagement activities too soon or carrying them out over too short a period of time. At the same time, consultees in these situations can pressure a nurse consultant to disengage before readiness is actually present.

Terminating a nursing consultation relationship too soon can have negative consequences for both the nurse consultant and consultees. When disengagement occurs too soon or is rushed, consultees are at risk for regressing to old patterns of behavior. When this occurs, everything that has been accomplished during the nursing consultation relationship can become undone. Once a nurse consultant leaves the client system, it is easy for the consultees to blame the nurse consultant for this "failure." When consultees return to business as usual with a current consultation problem unresolved, more problems are likely to follow because consultees have probably not incorporated problem-solving skills into daily behavior patterns (Kurpius et al., 1993).

Sometimes, disengagement does not begin soon enough or is stretched out over too long a period of time. Dependency needs on the part of either the nurse consultant or consultees are usually the forces behind this situation. For a nurse consultant, there is somewhat of a conflict of interest in disengagement because ending a consultation relationship means ending any consultation-related fees or benefits. Delaying disengagement, then, can reflect financial as well as psychological dependency needs. A nurse who is working as an internal consultant might be tempted to delay disengagement in order to prolong possible benefits such as better work hours, prestige, and avoidance of regular work responsibilities.

A key question to ask in regard to the timing of disengagement is whose and what needs are being met by the push to disengage or delay disengagement. In other words, is the timing of disengagement activities optimum for ultimate success of the nursing consultation relationship or does it reflect other issues and other needs?

Role-Related Dilemmas

Some difficulties that arise during the disengagement phase reflect the uniqueness of each nursing consultation situation as well as how a nurse has been enacting the consultant role.

For an external nurse consultant, disengagement and termination might be misinterpreted by consultees as meaning that the nurse consultant is no longer available to provide help with problems. Unless this is the message the nurse consultant intends, care must be taken that this is not the message that is inadvertently conveyed. Another difficulty

frequently faced by external nurse consultants is a lack of any opportunity to see the long-term consequences of their efforts. To some extent, this is simply inherent in the nature of any consultation relationship. However, formal post-termination follow-up can be built into both evaluation and disengagement plans. Also, less formal follow-up opportunities are generally present through networking, mutual acquaintances, and professional activities.

A nurse who has been functioning as an internal consultant generally has the opportunity to observe the outcomes of the nursing consultation relationship; the trade-off is that there is no real opportunity (other than quitting!) to exit the client system. This can create the dilemma of being perceived as continuously available for troubleshooting, problem solving, and giving advice. Initially, this may be somewhat flattering. Constant availability for problem solving, though, can foster dependency in both the nurse consultant and the client system. It can also create role conflicts and place substantial and generally uncompensated demands on the nurse consultant's time if it goes unchecked. Parameters of postconsultation availability need to be made explicit in the nursing consultation contract.

Nurse practitioners and other direct care providers who consult with patient groups or families need to be aware that disengagement and termination can be perceived as abandonment by consultees and clients. While disengagement activities should always be mutually planned and agreed on, it is especially critical that nurse practitioners communicate to their consultees and clients that it is only a specific problem-solving relationship, not the entire practitioner–patient or care provider relationship, that is the focus of disengagement. Completely terminating a care provider relationship with a patient involves its own specific and legally prescribed set of disengagement activities.

DISENGAGEMENT IN UNSUCCESSFUL NURSING CONSULTATION RELATIONSHIPS

Unfortunately, not all nursing consultation relationships are successful in terms of resolving the consultees' presenting problem. A disengagement phase still needs to occur in unsuccessful situations, but the disengagement task of maintaining change is replaced by the task of relationship review. In other words, the focus of disengagement in an unsuccessful nursing consultation relationship is determining what went wrong in the relationship.

To accomplish a relationship review, the nurse consultant and consultees should together review what happened during each phase of the nursing consultation process. Sometimes what is discovered is that elements from each phase of the consultation process contributed to the "failure" by having an additive effect. It is more likely, though, that some of the foundational conditions for a successful consultation relationship were missing. Box 14-3 presents questions a nurse consultant can use to guide the disengagement phase in an unsuccessful nursing consultation relationship.

There is a tendency by both a nurse con-

BOX 14-3   RELATIONSHIP REVIEW: THE DISENGAGEMENT PHASE IN UNSUCCESSFUL NURSING CONSULTATION RELATIONSHIPS

The focus of a relationship review is figuring out the reason for the unsuccessful consultation relationship by systematically reviewing what happened during each phase of the nursing consultation process. The following questions should be asked:

- Were the right conditions in place for the nursing consultation interaction pattern that was used?
- Were the implicit expectations of the nursing consultation relationship made explicit in the contract?
- Were the tasks of each phase in the nursing consultation process carried out completely?
- Was there an effective working relationship between the nurse consultant, the consultees, and other members of the client system? That is, had the nurse consultant achieved psychological entry into the client system?
- Were there quality data on which to base both conclusions about a problem's cause and feasible solutions?
- Was the problem definition accurate and owned by consultees?
- How ready and willing were the consultees and client system/community to problem solve and change?
- Were the system supports needed for change in place?
- Were the consultation goals and action plan jointly developed by the nurse consultant and consultees? Were the goals and action plan owned by the consultees? Were proposed goals meaningful and feasible for the client system?
- Did evaluation occur on an ongoing basis? Were the results used?

BOX 14-4   DOCUMENTATION CHECKLIST: THE DISENGAGEMENT PHASE

☐ Evidence of readiness to disengage—identify specific indicators, as well as who initiated disengagement

☐ Anticipated timeline for the disengagement phase

☐ Pattern of reduced involvement—describe, give rationale, document consultee reaction to this decision as well as reactions to subsequent interactions

☐ Intermittent follow-up activities—date, purpose, who initiated, what occurred

☐ Continuity supports—describe, give rationale

☐ Psychodynamics that occurred during disengagement—how they were responded to, results of nurse consultant's response

☐ Closure activities—date, describe activity and response, attach copy of final consultation report

☐ Difficulties encountered—how they were addressed, whether they were resolved

sultant and consultees to want to rush disengagement activities when a nursing consultation relationship has been unsuccessful. This reflects a cultural tendency to overvalue success and undervalue failure. Rushing through the disengagement phase of an unsuccessful nursing consultation relationship ignores that learning can occur in both positive and negative situations. What is learned from an unsuccessful consultation relationship can be used by a nurse consultant to increase the likelihood of success in future relationships.

DOCUMENTING THE DISENGAGEMENT PHASE

Because a nursing consultation relationship essentially ends once the tasks of the disengagement phase have been completed, it is tempting to overlook documentation responsibilities for this phase of the consultation process. However, documentation is as important in the disengagement phase as it is in earlier phases of the nursing consultation process, for what it can provide a nurse con-

sultant in terms of reminders (what has been done and what needs to be done next) and a learning device (what works and what doesn't). In addition, documentation can provide a nurse consultant with evidence to counter possible charges of premature or delayed closure of the consultation relationship or charges of abandonment. Box 14-4 is a checklist for documenting the disengagement phase of the nursing consultation process.

CHAPTER SUMMARY

The disengagement phase of the nursing consultation process is a time of letting go and an opportunity for a nurse consultant and consultees to celebrate success, acknowledge the problem-solving skills and relationships that have developed, secure the future, and learn from mistakes.

While the onset of the activities of the disengagement phase usually coincides with the presentation of findings from the summative evaluation of the nursing consultation process, the groundwork for disengagement is laid much earlier. The specific tasks of the disengagement phase—identifying readiness to disengage, developing strategies to maintain change, managing the psychodynamics of disengagement, and achieving closure—are intended to prevent dependency and ensure the continuity of changes and problem solving that have occurred. In an unsuccessful nursing consultation relationship, completion of the disengagement phase can provide a nurse consultant and consultees with insight about what needed conditions of a successful consulting relationship were lacking. When disengagement is thoughtfully planned and carefully implemented, both the nurse consultant and consultees should leave the consultation relationship with a sense of satisfaction about what has been accomplished.

APPLYING CHAPTER CONTENT

Develop a checklist of skills and outcome criteria needed for successful disengagement for a consultation scenario that is typical of those in which you are most likely to be involved. Compare your list to those developed by students in other practice roles. Which skills and effectiveness criteria seem to be universal and which seem to be role specific? How can you explain these differences?

References

Barron, A. (1989). The CNS as consultant. In A. Hamric & J. Spross (Eds.), *The clinical nurse specialist in theory and practice* (2nd ed.) (pp. 125–146). Philadelphia: Saunders.

Helvie, C. (1998). *Advanced practice nursing in the community.* Thousand Oaks, CA: Sage.

Kurpius, D., Fuqua, D., & Rozecki, T. (1993). The consulting process: A multidimensional approach. *Journal of Counseling and Development, 71,* 601–606.

Lippitt, G., & Lippitt, R. (1986). *The consulting process in action* (2nd ed.). San Diego: University Associates.

Monicken, D. (1995). Consultation in advanced practice nursing. In M. Snyder & M. Mirr (Eds.), *Advanced practice nursing: A guide to professional development* (pp. 183–195). New York: Springer.

Ross, G. (1993). Peter Block's Flawless Consulting and the Homunculus Theory: Within each person is a perfect consultant. *Journal of Counseling & Development, 71,* 639–641.

Schein, E. (1987). *Process consultation, volume II: Lessons for managers and consultants.* Reading, MA: Addison-Wesley.

PROFESSIONAL ISSUES
IN NURSING CONSULTATION

Legal Aspects
of Nursing Consultation

The more one considers some of the legal ramifications of the issues we've raised in this section, the clearer it becomes that most matters are not neatly defined. (Corey, Corey, & Calanan, 1984)

 ## KEY CONCEPTS:

liability, negligence, malpractice, reasonable prudence, duty, tort

 ## KEY TERMS FOR YOUR SEARCH ENGINE:

consultation and liability

INTRODUCTION

One of my first consulting experiences involved working with a physician to develop data collection strategies and plan data analyses for a research project about outcomes among women who had taken part in an inpatient substance abuse treatment program while they were pregnant. I wrote a letter agreeing to this opportunity (initial contact had been made over the telephone) and outlining my fees and reimbursement expectations for expenses. I then developed a series of data collection instruments (the women were to be followed for 18 months) that the consultee accepted. Following this, I traveled (a 400-mile round trip by car) to meet with the con-

sultee and other involved individuals to finalize study protocols. When I returned home, I submitted an itemized bill for my services and expenses to date. At the bottom of this bill were the words "Net 15 days," the same terms that had been stated in my original letter of understanding. Fifteen, thirty, sixty, and then ninety days passed without receiving payment. Over the next six months, I shared my frustrations with colleagues, made numerous telephone calls, and sent several registered letters to the consultee. Finally, I was paid. I have not heard from the consultee since.

So, what did I learn from this experience? First, I learned that despite my initial doubts, I

269

did have a legal contract with the consultee. Second, I learned to always have a mutually *signed* contract. Throughout this experience, however, I worried about liability issues related to confidentiality, breach of contract, abandonment, and fee collection. I also worried about the effect this incident would have on my reputation as a beginning nurse consultant.

Professional liability is a fundamental issue all nurse consultants must consider in order to be perceived as professionals as well as to protect professional and personal interests. While nurses working as external consultants are most likely to have concerns about these issues, the same issues, with just slight modification, also need attention by nurses who function as internal consultants.

This chapter introduces the legal issues with which nurse consultants are most likely to contend. The chapter begins by reviewing basic legal concepts and terminology, and applying these concepts to the practice of nursing consultation. The next section dis-cusses common causes of legal action against nurse consultants. Following this, issues about which a nurse consultant might initiate legal action against a consultee are considered. The final section explores self-protection strategies for nurse consultants. Think about the following questions as you read this chapter:

- How are the concepts of malpractice and confidentiality similar in clinical nursing practice and in nursing consultation? How are they different?
- In what ways are professional and legal standards of practice similar in clinical nursing practice and in nursing consultation? In what ways are they different?
- How are internal and external nursing consultation situations different in terms of risk of liability?
- How might self-protection strategies vary for internal and external nurse consultants?

BASIC LEGAL CONCEPTS AND TERMINOLOGY

Expanded roles in nursing practice, such as that of nurse consultant, promise increased autonomy for nurses. However, these roles also carry increased responsibility, accountability, and professional liability. As nurse consultants continue to gain recognition for their expertise and the positive contributions they make to health care delivery, they increasingly find themselves being held legally accountable for their specialized knowledge and problem-solving skills. The dilemma with this is that consultation in general, and nursing consultation in particular, is only an "emerging profession" (Dougherty, 1995). Thus, there are relatively few precedents to guide the courts when consultants encounter legal entanglements. Avoiding legal entanglements as a nurse consultant is facilitated by an awareness of the behaviors that can precipitate legal action. This requires an understanding of basic legal concepts and terminology.

Negligence and Malpractice

The terms *negligence* and *malpractice* are often used interchangeably. Negligence refers to the "omission to do something which a reasonable person guided by those ordinary considerations which ordinarily regulate human affairs, would do, or the doing of something a reasonable and prudent person would not do" (*Schneider v. Little Co.*, 1915, cited in Gardner & Hagedorn, 1997). Negligence, therefore, can take two forms: crimes of omission and crimes of commission.

Malpractice refers to professional negligence or to misconduct by a professional (Gardner & Hagedorn, 1996). In order for a charge of professional negligence or malpractice to be upheld, the plaintiff (e.g., a consultee) must establish each of the following four elements:

1. *Duty*—the obligation toward another to comply with a particular standard of conduct. Duty can be demonstrated by a contract or implied by the nature of a relationship. In nursing consultation, the nurse consultant's duty may be toward the consultee, the client, a patient or patient group that is a stakeholder, the contact person, or an organization or community as a whole. Because there are no clear-cut legal answers to the questions of liability in a nursing consultation relationship, the important question is whether a nurse–patient relationship exists, thereby invoking the duty of care. If such as relationship exists—and this would be a question of fact in a court of law—then liability attaches. If payment is received for consultation services or a nurse consultant interacts directly with clients, there is increased likelihood that a nurse–patient relationship (and therefore duty) exists (Barron & White, 2000). Chapter 16 discusses ethical dilemmas related to the concept of duty.
2. *Breach of duty*—failure to uphold a contract. The contract can be actual or implied. When a breach of duty occurs, a promise has essentially been broken. Negligence is one form of breach of duty since the "promise" to act as a professional is not upheld when negligence occurs.
3. *Harm or damages*—suffering some sort of loss. Loss can be physical, emotional/psychological, or financial.
4. *Causation*—the existence of a causal link between the breach of duty and the damages suffered by the plaintiff (Dougherty, 1995; Gardner & Hagedorn, 1997; McCarthy & Sorenson, 1993; Scott & Beare, 1993).

Embedded in the concepts of negligence and malpractice is the "reasonable person rule." That is, negligence represents departure of a defendant's behavior from that expected by a reasonably prudent person. In professional malpractice, the reasonably prudent person to whom a defendant is compared is another professional (in this case, a nurse consultant) who reflects the degree of knowledge and skill that is customary among other professionals practicing in the same area under the same or similar circumstances (Brent, 1997; Corey et al., 1984; Dougherty, 1995; Gardner & Hagedorn, 1997). It is important to note that reasonable prudence is not a static concept but, rather, reflects the circumstances of the professional relationship as well as current research, technology, and social expectations.

To summarize, in nursing consultation, professional negligence (i.e., malpractice) occurs when there is lack of "reasonable" or "ordinary" application of the nursing consultation process that results in injury to consultees, the client, or another member of the community or client system. Professional negligence can arise from two types of situations:

- A failure to possess the requisite skill and knowledge to fulfill an accepted consultation contract or not knowing what to do when a reasonably prudent nurse consultant would
- A failure to use judgment in applying one's knowledge and exercising one's skills in the implementation of the nursing consultation process or knowing what to do but not doing it, or doing it carelessly (Brent, 1997; Gardner & Hagedorn, 1996).

Tort Law, Civil Law, and Criminal Law

A tort is a legal wrong, not involving a breach of contract, that causes injury to another and for which the person committing the wrong can be held liable for damages in a civil suit. Professional negligence is the legal wrong that most often results in damages (Brent, 1997; Gardner & Hagedorn, 1997).

Civil actions differ from criminal actions in terms of purpose, the courts of law in which they are tried, and the standard of proof that is required. The purpose of a civil action is to obtain monetary compensation for damages suffered. In contrast, the purpose of criminal action is to punish the wrongdoer and deter repeated offensive conduct. Civil damages are awarded on the basis of a preponderance of evidence or certainty (of guilt) as established by an expert witness who is "competent and qualified to render such an opinion" (Gardner & Hagedorn, 1997). In nursing consultation, the expert witness would need to be another nurse consultant with similar expertise and credentials. By comparison, guilt in a criminal case requires proof beyond a reasonable doubt.

Professional negligence or malpractice reflects mistakes, inattention, and inexperience and is generally not considered a crime. In order to be considered a crime, malpractice needs to be accompanied by malice and/or wanton misconduct: that is, "an unconscious indifference to consequences" or "reckless disregard for the rights and safety of others" (Gardner & Hagedorn, 1997).

Statutes of Limitations

A statute of limitations is "the time limit during which a person, having a cause of action for damages due to professional negligence, is required to file a lawsuit" (Gardner & Hagedorn, 1997). After the statute of limitations has expired, a lawsuit may not be filed.

Time limits for statutes of limitations vary from state to state; most range from one to six years. The event to which the statute of limitations applies also varies by state. In some states, the statute of limitations is applied to the date of the activity that is alleged to have caused the injury. Other states apply the

statute of limitations to the date of discovery of injury.

Usually, the date of discovery refers to the date that the plaintiff first knew or should have known of the injury. In some states, however, the date of discovery is applied to the date on which the plaintiff learned of the cause of the injury—for example, that it was linked to the nurse consultant's actions (Gardner & Hagedorn, 1997). Because of variations in statutes of limitations as well as differences in terms of exactly to which event they apply, nurse consultants need to familiarize themselves with their state laws.

CAUSES OF LEGAL ACTION AGAINST NURSE CONSULTANTS

Currently, there are no records (i.e., case law and accompanying commentary) of legal action against nurse consultants. This could reflect several situations: (a) the actual lack of legal action against nurse consultants, (b) the possibility that nurse consultants identify themselves by other titles (e.g., management consultant, educator-trainer, or clinical nurse specialist), or (c) out-of-court settlement of threatened legal actions against nurse consultants. Regardless, areas that are legally problematic for other nurses in advanced and expanded roles and human resource consultants (i.e., consultants who work with schools and social service agencies) are instructive and applicable to nurse consultants.

Among human service consultants, lack of skill is the most common cause of malpractice (Dougherty, 1995). Other common causes of legal action against human service consultants are identified in Box 15-1. This list suggests that legal action can be brought against nurse consultants for behaviors related to implementation of the nursing consultation process as well as for behaviors related to the conduct of a nursing consultation (business) practice.

BOX 15-1   COMMON CAUSES OF LEGAL ACTION AGAINST HUMAN SERVICE CONSULTANTS

The following behaviors associated with legal problems for human service consultants can also create legal problems for nurse consultants:

- Use of improper assessment and diagnostic techniques
- Breach of contract
- Breach of confidentiality
- Misrepresentation of one's skills or credentials as a consultant
- Failure to consult with others about difficult cases
- Giving poor advice
- Failure to respect consultees' (or a community's) integrity and privacy
- Inappropriate public statements
- Lack of informed consent
- Poor record keeping
- Use of inappropriate methods to collect fees

Sources: Corey, G., Corey, M., & Calanan, P. (1984). *Issues and ethics in the helping professions* (3rd ed.). Pacific Grove, CA: Brooks-Cole; and Dougherty, A. (1995). *Consultation: Practice and perspectives in school and community settings* (2nd ed.). Pacific Grove, CA: Brooks-Cole.

Behaviors Related to Implementation of the Nursing Consultation Process

The nursing consultation process is a systematic way of working with consultees to help them resolve problems related to the health status of clients (individuals, a community, or an organization) and health care delivery. Although it has been stressed throughout this text that the consultees remain responsible for the outcome of the nursing consultation relationship, it is imperative that nurse consultants appreciate they are accountable for their practice relative to the consultation problem. The overall responsibilities of a nurse consultant can be summarized as gathering accurate data regarding the consultation problem or letting consultees know that data are not complete, making reasonable

recommendations, and giving good advice (Barron & White, 2000). Conscientiously attending to the details of the nursing consultation process increases the likelihood of successful problem resolution and adherence to professional standards of practice. Behaviors related to implementation of the nursing consultation process that can prompt legal action against nurse consultants include malpractice, breach of contract, and breach of confidentiality.

Malpractice

Charges of malpractice can be brought against a nurse consultant when incomplete, ineffective, or inappropriate implementation of the nursing consultation process has resulted in harm to the plaintiff. As mentioned earlier, the plaintiff in a malpractice suit against a nurse consultant could be the consultees, the client, the client system (e.g., a community or organization), or a stakeholder. Because one of the conditions necessary for a charge of malpractice to be valid is breach of contract, a malpractice suit is usually initiated by whomever signed the contract as the "consumer" of the nursing consultation services. Contracts, however, do not necessarily need to be written and can be implied by the nature of a professional relationship (e.g., giving some sort of professional help). This opens up the possibility of malpractice charges by additional parties involved in the nursing consultation relationship.

Novice consultants are at particular risk for malpractice stemming from ineffective implementation of the nursing consultation process. This is because expertise in a clinical specialty area does not necessarily translate into expertise in the process or human process issues of nursing consultation (Alvarez, 1993). Malpractice can result from actions or "misactions" during any phase of the nursing consultation process. Examples of actions in each phase of the nursing consultation process that could result in a charge of malpractice include the following:

• Gaining entry—contracting for consultation projects for which one is not qualified
• Problem identification—incomplete data collection, incomplete analysis, or inaccurate interpretation of assessment data
• Action planning—giving bad advice or proposing problem solutions that would cause harm to the client system if implemented (this often results from failure to assess or take into consideration the resources and culture of the client system)
• Evaluation—failure to monitor the consultation process (particularly for side effects) or to revise the nursing consultation process on the basis of evaluation feedback
• Disengagement—abandoning the consultee or client system without warning, failure to put continuity supports into place

Box 15-2 provides an example of ineffective implementation of the nursing consultation process.

Another potential source of malpractice action against nurse consultants is behaviors that reflect a possible confusion between ethical and legal duties. Activities that are legal or legally required may not seem ethical. Conversely, activities that seem ethical may not be legal. If a legal mandate applies to a problem or issue, however, it takes precedence over ethical or other concerns (McCarthy & Sorenson, 1993). Ethical dilemmas in nursing consultation are discussed in Chapter 16.

Breach of Contract

Failure to adhere to the terms of the nursing consultation contract can also prompt legal action against a nurse consultant. Breach of contract may or may not constitute malpractice since negligence is only one form of breach of contract. Typical situations that result in claims of breach of contract (which would not be considered negligence or malpractice) include:

• Failure to adhere to the timeline specified in the nursing consultation contract
• Cost overruns
• Failure to achieve promised results such as specified savings or increased productivity
• Failure to implement the nursing consultation process in the manner outlined in the contract; for example, not involving consultees when such involvement was specified in the contract

These situations point to the need for a contract to be written with some degree of flexibility rather than in absolute terms—for example, citing estimated or a range of costs and time needed. These situations also reinforce the need for including a revision clause in the contract and for regular progress reports to a designated person within the client system.

BOX 15-2   AN EXAMPLE OF INEFFECTIVE IMPLEMENTATION OF THE NURSING CONSULTATION PROCESS

A nurse consultant accepts a contract from a home health care agency to develop a protocol for the assessment and management of clients on tocolytic therapy for preterm labor. At the time of the contract, the agency stated they were in the process of hiring staff with experience in obstetrical nursing. The nurse consultant developed a protocol based on the assumption that the nurses who would be caring for these patients would have obstetrical nursing backgrounds. Part of the protocol consisted of specifying situations in which a patient's physician should be notified immediately.

An agency nurse who did not have a background in obstetrics made a home visit to a woman on tocolytic therapy. She utilized the assessment protocol but made an inappropriate decision in terms of failing to notify a patient's physician. This resulted in an emergency situation for the patient.

The agency claimed that the nurse consultant had not specified that the protocol could only be effectively implemented by nurses with obstetrical experience. The agency also stated that at the time the protocol was written, most of their nurses providing care to perinatal patients did not have a clinical background in obstetrics. They also said they had wanted a protocol that could be used by any home health care nurse since they did not have specialty teams.

In this case, the base line knowledge and skills of agency staff who would be implementing the protocol were not adequately assessed. As a result, the nurse consultant did not have full information on which to develop the protocol. Furthermore, the nurse consultant had failed to communicate with the consultation contact person to verify what the agency really wanted. As a result, a patient was placed in danger, and the nurse consultant could be held legally responsible.

Breach of Confidentiality

Breach of confidentiality as a cause of legal action against nurse consultants deserves special mention. Confidentiality is an ethical and professional as well as an actionable legal principle. In most states, breach of confidentiality is viewed as unprofessional conduct and can be grounds for revocation of certain types of professional licenses (McCarthy & Sorenson, 1993). Nurse consultants need to be familiar with how the issue of confidentiality is addressed by both their state Nurse Practice Act and by any other licensing regulations under which they may be practicing (e.g., dual licensure as a nurse practitioner, counselor, consultant, or social worker).

Nurses who are working as consultants also need to keep in mind and inform their consultees that confidentiality is not absolute. Disclosures may be both appropriate and required, as is the case with child abuse reporting requirements. In cases of known or suspected abuse, a nurse consultant's duty is to disclose information that was given in confidence; failure to disclose this information could precipitate legal action against the nurse consultant. Nurse consultants who work with parent or child consultee groups need to be particularly aware of this issue.

Nurse consultants who work with individual nurse or organizational or community consultees can also become privy to information (e.g., ongoing fraud or plans for a strike) that, if not disclosed, could harm clients or other members of the client system. In this situation, however, confidentiality is an ethical rather than a legal obligation. That is, a nurse consultant is not duty bound to disclose this information. In situations such as this, which are probably more common in nursing consultation, the nurse consultant needs to weigh the risks and benefits of protecting and violating confidentiality. Chapter 16 discusses the ethical considerations related to confidentiality.

Behaviors Related to Conduct of a Nursing Consultation Practice

Legal action can also be brought against a nurse consultant because of consultee (or client or client system) dissatisfaction with the way in which a nurse consultant conducts the business aspect of nursing consultation. Misrepresentation and issues related to fees and their collection are particularly likely to create business-related legal entanglements for a nurse consultant.

Misrepresentation

Misrepresentation is analogous to false advertising. Misrepresentation occurs when a nurse consultant gives inaccurate information about his or her credentials as a consultant, skills and abilities, and/or experience and "track record" as a consultant. Misrepresentation can create problems because it can lead a consultee to hire the wrong consultant for a project. For a nurse consultant, misrepresentation increases the likelihood of accepting a contract for which one is not qualified and setting in motion events that can ultimately lead to charges of professional negligence.

Another dimension of misrepresentation is inaccurately portraying how one conducts the nursing consultation process, including how charges are generated for services. For example, a nurse consultant could misrepresent a fee structure by quoting a "package price," but then billing extra for travel and other expenses.

Fees and Their Collection

Misrepresentation is one way in which fees can create legal entanglements for nurse consultants. Fees can also prompt legal action when a nursing consultation relationship is terminated prematurely or when fee collection becomes problematic.

When a nursing consultation relationship is terminated prematurely, fees are generally prorated or otherwise based on work that has been completed to date. Difficulties with collection arise when there is disagreement or dissatisfaction about the calculation of "early termination fees," usually because there is disagreement about activities for which the nurse consultant should actually be reimbursed. Efforts can be made to prevent this situation by including a clearly written termination clause in the consultation contract, including specification of who will be responsible for prorating fees and determining what activities will be chargeable in an early termination situation. In a consultation relationship that will involve a longer period of time, a nurse consultant may want to bill consultees or the fee payer on an ongoing basis rather than wait until the completion of the contract. This strategy helps a nurse consultant minimize losses should the consultation relationship end prematurely.

Fees can also create legal entanglements for nurse consultants when consultees are dissatisfied with the collection methods being used (e.g., a consultant expecting reimbursement within 15 days). This issue reinforces the need for a nursing consultation contract to clearly identify consultees' responsibilities in regard to fees and for adherence to the terms of the contract. Consultees' (or a community's) dissatisfaction would be warranted if, for example, a contract merely stated that charges would be billed at the completion of the project without specifying a "due and payable" time frame, but the consultee received a statement that specified "net due in 15 days" and was expected and pressured (e.g., charged interest or threatened with referral to a collection agency) to adhere to that time frame.

NURSE CONSULTANTS AS PLAINTIFFS

Thus far, this chapter has focused on behaviors that can prompt legal action against nurse consultants. However, nurse consultants can also find themselves in situations in which they are considering initiating legal action against consultees or a client system. The situations in which nurse consultants are most likely to find themselves giving consideration to assuming the role of plaintiff involve issues related to consultee breach of contract, fees and their collection, and rights to materials generated in the course of the nursing consultation relationship.

Breach of Contract

A nursing consultation contract specifies behavioral expectations and responsibilities for all parties involved in the nursing consultation relationship. Thus, consultees and other members of the client system as well as the nurse consultant have duties in regard to the nursing consultation relationship. Failure on the part of any party involved in the nursing consultation relationship to carry out agreed upon duties constitutes breach of contract.

Failure to make available previously agreed upon information is one situation that could prompt a charge of breach of contract against consultees or a client system. Withholding information can create problems for a nurse

consultant because it means that problem identification and action planning is carried out without full knowledge of both the problem situation and the characteristics of the problem setting. This can cause a nurse consultant to formulate ineffective, and possibly harmful, problem solutions. Failure to provide promised resources (e.g., personnel, meeting time, supplies) that are needed for completion of the nursing consultation contract also constitutes breach of contract.

While nurse consultants may not be able to prevent a breach of contract on the part of consultees or the consultation contact person, they can avoid problems such as malpractice that can arise from the breach by terminating the nursing consultation relationship when a breach occurs, assuming the contract allows for this. Nurse consultants are probably most likely to initiate legal action for breach of contract only as a countersuit strategy against a consultee who has initiated malpractice charges. In other instances, breach of contract results only in termination of the nursing consultation relationship and legal action is avoided because of the possible negative effect it can have on the nurse consultant's reputation.

Fees and Their Collection

Consultees' failure to pay agreed upon fees or to adhere to an agreed upon payment schedule is another form of breach of contract. Problems with fee collection can be referred to a collection agency or pursued through small claims court. Collection agencies are sometimes perceived by consultees as having more "clout" than a nurse consultant in terms of enforcing payment. Use of a collection agency also enables a consultant to avoid the time and hassle of repeated and often increasingly unpleasant follow-up telephone calls and letters. Collection agencies, however, charge for their services and generally keep 50 percent of whatever they collect for themselves.

After other collection strategies have been exhausted, nurse consultants can pursue collection of delinquent accounts through small claims court. Because of attorney expenses and the time away from work that court action entails, most nurse consultants opt not to pursue fees in this manner. Taking consultees to small claims court is also associated with a certain amount of negative publicity that can adversely affect a nurse consultant's practice.

Most consultants accept that they will fail to collect on 10 percent of their accounts (Tepper, 1985). Collection tends to be less of a problem in consulting than in other professions because failure to pay can have negative effects on both the reputation of the client system and the willingness of other consultants to work with them in the future. Strategies for avoiding collection problems are presented in Chapter 17. Billing consultees more frequently for smaller amounts is a particular strategy a nurse consultant can use for "testing" the client system. This practice also results in smaller losses for a nurse consultant if problems with fee collection do arise. A nurse consultant can also avoid escalating losses by stopping work on a project if an agreed upon payment plan is not adhered to. In general, despite the availability of legal recourse for collection problems, most consultants tend to take a loss as a bad debt and move on, wiser for the experience (Lewin, 1995; Tepper, 1985).

Rights to Materials

The third situation that may cause a nurse consultant to consider initiating legal action against consultees or a client system is disagreement about the ownership of materials (e.g., assessment tools and educational materials) generated by the nurse consultant during the course of completing a consultation project. The typical point of disagreement is whether such material belongs to the nurse

consultant as their creator or to the consultees or community/client system who paid the nurse consultant to solve the problem that necessitated the development of such materials. This dilemma arises when the consultation contract fails to identify to whom these materials belong after the consultation relationship is terminated. Nurse consultants who generate materials over which they want to maintain control in terms of access and use can consider copyrighting these materials (Lewin, 1995).

The issue of rights to materials becomes more complicated when a subcontractor is involved in the nursing consultation relationship. Subcontractors are individuals hired by a nurse consultant to assist with a specific component of a consultation project. Subcontractors are generally used to "fill gaps" in the skills needed to complete the project. The issue of rights to materials arises when a subcontractor is hired to create materials for use in the project. The typical point of contention is whether these materials are the property of the subcontractor, the nurse consultant, or the client system. Nurse consultants should deal with this issue proactively by generating a contract or letter of agreement with the subcontractor that addresses this issue (Lewin, 1995).

SELF-PROTECTION STRATEGIES

Things can go awry during even the most carefully planned and implemented consultation relationship. Although consultation is a contracted and service-related relationship, it is also a human relationship. There will always be misunderstandings and disappointed consultees or client systems who blame the nurse consultant for an inevitable or unforeseen outcome, no matter how well a contract has been written. Depending on the consultees, these disappointments may result in litigation or in behavior that causes a nurse consultant to consider legal action against the consultees. In order to protect professional and personal interests in a litigious society, nurse consultants need to engage in self-protection strategies. Self-protection strategies for nurse consultants include preventive measures, legal counsel, and liability insurance.

Preventive Measures

A priori preventive strategies have been emphasized over after-the-fact legal action throughout this chapter. The recurring themes of strategies for avoiding legal entanglements are the following: Establish and maintain open communication and a good working relationship with consultees, know one's limits, have a written contract, incorporate evaluation activities throughout the nursing consultation process, and maintain records of all consultation activities (Alvarez, 1993; Barron & White, 2000; Reinert & Buck, 1989). Specific preventive measures related to these themes are presented in Box 15-3.

Open Communication

Maintaining open communication and a positive working relationship with consultees and

---

BOX 15-3   AVOIDING LEGAL ENTANGLEMENTS AS A NURSE CONSULTANT

Experts agree that the following strategies are helpful for preventing legal action against consultants:

- Always act within your scope of competence, your job description, and your state Nurse Practice Act; know your limits and seek consultation or make referrals appropriately.
- Be sure that any promotional materials provide current and accurate information.
- Be aware of local and state laws that limit your practice of consultation; be familiar with the policies of your employing agency and act within these sets of guidelines.
- Engender positive feelings between yourself and your consultees; be open in your communication with consultees and take an active interest in their welfare; establish a personal consulting policy of personal and professional honesty and openness.
- Establish realistic expectations.
- Be aware of and communicate any limits of confidentiality.
- Use a written and mutually signed contract to clarify your professional relationship with a consultee; present contract information in clear language.
- Discuss fees and their payment at the outset of the nursing consultation relationship.
- Systematically follow the nursing consultation process.
- Provide high-quality service and stand behind it; regularly seek and respond to feedback.
- Keep adequate records; check how long they need to be retained.
- Have access to an attorney for consultation in problematic matters.

Sources: Corey, G., Corey, M., & Calanan, P. (1984*). Issues and ethics in the helping professions* (3rd ed.). Pacific Grove, CA: Brooks-Cole; Dougherty, A. (1995). *Consultation: Practice and perspectives in school and community settings* (2nd ed.). Pacific Grove, CA: Brooks-Cole; and Reinert, B., & Buck, E. (1989). Issues in liability insurance and the nurse consultant. *Clinical Nurse Specialist, 7*(6), 331–334.

other members of a client system helps prevent legal problems that can arise as a result of simple misunderstandings. Consultation is more than applying expert knowledge; it is also the process of communicating that expert knowledge so that consultees understand it, appreciate its importance, and feel empowered enough to use the information independently in the future (Alvarez, 1993).

Communication issues can create problems for a nursing consultation relationship when consultees feel unheard and unserved. Open communication and a positive working relationship is facilitated by paying attention to the details of establishing psychological entry (see Chapter 9) during the gaining entry phase of the nursing consultation process. Open communication is further promoted by ongoing progress meetings with the consultees or community contact person.

Knowing One's Limits

Knowing and respecting one's limits as a nurse consultant and adhering to standards of practice for one's specialty area can help a nurse consultant avoid becoming involved in problem situations that could ultimately result in charges of malpractice due to lack of knowledge or skill (Barron & White, 2000). Knowing and respecting one's limits also means subcontracting, consulting, and referring when a consultation situation progresses beyond the point of personal effectiveness. Finally, knowing and respecting personal limitations helps the nurse consultant avoid legal entanglements that can occur as a result of temptation to misrepresent one's knowledge and skills and accept inappropriate contracts.

Contracts

A contract provides legal protection by clearly delineating the expectations of both parties for the nursing consultation relationship. Thus, a contract should clearly identify agreed upon outcomes as well as provide an opportunity to establish any limits of confidentiality, responsibilities of both the nurse consultant and consultees, and expectations related to fees and their payment. A written contract that is signed by both the nurse consultant and a consultee or designated representative of the community/client system provides evidence that these issues were discussed and agreed upon before the working part of the nursing consultation process got under way. Components and formats of contracts are discussed in Chapter 17.

Evaluation

Evaluation acts as a device for both quality control and legal protection. An evaluation plan and evaluation data can be used in the event of legal action to demonstrate professionalism and fulfillment of contract obligations as well as document a nurse consultant's effectiveness during a project. Documentation of routine peer evaluation of one's consultation practices can also serve as evidence of a nurse consultant's concern for quality service and practicing within one's limits (Reinert & Buck, 1989). Peer feedback in terms of the appropriateness of one's actions also helps establish adherence to professional, reasonable, and prudent standards of practice.

Legal Counsel

Nurse consultants should seek legal counsel whenever they are developing new documents such as contracts for use in their consultation practice. Legal counsel should also be sought when a nurse consultant encounters difficulty implementing or enforcing consultee implementation of the conditions set forth in a contract, especially if such difficulties cannot be resolved by negotiation between the nurse consultant and consultees or contact person. Finally, nurse consultants should obtain legal advice when adverse outcomes are expected to occur or do occur as a result of premature and unilateral contract termination. In this case, legal counsel should be sought before any legal action against a consultee is initiated.

Liability Insurance

Although professional liability insurance cannot prevent charges of malpractice from arising, when legal action does occur, liability insurance can help a nurse consultant avoid devastating financial loss. Insurance carriers view nurses who are practicing in advanced or expanded roles (such as that of consultant) as independent practitioners and raise premiums accordingly (Scott & Beare, 1993). The specific type and amount of insurance a nurse consultant will need depends on the structure of the nursing consultation practice.

Nurses who negotiate a contract for their consultation services and are paid directly are considered self-employed and generally need more extensive and expensive coverage. Nurse consultants who have independent consultation practices may also need business or premise liability insurance (e.g., to protect against a lawsuit that could result from injuries a consultee sustains in a fall on the nurse consultant's business premises) in addition to malpractice insurance (Reinert & Buck, 1989).

Nurses who are practicing as internal consultants may be covered by standard personal professional liability policies. Traditionally,

---

BOX 15-4   TERMS USED IN MALPRACTICE INSURANCE CONTRACTS

Claims-made insurance: This type of insurance policy offers protection against claims that are filed only while the policy is in effect, that is, only while the professional is practicing her or his profession. A "tail" must be purchased to provide coverage against claims based on incidents that occurred during the policy period but filed after the policy has terminated. Claims-made insurance is generally less expensive to purchase than is occurrence coverage since the insurance company is assuming risk only for the duration of the policy.

Occurrence coverage: This type of insurance policy covers claims if the policy was in effect at the time of the incident. The claim itself can be filed after the policy is no longer in effect (e.g., the policyholder has retired from practice or changes insurance carrier) and the policyholder will still be covered. Occurrence coverage is more expensive to purchase than is claims-made coverage since the coverage is inadequate to cover a claim requesting damages in current amounts.

Declarations: The section of an insurance policy that states the limits of liability and the amount of coverage per claim.

Insuring agreements: Identification of what specifically is covered by the policy.

Conditions: Events that must be satisfied before the insurer is obligated to pay for any losses.

Provisions for cancellation: Specification of how the insurance contract can be canceled by either the insured or the carrier.

Sources: Reinert, B., & Buck, E. (1989). Issues in liability insurance and the nurse consultant. *Clinical Nurse Specialist, 3*(1), 42–45; and Scott, L., & Beare, P. (1993). Nurse consultants and professional liability. *Clinical Nurse Specialist, 7*(6), 331–334.

standard professional policies have covered nurses for any duties that are assigned to them by their employer as long as they are functioning within the scope of their state Nurse Practice Act, professional scope of practice, and institutional policies and procedures (Scott & Beare, 1989). It is important, however, that nurse consultants working in the same organization as their consultees (i.e., as an internal nurse consultant) recognize that they have a higher degree of accountability in relation to the situations for which they are providing consultation than do external nurse consultants. Internal nurse consultants are expected to follow through on urgent concerns and problem situations that an external consultant might not be aware of (Barron & White, 2000). Internal nurse consultants need to be familiar with the community or organizational structure within which they are consulting. Internal nurse consultants also need to be sure their consultation responsibilities are consistent with their overall job description and are congruent with their state Nurse Practice Act (Barron & White, 2000).

The laws relating to nursing practice and the availability of malpractice insurance and what it covers are changing rapidly as the health care environment is undergoing reforms. Nurses who are practicing in expanded or advanced practice roles need to check the parameters of their coverage with their carrier. Box 15-4 presents common terms that are used in malpractice insurance contracts. Liability insurance designed specifically for consultants in other disciplines does exist. This insurance is usually available through professional organizations such as the American Psychological Association and the American Management Association. Some nurse consultants hold membership in these or other professional organizations that specifically include consultants so that they can take advantage of the group's malpractice insurance.

CHAPTER SUMMARY

In today's litigious society, nurse consultants are naive if they believe that they don't need to worry about legal entanglements. Protecting oneself from legal action directly and effectively involves taking preventive measures. Another dimension of professional and personal self-protection is knowledge of legal terms and appreciation of the types of situations most likely to prompt legal action. Because the health care and legal environments are constantly and rapidly changing, staying informed and adapting one's practice of nursing consultation are important means of maintaining professional standards of practice and avoiding legal entanglements.

APPLYING CHAPTER CONTENT

1. Analyze the scenario presented in Box 15-2. Critique the nurse consultant's actions and liability issues. Rewrite the scenario to adhere to suggestions for legally protective behavior.
2. Investigate the statute of limitations for professional negligence in your state. What is the time frame for the statue of limitations? To what extent is it applied?
3. Look at your own professional liability insurance policy. Would it cover you (a) as an internal nurse consultant and (b) as an external nurse consultant?

References

Alvarez, C. (1993). Potential liability in good consultative practice. *Clinical Nurse Specialist, 7*(6), 330.

Barron, A., & White, P. (2000). Consultation. In A. Hamric, J. Spross, & C. Hanson (Eds.), *Advanced practice nursing: An inte-*

grative approach (pp. 217–244). Philadelphia: Saunders.

Brent, N. (1997*). Nurses and the law: A guide to principles and applications.* Philadelphia: Saunders.

Corey, G., Corey, M., & Calanan, P. (1984*). Issues and ethics in the helping professions* (3rd ed.). Pacific Grove, CA: Brooks-Cole.

Dougherty, A. (1995). *Consultation: Practice and perspectives in school and community settings* (2nd ed.). Pacific Grove, CA: Brooks-Cole.

Gardner, S., & Hagedorn, M. (1997). *Legal aspects of maternal–child nursing practice.* Menlo Park, CA: Addison-Wesley.

Lewin, M. (1995). *The overnight consultant.* New York: John Wiley & Sons.

McCarthy, M., & Sorenson, G. (1993). School counselors and consultants: Legal duties and liabilities. *Journal of Counseling and Development, 72,* 159–167.

Reinert, B., & Buck, E. (1989). Issues in liability insurance and the nurse consultant. *Clinical Nurse Specialist, 3*(1), 42–45.

Scott, L., & Beare, P. (1993). Nurse consultants and professional liability. *Clinical Nurse Specialist, 7*(6), 331–334.

Tepper, R. (1985*). Become a top consultant.* New York: John Wiley & Sons.

16

Ethical Issues
in Nursing Consultation

The complex nature of consultation requires a significant extension of even the most basic ethical principles. (Newman, 1993)

 KEY CONCEPTS:

professional ethics, moral philosophy, values, dual relationship, confidentiality, anonymity

---

 KEY TERMS FOR YOUR SEARCH ENGINE:

consultation and ethics

INTRODUCTION

Nurses are well accustomed to dealing with ethical dilemmas in clinical practice: being caught between the wishes of a patient or the patient's family and those of the attending physician, being asked by a parent to divulge information given in confidence by an adolescent, and using "floats" as a response to inadequate staffing. Nurse consultants deal with parallel dilemmas: being caught between the needs of consultees and those of the client system as a whole, being asked by an organizational contact person to divulge information given in confidence by a consultee, and being expected to solve a problem with inadequate resources. The common element in all

of these situations is the sense of unease and uncertainty about the "rightness" of one's decision. This sense of unease reflects that the decision means choosing between competing values. When a problematic situation has these characteristics, it is considered an ethical dilemma.

Members of the helping professions such as nurses and consultants are particularly likely to face ethical dilemmas because they work with individuals who are in somewhat vulnerable or needy positions. Ethical dilemmas also arise for both nurses and consultants because they work in situations involving more than one individual, each of whom has different needs and trusts that these needs will be met. Ethical dilemmas can be particularly burden-some for nurse consultants because of the potentially large number of people (e.g., a patient group, entire organization, or commu-nity) who can be directly and indirectly affected by the nurse consultant's values, interpretation of ethical principles, and deci-sions.

This chapter does not seek to provide answers to ethical dilemmas. Rather, it focuses on the ethical issues and dilemmas that nurse consultants are most likely to confront in prac-tice and offers suggestions for dealing with these dilemmas. The chapter begins with a brief overview of basic ethical concepts. Next, the ethics of consultation, specifically ethical guidelines for nurse consultants, are considered. The third section of the chapter explores the ethically problematic situations that are most likely to arise in a nursing consul-tation relationship. The chapter ends by offer-ing strategies nurse consultants can use to deal with ethical dilemmas. The following are

questions to think about as you read this chapter:

- What ethical obligations do nurse consul-tants have beyond those to their consul-tees?
- What examples can you think of in which legal and ethical obligations in nursing consultation might conflict with one another?
- In what ways are nurse consultants most likely to violate the rights of consultees? Why do you think this might occur?
- To what extent is the American Nurses Association's Code for Nurses useful as a guide to ethical behavior in nursing con-sultation? What are its limitations?
- What system of beliefs do you use to guide decisions when faced with an ethical dilemma? What implications might this have for your practice of nursing consulta-tion?

BASIC ETHICAL CONCEPTS

Ethics is the study and definition of values concerning how one ought to live (Kim-brough, 1985). Because ethics focuses on "oughts," it encompasses norms and beliefs about right and wrong as well as good and bad behavior. The ethics of any group has its roots in the group's value system. Ethics defines for members of a group the everyday judgments they are expected to make in terms of behavior, apart from the provisions of the law and written policy (Kimbrough, 1985).

Professional ethics is the system of moral principles or standards that govern profes-sional conduct (Dougherty, 1995). Profes-sional ethics, therefore, defines professionally acceptable behavior. A professional is consid-ered "ethical" when his or her behavior con-

forms to the standards of conduct of the par-ticular professional group.

The ethics of any group is characterized by recurring themes of expectations, or obliga-tions of form. (Kimbrough, 1985). Obliga-tions of form can be worded as "thou shalt" statements or ethical propositions—specific statements about duties, obligations, and responsibilities toward others. Obligations of form for consultants in general and for nurse consultants in particular are discussed in a later section of this chapter.

Ethical Dilemmas

An ethical dilemma is said to exist when a decision necessitates choosing between com-peting needs and values. For example, the ethical dilemma in the clinical nursing situa-tion of being asked by a patient not to reveal a diagnosis to her or his family reflects the tension between supporting values concerning autonomy, privacy, and others' rights to know. Nurse consultants can experience this same type of tension, and thus experience an ethical dilemma, when a consultee shares information in confidence (as an extreme example, knowledge of embezzlement) that has implications for the entire community or client system.

Ethical dilemmas are often manifested as a sense of unease or uncertainty about the decision one needs to make. This reflects that ethical dilemmas frequently represent a "gray zone" in which there is no absolutely right or wrong solution. This sense of unease also reflects that responses to ethical dilemmas threaten compliance with a group's obligations of form. Thus, ethical dilemmas present a "tug of war" between competing perspectives of what constitutes right and wrong behavior and a good or bad outcome.

Ethical Decision Making

Most, if not all, decisions in nursing consultation have an ethical component. That is, decisions made in nursing consultation, like those in clinical nursing, involve applying one's values and making value judgments about what constitutes "best" behavior and outcomes. The process of ethical decision making entails applying one's personal values, those core beliefs that "one holds most dear" and uses to guide behavior, as well as the values reflected in the ethics of one's profession, to the decision at hand.

Most of us can readily articulate at least some of our personal values—honesty, fairness, and service to others, for example. However, even these values can have different interpretations and applications: What is "fair" in one situation may not seem fair in another or may not be perceived as fair by everyone in the same situation. How one applies one's values reflects a more fundamental and overarching belief system that is influenced by family and friends, life experiences, reading, and contemplation. This overarching belief system constitutes one's moral philosophy—the most fundamental beliefs about how one ought to live, what counts as good reasons for acting one way or another, and what constitutes a good life for human beings (Norman, 1983).

Understanding one's own moral philosophy as well as that which shapes the ethics of one's profession provides one with decision criteria for responding to ethical dilemmas and making routine decisions (see Figure 16-1). Understanding one's moral philosophy is important because it reveals the biases one brings to problem situations. Traditionally, six major schools of moral philosophy have been recognized; these are summarized briefly in Box 16-1.

ETHICS AND CONSULTATION

Human service professionals such as nurses and consultants are expected by society to interact with their consumers (patients and consultees) according to certain standards of behavior. These standards of conduct are made explicit in each state's Nurse Practice Act and in the standards of practice and codes of ethics developed by different professional organizations. Codes of ethics make explicit the values, assumptions, and expectations a profession has about the form the behavior of its members should take.

Obligations of Form

Obligations of form were defined earlier in this chapter as the recurring themes in a group's ethics. Obligations of form reflect general rules of behavior that are stated more specifically in a profession's code of ethics. The following obligations of form can be identified in codes of ethics (and state Nurse Practice Acts) for nurses and consultants:

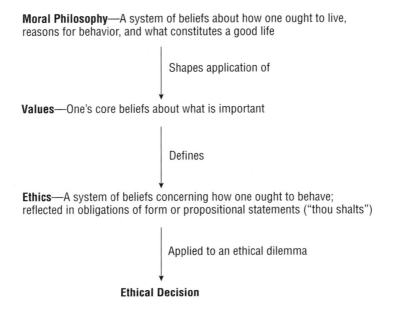

Moral Philosophy—A system of beliefs about how one ought to live, reasons for behavior, and what constitutes a good life

Shapes application of

Values—One's core beliefs about what is important

Defines

Ethics—A system of beliefs concerning how one ought to behave; reflected in obligations of form or propositional statements ("thou shalts")

Applied to an ethical dilemma

Ethical Decision

Figure 16-1   Relationship Between Moral Philosophy, Values, Ethics, and Ethical Decision Making.
One's moral philosophy is the foundation of ethical decision making because it shapes the application of one's values and defines how these values will be packaged into a system of beliefs about obligations and how one ought to live.

- The duty to uphold human rights
- The duty to fulfill commitments
- The duty to practice one's profession competently

Upholding Human Rights

The profession of nursing recognizes the basic human rights of self-determination, freedom from harm, privacy, and fair treatment (American Nurses Association [ANA], 1985).

Self-Determination. Self-determination is the right of an individual to have a say in his or her own future (ANA, 1985). Self-determination encompasses the concepts of willing participation and informed consent. In nursing consultation, the right to self-determination translates into freedom to choose to be a part of the consultation relationship and understanding what involvement in the relationship will entail. In

nursing consultation, the consultation contract is the primary vehicle for informed consent.

Freedom from Harm. Freedom from harm is the right of consultees to expect that things will not get worse as a result of participation in the nursing consultation relationship. Nurse consultants need to consider possible physical, emotional, and financial harm to consultees. Consideration needs to be given to harm or side effects that are more likely to be immediate as well as to those that might be delayed. This obligation of form ("do no harm") intertwines with that of self-determination in that part of informed consent involves making consultees aware of possible adverse side effects of the nursing consultation relationship.

In nursing consultation, consideration of a risk–benefit ratio often replaces the absolute obligation to do no harm. For example, a community agency may choose to incur a

BOX 16-1   MAJOR SCHOOLS OF MORAL PHILOSOPHY

Idealism: "Right" behavior is behavior that "naturally" brings happiness; according to idealists, ends justify means.

Kantian ethics: Behavior should be guided by categorical imperatives or independent moral obligations that are derived from pure reason and reflect duty and conscience; behavior is judged right or wrong independent of its consequences.

Utilitarianism: Proper decisions, actions, or behaviors are those that bring the greatest good to the greatest number; moral values are those that maximize pleasure and minimize pain.

Situation ethics: Ethical decisions reflect the spirit of the loving and caring thing to do.

Ethical relativism: There is no one set of ethics that is correct for all societies; what is good or right is determined by the cultural context in which a decision is being made.

Ethical egoism: Good acts are those that promote a person's self-interest.

Sources: Kimbrough, R. (1985). *Ethics: A course of study for educational leaders.* Arlington, VA: American Association of Counseling and Development; and Norman, R. (1983). *The moral philosophers: An introduction to ethics.* Oxford: Clarendon Press.

---

short-term financial loss while planning and implementing a new program in the hopes of attracting more patients, and perhaps state funding, in the long run.

Privacy. The right to privacy addresses expectations about sharing information. Confidentiality is an explicit promise to reveal nothing about an individual except under conditions the individual has agreed to (Corey, Corey, & Calanan, 1984; Dougherty, 1995). The intent of the right to privacy and confidentiality is to protect individuals from harm.

Fair Treatment. Fair treatment refers to providing services that protect human dignity. In nursing consultation, fair treatment encompasses fostering consultees' self-sufficiency rather than dependency and acting in the consultees' best interest rather than promoting one's own interests.

Fulfilling Commitments

The second obligation of form for nurse consultants is the responsibility to fulfill commitments. In other words, nurse consultants are ethically bound to fulfill the terms set forth in the consultation contract. From an ethical perspective, fulfilling a contract overlaps with consultees' rights to fair treatment. As discussed in Chapter 15, this obligation of form also has a legal component.

Competence

Nurses and consultants are expected to practice their professions competently. This obligation of form encompasses the expectation that nurse consultants participate in continuing education as well as in ongoing evaluation of their practice (ANA, 1985). A second dimension of the expectation of competence is knowing one's limitations and restricting consultation activities to those compatible with one's skills and expertise.

Ethical Guidelines for Consultants

A profession embodies its obligations of form in its code of ethics and standards of practice. A code of ethics provides general guidelines for acting as a professional and fulfilling the responsibilities associated with being a professional. Ethical codes provide professionals with minimal appropriate behavioral standards for their conduct and relationships with others in carrying out their professional role. By adhering to one's professional code of ethics, one should be safe from both legal action and professional censure (Corey et al., 1984). A code of ethics signifies the maturity of a profession and its attempts to engage in self-regulation. A code of ethics prevents a professional from bending behavior with the exigencies of volatile economics, difficult consultees, and "crass opportunism" (Lewin, 1995).

Like other professions, consultation has an ethic, or sense of right and wrong, of its own. Consultation, however, lacks a codified body of knowledge or a quality control body (Metzger, 1993). This situation stems, in part, from the fact that consultation is generally regarded as an "emerging" profession. It also reflects that consultants come from many disciplines and that consultation encompasses a variety of services provided to individuals and groups with diverse problems across a range of settings. Consequently, many consultants argue that no single code of ethics will ever work for all consultants. Nurse consultants are left, then, with applying and adapting the code of ethics of the nursing profession (including the standards of practice established by its specialty organizations) and ethical codes from other helping professions to situations and types of relationships that differ from those for which the codes were intended (Dougherty, 1995).

Some professional organizations such as the American Psychological Association, the American Society for Training and Development, the Institute of Management Consultants, and the American Association of Counseling and Development do provide specific guidelines for consultation activities that organizational members might undertake. Selected statements from the ethical codes of these non-nursing helping organizations are shown in Box 16-2.

The American Nurses Association's Code for Nurses (1985) offers guidelines primarily for direct care nursing activities. As discussed in Chapter 1, however, nursing consultation is an indirect care activity, and only selected statements from the ANA Code seem particularly applicable to nursing consultation activities. These statements and their application to nursing consultation are highlighted in Box 16-3.

To summarize, formal guidelines for the ethical practice of consultation, specifically nursing consultation, are not currently available. At the same time, existing codes of ethics provide only limited guidance for the practice of nursing consultation. As a result, nurse consultants bear heavy personal responsibility for the consequences of their decisions and actions as professional nurse consultants (Newman, 1993).

ETHICALLY PROBLEMATIC SITUATIONS FOR NURSE CONSULTANTS

Consultation relationships are tripartite, voluntary, peer relationships that focus on work-related rather than personal problems of consultees. These characteristics of nursing consultation relationships give rise to ethical dilemmas about responsibility, power, and dual relationships.

Responsibility Dilemmas

The tripartite nature of a consultation relationship can create problems in terms of determining to whom the nurse consultant's responsibility extends. Responsibility dilemmas reflect tension in terms of fulfilling obligations of form related to protecting human rights, freedom from harm, and fair treatment.

BOX 16-2   ETHICAL STANDARDS FOR NURSE CONSULTANTS: GUIDELINES FROM NON-NURSING HELPING PROFESSIONS

Statements from the codes of ethics of non-nursing professional organizations offer the following guidelines for implementing the consultant role:

1. Consultants put the welfare and needs of their consultees and clients ahead of their own.
2. Consultants inform consultees about the nature of the consultation process, including its risks and benefits.
3. Consultants do not accept contracts for activities for which they lack skill or training.
4. Consultants avoid dual relationships that create conflicts of interest and interfere with their effectiveness.
5. Consultants avoid manipulating consultees and creating dependency. Instead, they assist a consultee to develop autonomy in problem solving.
6. Consultants establish contracts with well-defined limits and adhere to their contracts.
7. Consultants clarify the nature and purposes of data-gathering activities at the outset of the consultation relationship.
8. Consultants choose assessment strategies that are consistent with the needs and purposes of the consultee.
9. Consultants only propose actions for consideration. These actions should fit the needs, values, and resources of the client system.
10. Consultants evaluate the outcomes of their services. They ask for feedback from consultees and peers on a regular basis.
11. Consultants respect the privacy of consultees. This entails informing them of confidentiality and its limits. This also means that participation in consultation activities is voluntary.
12. Consultants respect a consultee's freedom to decline involvement in activities that require disclosure of feelings, values, and personal issues.
13. Consultants are continually involved in professional and personal development activities for the purpose of increasing their knowledge and skills.

Source: Corey, G., Corey, M., & Calanan, P. (1984). *Issues and ethics in the helping professions* (3rd ed.). Pacific Grove, CA: Brooks-Cole.

Usually, a nurse consultant's primary responsibility is considered to be to the consultees with whom the consultant is directly working in the consultation relationship. It is often difficult to conceptualize responsibility to a client since the client may be an entire community or organization and its individual members do not usually take an active part in the consultation process and do not have an opportunity to voice and advance their goals and priorities. In cases in which the client is an individual patient or type of patient (e.g., a group defined by a particular illness), it is unlikely that the client is even aware that consultation on his or her behalf is taking place. Clients are affected by consultation then, but usually without the benefit of participating in the consultation process (this creates an

BOX 16-3   ETHICAL STANDARDS FOR NURSE CONSULTANTS: GUIDELINES FROM THE AMERICAN NURSES ASSOCIATION'S CODE FOR NURSES

The following statements from the American Nurses Association's Code for Nurses (1985) seem particularly applicable as guidelines for implementing the role of nurse consultant:

The nurse provides services with respect for human dignity and the uniqueness of the client . . .

Application to Nursing Consultation

- Involve consultees in the nursing consultation process.
- Provide informed consent about what the consultation relationship will involve.
- Individualize consultation activities.
- Foster consultees' self-reliance.

The nurse safeguards the client's right to privacy by judiciously protecting information of a confidential nature.

Application to Nursing Consultation

- Be clear about limits of confidentiality.
- Use professional judgment and discretion.
- Provide anonymity when information must be shared.

The nurse assumes responsibility and accountability for individual nursing judgments and actions.

Application to Nursing Consultation

- Areas of responsibility for a nurse consultant are problem identification, action planning, evaluation, and disengagement.
- Be aware of the limits of one's competence.
- Evaluate the effectiveness of one's performance as a nurse consultant as well as the effectiveness of specific interactions and interventions.

The nurse maintains competence in nursing.

Application to Nursing Consultation

- Engage in personal and professional development activities.
- Seek feedback from peers about one's skills.

The nurse exercises informed judgment and uses individual competence as qualifications and criteria in seeking consultation and accepting responsibilities.

Application to Nursing Consultation

- Know and respect personal limits in knowledge and skills.
- Seek consultation and refer when appropriate.
- Avoid misrepresentation of abilities and qualifications.

Source: American Nurses Association. (1985). *Code for nurses with interpretive statements.* Kansas City, MO: Author.

additional dilemma around the right to self-determination).

One response or view to responsibility dilemmas is that a consultant's responsibility extends to clients as well as to others who may be victims or beneficiaries of the nursing consultation relationship. This view of responsibility is consistent with that proposed in Chapter 1. That is, nurse consultants need to consider the risks and benefits of any nursing consultation action on actual and potential health care consumers, because health care consumers—who can be either clients or stakeholders—are always the ultimate beneficiaries of a nursing consultation relationship. The ethical dilemma associated with this view of responsibility is determining how much responsibility is then owed to consultees. Also, if health care consumers are only stakeholders, how much responsibility is owed to them as compared to the client (who might be an entire organization or community)?

Another view of responsibility in nursing consultation is that a consultant's primary responsibility is to the client and that responsibility to consultees and stakeholders (including health care consumers) is only a secondary obligation. The situation becomes even more confusing when the consultation has been arranged by a contact person such as an administrator in the client community or organization. In these situations, is the nurse consultant responsible to the contact person, the organization/community, or the consultees?

In summary, the implications and difficulty of the tripartite nature of nursing consultation relationships is that nurse consultants are responsible for the impact of their services on individuals with whom they may have little contact (Herlihy & Corey, 1992). The nature of the nursing consultation relationship can create ethical dilemmas in terms of target of responsibility. These dilemmas occur because of tension upholding the human rights of fair treatment and freedom from harm.

Misuse of Power

The power relationship between a nurse consultant and consultees is complex. The consultation relationship is intended to be one of peers: A nurse consultant shares expertise and knowledge and works with consultees to resolve a problem. At the same time, the nurse consultant–consultee relationship is inherently one of unequal power. The fact that a contact person or consultees are seeking help implies that the consultees are lacking and in need of something (knowledge or skills) that the nurse consultant has (Herlihy & Corey, 1995; Sneed, 1991). Nurse consultants need to be aware of the potential for misusing their power and the possibility of manipulating and inappropriately influencing needy consultees' attitudes and behavior. Misuse of power can create dependency and conflicts of interest and create tension in terms of satisfying obligations of form related to providing fair treatment, freedom from harm, and fulfilling commitments.

Recall from Chapter 6 that nurse consultants are most likely to have expert power (related to specialized and needed knowledge and skills) and personal power (related to the ability to develop followers through personal characteristics such as charisma and friendship tactics). These forms of power can be blatantly as well as more subtly misused.

Misuse of Expert Power

Perceived expertise is usually the reason for asking a specific nurse to provide consultation. The appropriate and ethical use of expertise is to help consultees increase their own problem-solving abilities. Expertise is misused when knowledge of problem-solving skills is withheld to keep consultees in a dependent position.

Nurse consultants may also foster consultee dependency and prolong a consultation relationship in order to meet their own financial needs or to gain personal gratification through a sense of significance (Corey et al., 1984; Newman, 1993). These actions violate obligations of form related to self-determination, fair treatment, freedom from harm, and fulfilling contracts. Professional codes of ethics (e.g., those of the American Association of Counseling and Development) speak specifically against creating dependency.

Expert power can create further ethical dilemmas due to its "halo effect." That is, consultees (and nurse consultants themselves) may generalize a consultant's expertise in one area to other areas. This violates obligations of form related to competence. Expert power is also misused when nurse consultants allow their qualifications to be misrepresented or attempt to intervene in areas outside their scope of competence. In addition to being unethical, attempting to exercise expert power in areas outside of one's actual range of expertise can backfire and decrease a nurse consultant's perceived power if consultation efforts are unsuccessful (Sneed, 1991). Furthermore, as mentioned in Chapter 15, practicing nursing consultation in areas outside of one's expertise can result in legal action against a nurse consultant for malpractice or breach of contract. Box 16-4 presents a scenario illustrating the problem of the halo effect.

Misuse of Personal Power

A second source of power for nurse consultants is personal power. Personal power is useful in nursing consultation because it facilitates the establishment of trust and rapport between a nurse consultant and consultees. Personal power is misused, however, when a nurse consultant uses charisma and friendship tactics to enter into or use a consultation relationship for reasons of self-interest. These actions create a conflict of interest and may cause a nurse consultant to lose objectivity about the consultation situation. Misusing one's personal power to advance self-interests in a nursing consultation relationship violates obligations of form regarding self-determination, protection from harm, fair treatment, and fulfilling commitments. Box 16-5 presents a situation that involves a potential misuse of personal power.

Dual Relationships

A dual relationship occurs when "a professional assumes two roles simultaneously or sequentially with a person seeking help" (Herlihy &

BOX 16-4 A POTENTIAL MISUSE OF EXPERT POWER: THE "HALO EFFECT"

A family nurse practitioner (FNP) is asked to provide consultation to a school district about a comprehensive health education curriculum. The curriculum is to include topics such as AIDS, eating disorders, violence, substance abuse, depression, and suicide. The school district also wants the FNP to identify and develop teachers for this curriculum. The FNP was offered this opportunity because of a reputation of being a skilled and empathetic clinician who is "good with teens." The FNP accepts the consultation opportunity because of a desire to help.

- *Was there a misuse of expert power in this situation?*

BOX 16-5   POTENTIAL MISUSE OF PERSONAL POWER: PROMOTING SELF-INTERESTS

A nurse consultant is working with the nurse-managers in a large health maintenance organization (HMO) to help them develop a telephone triage system. Over the course of several weeks, the nurse consultant develops rapport and a friendly, trusting relationship with several of the nurse-managers. While the nurse consultant and the nurse-managers are having coffee after one of the work sessions, one of the nurse-managers reveals rumors about the impending resignation of two top administrators at the same time that an opening is planned for a major satellite clinic in the HMO system. Based on this information, the nurse consultant schedules an appointment with the chief administrative officer of the HMO to discuss interest in pursuing administrative level full-time employment in the system.

- *Was there a misuse of personal power in this situation?*

Corey, 1992). Assuming a dual role reflects trying to accommodate a professional role plus a personal, social, or financial relationship, or to fill two conflicting professional roles. It is easy for nurse consultants to end up in dual relationships because consultation interventions can be difficult to define and often encompass a variety of intertwined needs and issues. Dual relationships tend to create conflicts of interest and, therefore, violate obligations of form related to protection from harm, fair treatment, and fulfilling commitments.

Dual relationships also cause incompatible behavioral expectations for both consultees and the nurse consultant. Combining a social or financial relationship with a professional relationship such as that of nurse consultant, for example, can result in decisions and actions that promote the consultant's self-interest but collide with what would be in the best interest of consultees or the client. Dual relationships can cause low morale within a consultee group if one group member is singled out for special treatment by the nurse consultant. Dual relationships can also undermine the credibility of the nurse consultant (and the entire profession) if they are per-

ceived as "cheating" the client system of full attention and loyalty (Herlihy & Corey, 1992). The dual relationships that are particularly likely to be problematic for nurse consultants are those of consultant/supervisor, consultant/counselor, and consultant/clinician (caregiver).

Nurse Consultant/Supervisor.
The potential for a nurse consultant to take on a second role as supervisor exists because it is often hard to determine when the feedback given to consultees as a part of the nursing consultation process becomes supervisory evaluation (Herlihy & Corey, 1992). This can be especially problematic in internal consultation situations because an internal nurse consultant often holds an administrative or managerial role within the client system.

Assuming a supervisory role while providing nursing consultation services violates the peer nature of the consultation relationship because supervision involves making judgments about and having control over a supervisee (Dougherty, 1995). By the same token, a consultation relationship is built on values of consultee growth and formative evaluation and feedback.

The dual role of nurse consultant/supervisor creates further dilemmas because a supervisor is expected to serve not only the supervisee's interests (such as fair performance evaluation and facilitation or protection of continued employment) but the interests of the employing agency and the public (such as safe practice and cost containment). Finally, the dual role of nurse consultant/supervisor creates an ethical dilemma related to expectations to share information with parties at interest and yet maintain the confidentiality of the consultation relationship (Herlihy & Corey, 1992).

Nurse Consultant/Counselor. Because nurses have a personal helping orientation, it can be difficult for them to draw the line between consulting and counseling when they are acting as nurse consultants. Indeed, there is often a fine line between consultation interventions and counseling. When, for example, does acknowledging consultees' negative emotions become counseling about these emotions? Also, in many nursing consultation situations, the boundaries between personal and work-related issues are blurred. The problem of blurred boundaries and a potential dual relationship is illustrated in the scenario presented in Box 16-6.

Assuming a dual role as nurse consultant and counselor can be problematic for several reasons. First, focusing on consultees' emotional needs and issues tends to disrupt the peer relationship on which effective consultation practice is built and emphasizes instead the neediness and vulnerability of the consultees; this creates a hierarchical or uneven relationship. Secondly, adding the role of counselor to that of nurse consultant contaminates, deemphasizes, and possibly dislocates the work-related focus of the consultation relationship. In some cases, this change in emphasis from work-related to personal problems can be interpreted as a breach of contract and as cheating a client system of the work-related problem-solving services for which it contracted. This type of dual relationship, therefore, violates obligations of form related to fulfilling commitments.

BOX 16-6   "BLURRED BOUNDARIES" IN NURSING CONSULTATION

A nurse consultant in independent practice who has a background in management and psychiatric nursing (including experience with group therapy) is hired to facilitate a team-building retreat with the nursing staff of two recently merged air ambulance services. As the retreat gets under way and the nurse consultant is assessing the needs of the group, it becomes apparent that many of the nurses have unresolved feelings about the merger and how it has affected them on a personal level. For some workers, feelings of grief over loss of former co-workers has triggered unfinished business in regard to grieving other losses. For other nurses, the key issues have to do with loss of trust, betrayal, financial impact of decreased work hours, and job insecurity. The nurse consultant decides it is more important to focus on these individual needs rather than on team building. During the remainder of the retreat, the nurse consultant meets with staff individually and in small groups to deal with these issues.

- *Did this nurse consultant take on a dual role? If so, was it justified?*

Nurse Consultant/Clinician. Nurse consultants who are providing consultation about patient care issues may face the dilemma of needing to determine when it is appropriate and inappropriate to assume the simultaneous role of clinician and direct caregiver. While a nurse consultant usually needs to step back and help nursing staff learn to problem solve a patient care problem on their own, there are times when patient safety issues warrant stepping in and taking on this dual role. In consulting situations in which patient care is seriously compromised and a nurse consultee is not able to make the decisions or provide the care needed, the nurse consultant is legally and ethically bound to step in and assume clinical responsibility for the patient (Barron, 1989). Box 16-7 illustrates an extreme situation in which a nurse consultant needs to assume a dual role on a temporary basis.

Confidentiality

While confidentiality is a professional expectation and obligation of form for consultants, how it is enacted is increasingly being deter-mined by the law. Child abuse reporting laws and the duty to warn and protect potential victims are just two of the legal limits that have been set in regard to confidentiality. In nursing consultation situations, any limits to confidentiality should be explicitly identified in the nursing consultation contract. The contract should identify what information can be shared and how it is to be shared (e.g., only verbally), as well as with whom it can be shared and under what circumstances (e.g., only "in emergency" or at the completion of the consultation engagement).

Confidentiality can present a nurse consultant with the ethical dilemma of having important information but not being able to use it. It is not uncommon that during the course of a nursing consultation relationship, consultees will develop enough trust and rapport with a nurse consultant that information is shared on a private basis. Accepting information under these conditions may place a nurse consultant in the uncomfortable position of having information that is important to the consultation process or the well-being of the client system but not being able to use it. Accepting this information also supports a

---

BOX 16-7   AN ETHICALLY MANDATED DUAL RELATIONSHIP

A clinical nurse specialist (CNS) is asked by nursing staff to help them develop interventions for dealing with a post–myocardial infarction patient's delirium and disorientation. The staff insist these conditions are just normal psychological reactions to adjusting to the seriousness of the medical condition. The staff further insist that the patient is medically stable and just needs some cognitive interventions such as "those that are used in nursing homes." The CNS, however, recognizes that these reactions of the patient may signal a change in medical condition or an adverse reaction to a medication the patient is taking. Accordingly, the CNS immediately orders some laboratory studies, conducts a neurological screening assessment, and contacts the patient's physician rather than proceed to work with staff to develop cognitive interventions.

• *Was assuming a dual role justified in this situation?*

system's norm of secrecy and is antithetical to the desired openness of the nursing consultation relationship. On the other hand, if the information is rejected, a nurse consultant may miss valuable information and compromise the trust relationship that has been established with the consultees.

To deal with this type of dilemma, consultants frequently substitute a promise of anonymity for one of confidentiality. Anonymity allows information to be used as long as its source is protected (Dougherty, 1995). Anonymity, therefore, has the advantage of facilitating the flow of information critical to successful consultation. A typical dilemma presented by obligations of form related to confidentiality forms the basis for the scenario presented in Box 16-8.

Informed Consent and Voluntary Participation

Informed consent means that participation in a nursing consultation relationship is voluntary and based on full awareness of the purpose, nature, risks, benefits, and potential outcomes of the relationship (Newman, 1993). Informed consent implies the freedom to choose from among alternatives, including nonparticipation. As mentioned earlier, the nursing consultation contract is the primary vehicle for informed consent in a nursing consultation relationship. Two types of liability can arise from failure to obtain informed consent: negligence/malpractice and breach of contract (Corey et al., 1984).

Trying to uphold obligations of form related to informed consent and self-determination can create ethical dilemmas for a nurse consultant. For example, in organizational consulting situations (in which the organization is the client and initial contact has been made by someone in the administrative hierarchy of the organization), administration may require personnel (consultees) to participate in the nursing consultation process. Personnel (e.g., nursing staff) fear negative consequences if they refuse, so they participate when they

---

BOX 16-8   AN ETHICAL DILEMMA ASSOCIATED WITH CONFIDENTIALITY

A nurse consultant is asked to work with the personnel (many of whom are volunteers) in a community agency to help them implement a plan for restructuring the organization. Specific interventions include working with the personnel to develop communication, decision-making, and delegation skills. At the outset of the consultation, it was agreed that the nurse consultant would not be asked to give opinions about the performance of any of the consultees. It was also agreed that all aspects of the consultation would remain confidential.

A couple of months into the consultation relationship, the chairperson of the agency's board of directors (who was the initial contact for the consultation and who signed the contract) asks the nurse consultant about the performance of one particular individual to whom they are considering offering a promotion. The chairperson assures the nurse consultant that this information will go no further. When the nurse consultant reminds the chairperson that sharing this type of information is strictly precluded by the consultation contract, the chairperson becomes angry, demands that the information be shared, and threatens to terminate the consultation relationship if it is not.

would rather not. Nurse consultants who decline a consultation opportunity in this type of situation forego the opportfunity to become involved in helping (and learning from helping) the consultees and client system. On the other hand, proceeding with a nursing consultation engagement in a situation where consultees are not truly voluntary participants undermines the obligation of form related to self-determination. It also creates the challenge of needing to overcome consultee resistance in order to develop an effective problem-solving relationship. In situations where there is less than voluntary participation in the nursing consultation process, a nurse consultant should, at the very least, openly acknowledge the dilemma and discuss the accompanying issues with the consultees.

In nursing consultation, informed consent and self-determination also mean that consultees have the freedom to do whatever they wish with a nurse consultant's opinions and recommendations. The positive aspect of self-determination and informed consent is that it relieves a nurse consultant of any responsibility for consultees' behavior. This relief may be more perceived than real, however. For example, what (and to whom) is a nurse consultant's responsibility when consultees' refusal to participate could bring harm to the client or client system?

DEALING WITH ETHICAL DILEMMAS

Thus far, the discussion in this chapter has focused on "consciousness-raising" or increasing awareness about the types of situations that can create ethical dilemmas for nurse consultants. Unfortunately, there is no way of avoiding these situations and dilemmas and there are no absolute strategies for resolving them. Nurse consultants can, however, rely on some general guidelines—in addition to state Nurse Practice Acts, standards of practice,

and existing professional codes of ethics—when formulating a response to an ethical dilemma.

Earlier in this chapter, an ethical dilemma was defined as occurring when the need to make a decision about an appropriate course of action arouses feelings of unease or uncertainty because the decision entails choosing between competing values. The following steps can be used to facilitate decision making in these situations:

1. Identify the problem or dilemma.
2. Identify the ethical issues involved. Specifically, what obligations of form are being threatened?
3. Review relevant professional guidelines (e.g., state Nurse Practice Acts and organizational policies).
4. Identify possible courses of action and the most likely consequences of each.
5. Obtain consultation from a colleague.
6. Determine the best course of action for the circumstances (Corey et al., 1984; Dougherty, 1995).

From a legal perspective, the fifth step in this process ("consult with a colleague") is particularly important. If a colleague agrees with the course of action that has been taken, there is an increased likelihood of being able to demonstrate that a decision was both made in good faith and was reasonably prudent.

Lewin (1995) offers additional "tests" that can be applied when one has doubts about actions in regard to an ethical dilemma. First, validate actions for consistency with one's professional codes. If uncertainty about one's actions remains, apply the "*New York Times* Rule": Don't do anything you wouldn't want to read about in the banner headlines of the *New York Times*. If, after this test, "right" or "best" actions are still ambiguous, err on the side of omission rather than commission. That is, don't do something that might be interpreted as ethically ambiguous. As a final guideline for dealing with ethical dilemmas, the following is worth keeping in mind:

> The ethical basis of consulting boils down to the eternal Golden Rule: Do unto others as you would have them do unto you. That means show your clients [consultees] respect, discretion, honesty, and appropriateness as we would have them do unto us. (Lewin, 1995)

A nurse consultant can minimize the likelihood of making an inappropriate or unethical decision by objectively confronting each consultation task and situation. Incorporating values of consultee self-determination, growth, and learning into one's practice of nursing consultation can help to prevent the misuse of power, creation of dependency, and manipulation of consultees and consultation relationship for personal gain. Making use of all available resources, including assessment data and consultation with colleagues, to help determine an appropriate course of action can help a nurse consultant identify the issues and consequences associated with different behaviors and interventions. Finally, engaging in reflection of one's own moral philosophy, self-evaluation, and professional growth activities sensitizes a nurse consultant to personal values and biases that can precipitate an ethical dilemma (Lippitt & Lippitt, 1986).

CHAPTER SUMMARY

In nursing consultation, ethical dilemmas arise because consultation is a tripartite helping relationship that entails competing needs of consultees, clients, stakeholders, and the nurse consultant. Ethically problematic situations rarely occur in isolation and instead tend to arise from and present as a set of intertwined issues and dilemmas. Likewise, ethical obligations can intertwine or conflict with other professional and legal obligations. Nurse consultants are faced with dealing with ethical dilemmas by translating and applying ethical standards from related helping professions and the direct care–oriented Code for Nurses, seeking consultation from peers, and assuming personal values of self-evaluation and professional growth.

APPLYING CHAPTER CONTENT

1. Analyze the scenarios presented in Boxes 16-4, 16-5, 16-6, 16-7, and 16-8, and answer the following questions:
   - What are the specific ethical issues, potential violations of obligations of form, and other potential problems in the scenario?
   - Critique the nurse consultant's response to the situation. Identify the moral philosophy that is reflected in the response.
   - What possible harm could result from the nurse consultant's response?
   - Develop an ethically acceptable alternative course of action. Identify the moral philosophy that underpins this course of action.

2. What potential ethical issues and dilemmas are you most likely to face in your own practice of nursing consultation? What kind of harm might arise from these issues? How would you respond to these dilemmas?

References

American Nurses Association. (1985). *Code for nurses with interpretive statements.* Kansas City, MO: Author.

Barron, A. (1989). The CNS as consultant. In A. Hamric & J. Spross (Eds.), *The clinical nurse specialist in theory and practice* (2nd ed.) (pp. 125–146). Philadelphia: Saunders.

Corey, G., Corey, M., & Calanan, P. (1984). *Issues and ethics in the helping professions* (3rd ed.). Pacific Grove, CA: Brooks-Cole.

Dougherty, A. (1995). *Consultation: Practice and perspectives in school and community settings* (2nd ed.). Pacific Grove, CA: Brooks-Cole.

Herlihy, B., & Corey, G. (1992). *Dual relationships in counseling.* Alexandria, VA: American Association of Counseling and Development.

Kimbrough, R. (1985). *Ethics: A course of study for educational leaders.* Arlington, VA: American Association for School Administrators.

Lewin, M. (1995). *The overnight consultant.* New York: John Wiley & Sons.

Lippitt, G., & Lippitt, R. (1986). *The consulting process in action* (2nd ed.). San Diego: University Associates.

Metzger, R. (1993). *Developing a consulting practice.* Newbury Park, CA: Sage.

Newman, J. (1993). Ethical issues in consultation. *Journal of Counseling and Development, 72,* 148–156.

Norman, R. (1983). *The moral philosophers: An introduction to ethics.* Oxford: Clarendon Press.

Sneed, N. (1991). Power: Its use and potential for misuse by nurse consultants. *Clinical Nurse Specialist, 5*(1), 58–62.

17

The Business of Consulting: Marketing, Fees, and Contracts

Areas of growth in nursing are to be found at the edges of traditional practice. (Doughty & Keller, 2000)

 KEY CONCEPTS:

marketing, promotion, market segment, contract

 KEY TERMS FOR YOUR SEARCH ENGINE:

professional and marketing

INTRODUCTION

One of the underlying premises of this book is that when a health care delivery system is driven by a community perspective, all nurses, regardless of their level of educational preparation, functional role, and clinical specialty, will find themselves practicing consultation. Many nurses currently practice consultation on a more or less informal and incidental basis; they give advice and help people solve work-related problems but don't consider themselves consultants or consciously think about the consultant role. Increasingly, however, nurses—particularly nurses practicing in an advanced role and those with higher levels of education, experience, or expertise—are recognizing and taking advantage of

opportunities to practice consultation on a more formal basis. That is, they are representing themselves and establishing businesses as nurse consultants.

Success in developing a practice as a nurse consultant, regardless of whether that practice is "moonlighting," part time, or full time, demands additional knowledge and skills. More specifically, nurses who are formally practicing nursing consultation, as either internal or external consultants, need "business savvy"—knowledge and skills in marketing, setting and collecting fees, and developing contracts—if they are to be perceived as professionals and able to protect their personal and professional interests. This information is

303

useful for nurses who practice consultation on an informal and incidental basis as well.

This chapter focuses on "business basics" for nurse consultants. The chapter begins by presenting basic marketing principles and strategies for promoting oneself as a nurse consultant. Next, issues related to setting and collecting fees are considered. The final section of the chapter discusses developing consultation contracts. As you read this chapter, think about the following questions:

- What professional and public responsibilities does presenting oneself as a nurse consultant entail?

- What specific skills, experiences, and interests could you use to build a nursing consultation practice?
- Which promotional strategies would you prefer to use to present yourself as a nurse consultant? How might these preferences enhance or limit consultation opportunities?
- What feelings do you have about charging for your services? How might these feelings affect your practice as a nurse consultant?

MARKETING AND PROMOTING NURSING CONSULTATION SERVICES

As much as 75 percent of a consultant's business activity comes from referrals and repeat business (Cosier & Dalton, 1993). As a result, developing and maintaining a business as a nurse consultant requires establishing positive working relationships, nurturing a favorable reputation, and developing supporters and alliances (Barron, 1989). In a very real sense, every consultation engagement needs to be considered an opportunity for marketing and promoting oneself as a nurse consultant.

The terms *marketing* and *promotion* are often used interchangeably. Though they are interrelated, marketing and promotion are distinct activities for generating business. Marketing refers to determining what potential customers (consultees) want and/or need and designing and offering a service that will meet those needs (Lachmann, 1996). Marketing is about meeting the needs of clients and positioning one's services in a competitive marketplace (Doughty & Keller, 2000). Thus, marketing is aimed at locating an opportunity and developing a business around that oppor-

tunity. Promotion, on the other hand, is the part of marketing that focuses on telling potential consumers (consultees) about a service. Promotion can be thought of as selling or advertising a service. Marketing is driven by three principles: service differentiation, market segmentation and analysis, and product promotion (Longworth & DiNardo, 1995). These principles define the issues that are addressed in the marketing process.

Service Differentiation

Service differentiation involves identifying how the products or services one proposes to offer are unique. It means identifying aspects of a service that are valued by clients yet unmatched by others providing the same service (Doughty & Keller, 2000). Service characteristics that are typically considered in the process of service differentiation include quality, features, options, packaging, service parameters, warranties, and cost (Lachmann, 1996). When applied to nursing consultation services, service differentiation entails defining how these characteristics are apparent in both the proposed consultation services and the nurse consultant as the service provider. Examples of how these characteristics might be used to define and differentiate nursing consultation services include the following:

- *Specific nature of service or area(s) of expertise*—for example, management, team building, data analysis, program planning, work redesign, health-related needs of a specific population group, information management, legal expertise, and so forth
- *Quality indicators*—success stories, specialty qualifications and education, certifications
- *Features*—skills, approach to the consultation process, specific creative innovations (e.g., use of computer technology or education strategies)
- *Packaging*—means of delivering services (e.g., seminars, retreats, education and training sessions)
- *Options*—on-site or off-site work, individual or group work
- *Service parameters*—follow-up, limitations in skills or services (e.g., a nurse legal consultant might specify unavailability for courtroom appearances)
- *Price*—demand for services, competitors' prices, and the actual cost of doing business; this is set in large part by the marketplace (issues related to setting fees for nursing consultation services are discussed in a later part of this chapter)
- *Warranties*—outcomes a nurse consultant wants to ensure such as increased productivity, more effective communication, cost savings, increased patient satisfaction, and so forth

Market Segmentation and Analysis

Market segmentation is the process of dividing the market (all potential consultees) into groups or "niches" according to factors or characteristics that influence selection and use of services (Doughty & Keller, 2000;

Lachmann, 1996). For example, the potential market of all primary care providers might be segmented as follows: solo practices, group practices, urban versus rural practices, practices that offer versus those that do not offer obstetrical care, and so on. These groups are then analyzed in terms of their current and future needs. The following are questions a nurse consultant can use to direct the market segmentation and analysis process:

- Who are my intended consultees? What group am I most interested in working with?
- What needs does this group have or are they likely to have?
- What does this group buy (e.g., education, support services, troubleshooting)?
- When do they tend to buy? That is, are they reactive or proactive? (Franck, 1991)

This list of groups and their needs is then compared to a nurse consultant's proposed services. If a nurse consultant's proposed services are a good fit with the market niche of interest, there is an increased likelihood of service and business viability. On the other hand, if there is a poor fit between proposed services and preferred market niche, the nurse consultant can either change "product" characteristics to better meet the needs of the preferred market niche or target a different market niche whose needs are more compatible with the proposed services. Market segmentation and analysis, therefore, helps a nurse consultant identify to whom to promote proposed consultation services. Examples of niche marketing by nurse consultants include offering team-building services to organizations that are undergoing restructuring, providing medication and symptom management consultation services to families of individuals with schizophrenia, and providing research development consultation services to primary care providers.

Product Promotion

The third principle of the marketing process is product promotion. In nursing consultation, product promotion includes all of the activities a nurse consultant undertakes to inform the target market or niche about the availability of services (Longworth & DiNardo, 1995). Product promotion includes personal selling, advertising, and all types of publicity. The goal of a nurse consultant's promotional activities is gaining recognition and having an image and reputation that attracts referrals and is known for producing results (Lachmann, 1996). Promotion strategies can be either direct or indirect.

Direct Promotion Strategies

Direct promotion is analogous to advertising. Nurse consultants engage in direct promotion when they directly approach a potential consultee and inform them about one's consultation services. Direct promotion can involve face-to-face appointments ("cold calls"), telephone solicitation, and mailings. Occasionally, a consultant will host an informational meeting (usually with a meal) for a group of consultees (Lippitt & Lippitt, 1986; Metzger, 1993). However, because the time involved in hosting meetings is not income-generating and because relatively few potential consultees can be reached at any one meeting, most consultants use targeted mailings as their primary direct promotion strategy. Mass mailings are generally avoided because of their low cost–benefit ratio; a mass mailing to 10,000 potential consultees will most likely yield only 200 inquiries and only one contract (Lewin, 1995). Consultants tend to rely on the following four types of printed materials for direct promotion: announcements of services, brochures, a consulting vita, and capability statements.

An announcement of services (Figure 17-1) is generally sent to potential consultees at the time a nurse consultant first establishes services, moves services from one location to another, or changes the focus of offered services. The announcement is in the form of a letter that defines the nurse consultant's overall objective and describes typical situations for which her or his services are appropriate. The announcement should be printed on good-quality letterhead stationery, addressed to the specific potential consultee, and personally signed by the nurse consultant. A nurse consultant should enclose a professionally produced business card or telephone index card with the announcement of services. Art departments of local colleges are often a good source of reasonably priced help for designing a letterhead and logo.

An announcement of services is frequently accompanied by a brochure, consulting vita, or capability statement. A brochure (Figure 17-2) should include a brief statement about the nature of the consultation services being offered, the consultant's background and experience, and a description of how assignments are conducted (Lewin, 1995). An effective brochure is characterized by a professional layout and attention to readability. A brochure needs to make a potential consultee aware of the services being offered in three seconds of reading time or less if it is to be given any attention (Lewin, 1995).

A consulting vita (Figure 17-3) highlights a nurse consultant's experiences and qualifications that directly support or demonstrate the ability to offer the advertised consultation services. The goal of a consulting vita is to concisely convey a nurse consultant's credibility (Metzger, 1993). Most consulting vitae also list a "few other interesting things" (e.g., hobbies) about the nurse consultant in an attempt to demonstrate balance and establish identity with potential consultees (Lewin, 1995).

A capability statement (Figure 17-4) is a fourth type of promotional material that nurse consultants find useful. A capability statement lists the specific skills and abilities that undergird or are a part of a nurse consul-

Perinatal Solutions, Inc.
Nursing Consultation Services
Partners for promoting healthy mothers, babies,
families, and communities

Leslie Norton, RNC, MSN
12703 125th Avenue, SE
Bellevue, WA 98772

Phone: (208) 546-9808
Fax: (208) 546-9888
e-mail: peri.1342@aol.com

Dr. Sandra Davison
Director of Obstetrical Services
Mercy Medical Center
1720 NW Mountain Blvd.
Bellevue, WA 98605

January 15, 2002

Dear Dr. Davison,

I have recently established a consulting practice to share my twenty years of experience in obstetrical nursing and ambulatory health care. My primary objective is to help care providers meet the challenge of providing safe and cost-effective family-centered obstetrical care in today's health care environment of managed care, higher-risk clients, and increasing malpractice costs. The strength of my practice is the breadth and depth of my experience, my extensive knowledge of both obstetrics and health care systems, as well as my creativity and passion for my work. Below are a few of the situations in which my services are most likely to be useful.

- Facility design or redesign (inpatient or outpatient) to enhance productivity while maintaining safe, family-centered care

- Developing perinatal and obstetrical care programs (protocols, fees schedules, and so forth) for nonobstetrical providers such as family practice physicians, home health care agencies, and community-based clinics

- Staff development—inpatient cross-training, perinatal home care services

- Market research regarding the need for services or satisfaction with services

- Development of documentation and evaluation systems

- Expert testimony

Should you learn of or encounter any situations in which my services may be of help, please call. All consultations are strictly confidential and a preliminary meeting is free of charge or further obligation. I have enclosed a telephone index card for your convenience.

Sincerely,

Leslie Norton

Leslie Norton, RNC, MSN

Figure 17-1   Sample Announcement of Nursing Consultation Services.
An announcement of services is used to notify potential consultees of new, relocated, or revised consultation services.

WHAT WE DO...

We sit down and work with you to clearly envision your future.

We gather information on what changes you would like to see take place. We work with you to identify causes of current problems or reasons for making a proactive change in services. We also identify your internal resources, the harnessing of which will reduce your costs and enable you to maintain any implemented changes.

We include you in the problem-solving process.

We recognize that *you* are the expert about what will and will not work in your system. We rely on your input and insight to help us develop problem solutions that will be meaningful, feasible, culturally sensitive, and long-lasting.

We do the legwork and negotiation.

Often, change and problem solving involves negotiating and working with other parties such as insurance providers, other care provider systems, equipment vendors, and the legislative/political system. We will contact these people on your behalf and introduce you to key players. We want to facilitate change for you and enable you to maintain the change on a long-term basis.

We empower you!

Our role is to facilitate change and ensure that change is long-lasting. We recognize that change will be long-lasting only when you can maintain it after we leave. To this end, we provide you with the training and support needed to manage change on an ongoing basis. We will also work with you to develop system supports such as policies, protocols, and reward (salary and benefit) structures.

We won't leave you high and dry.

Too often, consultants end up abandoning consultees at the end of a contract. We are always available for follow-up, support, and troubleshooting.

WHO WE ARE ...

Perinatal Solutions, Inc. was founded to help health care providers meet the challenges of providing safe and cost-effective family-centered obstetrical care in today's rapidly changing — and challenging — health care environment. Our goal is to promote the health of mothers, babies, families, communities, and society. We are a group of expert perinatal nurses who have combined our extensive and varied experiences into a system that helps providers solve a range of problems and plan for the future as an obstetrical care provider. Our services include the following:

- Inpatient or outpatient facility design or redesign
- Program development, including perinatal curriculum for educational systems
- Staff development
- Market research
- Development of quality assurance programs
- Expert testimony

Perinatal Solutions, Inc. was founded by Leslie Norton, RNC, MSN. Ms. Norton has more than 10 years experience as a consultant and over 20 years experience in perinatal nursing. She is also a Women's Health Care Nurse Practitioner. Ms. Norton holds courtesy faculty appointments in both the School of Business and the College of Health Professions at Northwest Washington University.

Ms. Norton is a member of a variety of professional and civic organizations and is certified by the Association of Health Care Consultants and the American Nurses' Credentialing Center. In her spare time, she designs quilts and raises Labrador retrievers.

Perinatal Solutions, Inc.
Nursing Consultation Services

Partners for promoting healthy mothers, babies, families, and communities

12703 125th Avenue, SE
Bellevue, WA 98772

Phone: (208) 546-9808
Fax: (208) 546-9888
e-mail: peri.1342@aol.com

Figure 17-2   Sample Brochure for Nursing Consultation Services.
A brochure needs to be professional and readable. It needs to make a potential consultee aware of the services being offered within three seconds of reading.

Leslie Norton, RNC, MSN
Founder and President
Perinatal Solutions, Inc.

Leslie Norton is founder and president of Perinatal Solutions, Inc., a local consulting firm that has served the health care industry throughout the Northwest for more than 10 years. Ms. Norton has worked with hospitals, HMOs, home health care agencies, and private care providers to develop creative ways of delivering perinatal services in today's changing health care environment.

Ms. Norton is a member of the faculty of Northwest Washington University where she holds courtesy appointments in the School of Business and the College of Health Professions. She teaches courses in nursing consultation, marketing, health care policy, and evaluation research.

Ms. Norton began her career in health care as a registered nurse working in the labor and delivery unity of a Level 3 medical center. Her area of study for her MSN was Parent–Child Nursing. She has also worked in home health care and is a women's health care nurse practitioner. She regularly conducts research in health promotion during high-risk pregnancies.

Ms. Norton is a member of the National Academy of Nurse Consultants, the Association of Home Health Care Nurses, and the Association of Perinatal and Women's Health Care Nurse Practitioners. She holds specialty certifications from the Association of Health Care Consultants and the American Nurses' Credentialing Center.

Perinatal Solutions, Inc.
Nursing Consultation Services

Partners for promoting healthy mothers, babies,
families, and communities

12703 125th Avenue, SE
Bellevue, WA 98772

Phone: (208) 546-9808
Fax: (208) 546-9888
e-mail: peri.1342@aol.com

Figure 17-3   Sample Consulting Vita.
In contrast to a traditional academic curriculum vita, the consulting vita focuses only on experiences and qualifications that directly support the consultation services that are being promoted.

Capabilities of Leslie Norton, RNC, MSN, Founder and President of Perinatal Solutions, Inc. as a nurse consultant for high-risk obstetrics home health care services

- Conduct community assessments to determine the need for and feasibility of services

- Develop a marketing plan, including promotional brochures for services; this plan can be targeted to specific market segments such as physicians, hospitals, or consumers

- Develop protocols and standards of care for common high-risk obstetrical conditions

- Provide staff training and competency validation in regard to nursing knowledge and skills needed for effective delivery of high-risk obstetrical home health care services; this can be delivered in traditional or self-study formats

- Develop billing guidelines for services

- Identify equipment needs and purchasing options

- Assist with recruiting and interviewing for staff positions for high-risk obstetrical home health care services

- Develop risk management programs

- Work with staff to develop and implement an ongoing quality assurance program

- Conduct program evaluations, including cost effectiveness and satisfaction

- Serve as a clinical consultant to nursing staff and physicians in regard to problematic cases

Perinatal Solutions, Inc.
Nursing Consultation Services

Partners for promoting healthy mothers, babies,
families, and communities

12703 125th Avenue, SE   Phone: (208) 546-9808
Bellevue, WA 98772   Fax: (208) 546-9888
                                                 e-mail: peri.1342@aol.com

Figure 17-4   Sample Capability Statement.
A capability statement is a task-oriented listing of skills that informs a potential consultee about the nature of problem solutions a nurse consultant is qualified to implement.

tant's services. The intent of a capability statement is to give potential consultees ideas about the specific tasks and types of problem solutions the nurse consultant is capable of implementing.

Announcements of services and capability statements can be adapted into advertisements for placement in business and professional journals or for publication in telephone directories. The intent of all these direct promotion activities is to create a "mental hook" so that when potential consultees have a need for specific services, an immediate picture is formed of who should be contacted to provide those services.

Indirect Promotion Strategies

The focus of indirect promotion is to gain the attention of those who are in a position to help one's career as a nurse consultant. Indirect promotion activities increase one's visibility and educate specific as well as more general audiences about one's services. Speaking engagements, publishing, professional memberships, and volunteerism are common indirect promotion activities (Schulmeister, 1999).

Public speaking offers nurse consultants an opportunity to get their name and face and credentials in front of a lot of potential consultees in a short period of time. Whether the investment of the time spent in public speaking has a long-term payoff, however, depends on who is in the audience (e.g., administrators or staff nurses). A nurse consultant can also gain visibility by becoming a spokesperson about topics within their own area of expertise for local radio and television stations.

Publishing gives a nurse consultant an opportunity to build a reputation and establish credentials as an expert. Publishing establishes name recognition and can bolster market clout, generate consultation inquiries, and prompt invitations to speak at meetings and conferences. In addition to seeking publication opportunities in professional journals, a nurse consultant might also explore publishing in the lay press or writing a regular newspaper or newsletter column.

Attending professional meetings gives a nurse consultant the opportunity to network with colleagues. Volunteering, serving on community boards, and sponsoring selected community activities are other strategies a nurse consultant might use to gain name recognition. Finally, nurse consultants need to keep in mind that attention to personal presentation, maintaining professionalism in dealing with others, and the quality of their business cards, brochures, and stationery are ways of creating a professional image and enhancing one's reputation.

To a certain extent, the amount of time a nurse consultant spends on promotional activities limits the amount of time that is available to carry out income-generating consultation activities. A challenge for nurse consultants, then, is to maintain a balance between conducting business and creating new business opportunities. A one-to-four or two-to-three rule is used by many consultants to maintain this balance. More specifically, one or two days are spent on promotional activities for every three or four days of billable work (Lewin, 1995; Metzger, 1993).

Promotion Strategies for Internal Nurse Consultants

Nurses who work as internal consultants (e.g., clinical nurse specialists and nurse-managers) also need to engage in activities that will enhance their visibility and credibility as a nurse consultant. This is particularly important when the nurse consultant or consultant role is new to the client system.

Internal nurse consultants can begin the marketing process by meeting with the key people in the client system (e.g., nursing staff and administrators in a hospital, or community business and service leaders) to identify their potential service needs. These meetings also give a nurse consultant an opportunity to describe and garner support for the consulting role. These activities can help prevent two common causes of failure of the internal nurse consultant role: unrealistic expectations of potential contact persons or consultees and a distorted view of consultation (Barron, 1989).

Members of a client system can also be educated about the nurse consultant role through brochures and announcements similar to those an external nurse consultant would use. Consultation referral forms and telephone index cards are additional strategies an internal nurse consultant can use to increase name and service recognition.

MONEY ISSUES IN NURSING CONSULTATION

Typically, nurses have not been paid fees that are linked directly to the services they provide and are unaccustomed to charging others for their acquired skills, time, and talent. As a result, nurses who are establishing themselves as nurse consultants frequently find establishing and collecting fees to be a difficult task. However, the fees a nurse establishes for consulting services can have implications for the marketability of these services: Fees that are too low unintentionally discredit oneself and one's services, whereas fees that are too high can price oneself out of business. In addition, as discussed in Chapter 15, issues related to fees and their collection can be a cause of legal action against a nurse consultant. The challenge of establishing and collecting fees for nursing consultation services, therefore, is to balance self-interest, guilt, and other factors with consultee and client needs for one's services (Lanza, 1996).

Setting Fees: Guidelines and Options

The true value of one's work as a nurse consultant reflects both beliefs about the worth of one's time and skills and what the market will bear (Doughty & Keller, 2000; Metzger, 1993). A reasonable starting place for establishing fees is to find out the going rate. This information can be obtained from other consultants, individuals, or organizations that have recently used consultation services, and employment advertisements. If employment ads are used as a source of information, the fees or salary they quote needs to be adjusted (if one is practicing as an independent nurse consultant) to account for the costs of overhead and benefits (Finnigan, 1996). Typically, hourly fees or salaries cited for employment by a consulting agency are lower than what an independent nurse consultant would charge because benefits (insurance, vacation, etc.) are also received as part of an employment package.

Fees also need to take into consideration the actual cost of offering one's services, needed or desired income, and hours available for generating that income. Finally, the fees one can realistically establish for nursing consultation services are affected by the laws of supply and demand. That is, the value of one's nursing consultation services will decrease if the same service is also being offered by others (Finnigan, 1996). Consequently, nurse consultants must carefully differentiate their services and be aware of their competition as well as what the market will bear. Box 17-1 presents several common formulas for establishing consultation fees.

Many nurse consultants will vary their fees according to the nature of a consultation contract (e.g., whether the contract is for a few hours, a day, or an extended period of time). It is often helpful to get some sense of the nature and scope of a nursing consultation project before citing a definite fee. If a nurse consultant is pressed for a fee at the initial meeting with a consultee, it is often best to quote a range of fees with the explanation that actual fees depend on the specific circumstances and the nature and scope of consultation activities.

BOX 17-1 ESTABLISHING FEES FOR NURSING CONSULTATION SERVICES

Several simple formulas exist for helping nurse consultants (and other entrepreneurs) establish fees for their services.

Option 1

1. Identify base salary desired.
2. Divide this by 2,000 hours to get hourly rate.
3. To this number add 100% for overhead[a] and 100% of salary rate for profit ("take home" pay).

Option 2

1. Look at the fixed plus variable expenses in your business plan.
2. Add profit desired ("take home" pay).
3. Divide by expected billable time[b] to get service price.

Option 3

1. Establish income goal.
2. Add what is needed (by you personally) for benefits (includes vacation, sick leave, insurance, etc.).
3. Add overhead[a] from business plan.
4. Add desired percentage for profit.
5. Divide by billable hours.[b]

Option 4

1. Calculate days or hours available for consulting per year: Full time = 22 working days per month × 8 hours per day = 176 billable hours per month.
2. Subtract one third of these hours (176 × .33 = 58) for new business development plus 1 day per week for administrative time (32 hours per month).
3. Adjusted billable hours per month = 176 − 58 − 32 = 86.
4. Divide #3 into income desired from consultation hours = hourly fee.
5. To this add 40% to cover operating expenses.

---

[a]Most experts say "double the overhead." That is, in calculations for overhead enter double what was already calculated in your business plan.

[b]Billable hours = hours available for consultation activities.

Sources: Finnigan, S. (1996). Getting started in business: From fantasy to reality. *Advanced Practice Nursing Quarterly, 2*(1), 1–8; Lewin, M. (1995). *The overnight consultant.* New York: John Wiley & Sons; and Metzger, R. (1993). *Developing a consulting practice.* Newbury Park: Sage.

Other consultants suggest quoting a flat daily rate that can then be broken down by the hour (Schein, 1987). Most consultants identify a minimum billing time and bill in increments of an hour (e.g., "Fees are calculated in 15-minute increments; minimum billing time is 4 hours"). Some consultants also state a project maximum (e.g., "Fees will be calculated at the rate of $150 per hour, not to exceed $7,500 for the project").

In general, consultants bill for all preparation time as well as actual contact time with a consultee. Travel within a reasonable distance to a consultation workplace is usually not billed. Extensive travel is typically billed at 50 percent of the consultant's usual hourly rate, plus the cost of the travel itself (e.g., airfare, mileage). Some consultants will charge more for making a presentation (such as an in-service education offering) than they will for activities such as reviewing documents and attending meetings to help a consultee with process and communication issues (Schein, 1987).

As discussed in Chapter 9, consultants differ in terms of whether they charge for an exploratory meeting with a consultee or contact person. Some consultants advocate treating an initial meeting as a marketing strategy and a cost of doing business (Frings, 1991). Other consultants routinely charge for an initial meeting because they have found that often enough advice is shared during an initial meeting so that no further intervention is needed (Schein, 1987). If a nurse consultant decides to charge for an initial meeting, the amount needs to be agreed upon in advance rather than arbitrarily decided on by the nurse consultant after the meeting has taken place.

Just as nurse consultants may vary their fees with the nature of the nursing consultation contract, they may also vary them for different consultees. Nurse consultants must keep in mind, however, that discounting their work without valid reason in a manner that is inconsistent from consultee to consultee demeans their work (Frings, 1991). In the case of a truly needy consultee who cannot afford the nurse consultant's usual fees, a nurse consultant may accept or offer a contract for intangible payoffs such as the opportunity to gain or practice skills, work with a certain individual or group, or get a foot in the door for other possible paying opportunities. Some nurse consultants will reduce their fees for a needy consultee in exchange for having the client system be responsible for completion of specific tasks such as taking notes of meetings and making logistical arrangements for training sessions. Nurse consultants need to remember, however, that in the eyes of many potential consultees, a nurse consultant's worth is determined by cost (Frings, 1991). While a modest amount of discounted or free work can bring excellent results, too much can drive a nurse consultant out of business (Franck, 1995).

Because nurses who are working as internal consultants are usually engaged in consultation projects during their regular work hours, they are usually more time conscious than money conscious. For internal nurse consultants, involvement in a consultation project typically occurs in lieu of other work tasks. Internal nurse consultants do, however, need to be clear about the resources (time, personnel, equipment, etc.) they will need in order to complete a project. If time in addition to regular work hours will be needed for a project, the nurse consultant should arrange for compensatory time or for these additional hours to be paid at their regular rate of pay or as overtime. Some internal nurse consultants negotiate for "payment" to be the opportunity to attend a conference or to have the client system purchase educational material for his or her personal use.

Collection Issues

The use of inappropriate methods to collect fees is a frequent reason for legal action against consultants (this was discussed in Chapter 15). Regardless of how a nurse consultant decides to handle fees and billing and collection procedures, expectations should be discussed in advance with the consultee or contact person. Fees and collection issues must also be spelled out in the nursing consultation contract.

Most consultants bill a consultee as soon as the contracted service has been completed (Finnigan, 1996; Metzger, 1993). The bill should restate the fees and payment terms that were agreed to in the nursing consultation contract (e.g., "Terms: net 30 days"). Receiving payment for nursing consultation services is facilitated by getting to know the client system's payment processes such as the need for a purchase order, payment cycle, and who is responsible for paying the bills. Detailing exactly what is being billed (time,

travel, other reimbursable expenses) tends to prevent the client system's questioning of the charges (Box 17-2 identifies expenses that are usually billed to consultees). Many consultants find that their bill is less likely to be challenged if they present it in person and accompany it with a progress report (Lewin, 1995).

A nurse consultant who is going to be working with a consultee group over a prolonged period of time may want to get the client system to agree to a monthly itemized bill for "progress payments" (Metzger, 1993). A bill for a progress payment usually incorporates charges for supplies as well as the nurse consultant's time. Nurse consultants who are working with a group of consultees or a particular client system for the first time will sometimes ask for start-up supply costs as well as a down payment (one third to one half of the estimated total) on the actual nursing

BOX 17-2 CHARGING FOR EXPENSES

Expenses that are incurred while completing a consultation project are generally charged back to the consultee or client system. The following expenses should be itemized on the billing statement:

- Long-distance telephone calls to or on behalf of the consultee
- Printing and copying costs
- Overnight mail (not ordinary postage) charges
- Materials—binders, folders, and so forth (but not paper as this is covered in copying costs)
- Parking
- Airplane or public transportation costs
- Hotel and meal expenses
- Travel—50% of hourly rate plus mileage at current rates (local travel is generally not billed)
- Books, software, and so forth that are purchased for the consultee or are needed to complete the project, as preapproved
- Training needed to complete an assignment, as preapproved. If training is one-time and essential for a project, the consultee is usually charged 100% of incurred costs. If training can be applied to future consultation situations, the consultee is usually charged 50%.

Source: Lewin, M. (1995). *The overnight consultant.* New York: John Wiley & Sons.

consultation fees as evidence of "good faith" (Metzger, 1993; Tepper, 1985).

CONTRACTS FOR NURSING CONSULTATION SERVICES

The process of contracting in nursing consultation was discussed in Chapter 9. The focus of the discussion in this section is the components of formal contracts and the ways in which consultation contracts can be structured.

From a legal perspective, a contract is formed every time two parties come together and enter into an arrangement that involves (a) an offer (i.e., for a specific consultation service), (b) acceptance of the offer, and (c) consideration (Remley, 1993).

Consideration refers to something of value that is given in exchange for service. In external nursing consultation situations, consideration is usually money but can also be intangibles such as access to information or people. In internal nursing consultation situations, consideration is more likely to consist of intangibles such as release from usual duties, an office, travel, and so forth. Without consideration, or the exchange of something of value, a contract does not exist. However, nurse consultants need to realize that they have a legal contractual obligation even in many circumstances in which they are not being paid. In nursing consultation, a contract can be offered by either the nurse consultant or the consultee.

Contracts do not necessarily have to be in writing. In most cases, any time a verbal offer is made and accepted and consideration exists, there is a legal contract. In some states, common law requires that contracts that transfer property (money) must be in writing (Remley, 1993). Nurse consultants will want to check their state statutes regarding contract issues.

Nurses who are working as internal consultants should be aware that a legally enforceable contract does *not* exist when an individual in an organization agrees to provide nursing consultation services to a consultee within the same organization (Remley, 1993). Because all parties involved are paid by the same employer, consideration does not exist within an in-house consultation situation. However, a contract *does* exist in the practical sense of the word—there is an offer and its acceptance—and fulfillment of the contract can have implications for an internal nurse consultant's performance evaluation and salary adjustments. Consequently, in internal nursing consultation situations, a written statement of understanding should be developed and signed by the parties involved.

Why Contract?

A formal contract represents agreement between a nurse consultant and consultees or other representatives of the client system on key issues such as fees and their collection and goals for the nursing consultation relationship. As a result, a contract decreases the likelihood of future conflicts and legal problems arising from misperceptions and misunderstanding. A formal written contract also enhances a nurse consultant's image as a professional (Scott & Beare, 1993).

Contract Components and Formats

Regardless of the format used for a nursing consultation contract, it should address the purpose of the consultation, methods for achieving this purpose, ground rules, expectations, resources needed to complete the consultation, and a timeline (Kurpius, Fuqua, & Rozecki, 1993). Box 17-3 provides a checklist of contract components for nursing consultation contracts.

Some consultants believe that written contracts are too "legalistic" and signify a distrust between the consultant and consultees that is

BOX 17-3   CHECKLIST OF CONTRACT COMPONENTS FOR NURSE CONSULTANTS

A complete formal contract for a nursing consultation project should address the following elements:

- ☐ General statement of project goals
- ☐ Avoidance of guaranteeing outcomes
- ☐ Work to be done by the nurse consultant—services to be provided, methods to be used
- ☐ Consultee responsibilities—tasks, supplies/resources to be provided
- ☐ Timeline for consultation—number and length of sessions with consultee, desired date of final report
- ☐ Line of authority and to whom the nurse consultant is responsible; frequency of communication
- ☐ Procedures for auditing progress of work
- ☐ Criteria and methods of evaluation
- ☐ Confidentiality and its limits
- ☐ People and materials to which the nurse consultant has access
- ☐ Fees to be paid, reimbursement for expenses, terms of payment
- ☐ Process for modifying contract
- ☐ Process for terminating contract
- ☐ Signatures and date of acceptance

Sources: Dougherty, A. (1995). *Consultation: Practice and perspectives in school and community settings.* Pacific Grove, CA: Brooks-Cole; Remley, T. (1993). Consultation contracts. *Journal of Counseling and Development,* 72, 157–158; Scott, L., & Beare, P. (1993). Nurse consultants and professional liability. *Clinical Nurse Specialist,* 7(6), 331–334.

antithetical to a productive consulting relationship (Schein, 1987). However, contracts can vary in format from a relatively formal legal document with "legalese" (Figure 17-5) to a comparatively simple letter that is sent by one party (Figure 17-6) and signed and returned by the other (Figure 17-7). Most frequently, nurse consultants use a letter of agreement signed by both participants or a simple contract drafted by one party and signed by both (Remley, 1993). Letters of understanding and memos (Figure 17-8) are also useful contract formats for internal consultation situations. When using a less formal format of contract, it is often easy to overlook

the inclusion of essential contract components. The use of a checklist such as the one presented in Box 17-3 can help ensure that each contract has the components that are needed and appropriate for the specific consultation situation.

Contracts with individual consultees are less likely to be written formally. A nurse consultant should keep in mind, however, that verbal contracts are often inadequate backup for any misunderstandings that may develop in a nursing consultation relationship. Most consultants have learned from experience that a written agreement of some sort should be developed for every nursing

Perinatal Solutions, Inc.
Nursing Consultation Services

This is a contract between Mercy-West Home Health Care Agency, herein called the party of the first part, and Perinatal Solutions Inc., herein referred to as the party of the second part. This contract is entered into on the seventh day of September, 2002, as follows:

The party of the second part agrees to serve as a consultant between September 7 and October 19, 2002, by providing education and training concerning fetal assessment techniques for home health care nurses employed by the party of the first part. Specifically, the party of the second part agrees to serve as workshop facilitator and trainer for five days (each day from 9 AM to 4 PM): September 20, 25, 30, and October 5, 10 for a workshop to be entitled, "Teaching Home Care Nurses Fetal Assessment." The party of the second part further agrees to conduct evaluations of the workshop participants' learning relative to the goals of the workshop and, with the permission of the participants, to share those evaluations with the contact person designated by the party of the first part. The party of the second part agrees to uses Gladys Jackson, Director of Nurses at Mercy-West Home Health Care Agency, as the contact person for all matters pertaining to this consultation, including the possible use of additional consultants or the addition of other consultees as participants in the workshop.

The party of the first part agrees to pay the party of the second part a total of five thousand dollars ($5000) plus expenses for materials within 10 days of completion of the consultation services. The party of the second part also agrees to provide materials (including audiovisuals and handouts) as long as the request for such materials is made by September 15, 2002.

This contract is subject to renegotiation at any time and either party is free to terminate the agreement if either determines the consultation progress to be unsatisfactory. Fees (prorated) and expenses become immediately due and payable at such a time.

For Mercy-West Home Health Care Agency: For Perinatal Solutions, Inc.:

_____   _____

Title: _____   Title: _____

Date: _____   Date: _____

Perinatal Solutions, Inc.
Nursing Consultation Services

Partners for promoting healthy mothers, babies,
families, and communities

12703 125th Avenue, SE   Phone: (208) 546-9808
Bellevue, WA 98772   Fax: (208) 546-9888
                                      e-mail: peri.1342@aol.com

Figure 17-5   Sample Formal Contract.
This contract is an example of a formal contract that has been generated by a nurse consultant.

Perinatal Solutions, Inc.
Nursing Consultation Services

12703 125th Avenue, SE
Bellevue, WA 98772

Margaret Planter, RN
Director of Community Health Services
MountainView Women's Clinic
North Avenue and C Street
Boise, Idaho 95443

July 12, 2002

Dear Ms. Planter,

I have had a chance to look over the packet of material that you sent and am eager to pursue a role working with your organization on the breast health awareness project. I think that breast health is an important and timely issue for women and your project looks like a good way to provide information as well as clarify some myths. I applaud your efforts in undertaking a project of this scope and think it is especially commendable that you have included evaluation plans in the project design.

The data analyses for this project would be pretty straightforward. I would look not only at test scores but at their relationship to demographic characteristics of the participants. The relationship between mammography utilization, breast self-exam, and these other characteristics could also be explored. This would give you information for further educational efforts.

I reviewed the questionnaires that you sent. You will note that I proposed some changes in wording and some additional items that I think would be worth reviewing. I would be happy to work with you to incorporate any of these items into the survey as well as to help you with format so that data can be entered directly from the survey into the computer.

If you do choose to involve me in this project, I would be willing to do all of the data processing and analyses as well as write a summary interpretive report. I would, of course, return all of the raw data and computer printouts to you either at the completion of the project or on an ongoing basis. I would like to discuss fee considerations and other contract details with you on the phone. I understand your financial constraints and am certain that I can work within your budget. I will want a portion of the total fee agreed upon at the time that I receive the first set of questionnaires for analyses. The remainder of my fee would be due at the time of submission of my final report. The timeline you presented on the phone the other day would work out fine for me.

As you requested, I have enclosed a copy of my current curriculum vita. I look forward to hearing from you regarding this project. The best days to reach me in my office are Mondays and Tuesdays.

Sincerely,

Leslie Norton

Leslie Norton, RNC, MSN

Perinatal Solutions, Inc.
Nursing Consultation Services

Partners for promoting healthy mothers, babies,
families, and communities

12703 125th Avenue, SE   Phone: (208) 546-9808
Bellevue, WA 98772   Fax: (208) 546-9888
                                                e-mail: peri.1342@aol.com

Figure 17-6   Sample Offer of Nursing Consultation Services.
This offer of services is less formal than a formal contract but, like a contract, establishes the parameters of a nursing consultation relationship. It requires acceptance and consideration before it is considered a contract.

MOUNTAINVIEW WOMEN'S CLINIC

North Avenue and C Street
Boise, Idaho 95443

Leslie Norton, RNC, MSN
c/o Perinatal Solutions, Inc.
12703 125th Avenue, SE
Bellevue, WA 98772

July 25, 2002

Dear Ms. Norton:

This correspondence serves as a letter of understanding regarding your offer to provide statistical analyses and final reporting of same in support of MountainView Women's Clinic's Breast Health Awareness project. As discussed, this project is being funded by a grant that was awarded to us by the State Health Division for purposes of planning, facilitating, and evaluating a project of health education to increase awareness and education among women about the personal and economic efficacy of early detection of breast cancer through better breast health practices.

As summarized in your letter, your services would include the following activities:
• Formatting of the survey to facilitate data entry into your computer
• Data processing and analyses
• Provision of a written summary interpretive report

As we discussed, your fee for the above services is $2,500, one half to be paid at the time the first surveys are sent to you. The remainder of your fee will be paid to you at the time of our acceptance of your final written report. If these terms are acceptable, please sign below and return this letter to me. I will make certain that you receive a copy for your files.

Sincerely,

Margaret Planter

Margaret Planter, RN
Director of Community Health Services

I accept and agree to the conditions outlined in this Letter of Understanding.

Name: _____

Title: _____

Date: _____

Social Security #:   _____

Figure 17-7   Sample Letter of Understanding.
This letter is in response to an offer of services. Note that it delineates tasks and fees. The nurse consultant and consultee (or whoever signs the letter on behalf of the client system) should both keep a copy of this document.

Jeanne Paulson, RNC, MSN
Pediatric Clinical Nurse Specialist
Mercy Medical Center

Corrine Raye, RN, CS
Director of Patient Care Services
Mercy Medical Center
1220 NW Mountain Blvd.
Bellevue, WA 98605

March 15, 2002

Dear Ms. Raye,

This memo serves as a letter of understanding about the nursing consultation services I will be providing for Mercy Medical Center.

The purpose of this consultation project is to work with employees of Mercy Medical Center to develop a plan for on-site child care services. As I understand the situation, I am to first conduct a needs assessment/interest survey and compile results. I also will conduct focus group interviews as a way of obtaining more in-depth responses from employees.

Once employees' interest in on-site child care is verified and I have obtained a sense of needs and preferences, I will visit other facilities that have on-site child care to observe how they operate. Finally, I will form a committee that represents a cross-section of interests in regard to this issue. I will work with this committee to develop a proposal to submit to Mercy Medical Center's administration and Board of Trustees.

My understanding is that nine months have been allocated for this project and that I am to be released from my other responsibilities as Pediatric Clinical Nurse Specialist for up to 28 hours a week in order to provide this consultation. During these nine months, I will continue to receive my regular salary (including any pay increases to which I am entitled during that period). Mercy Medical Center will make any needed travel arrangements and provide needed supplies and secretarial support services. Also, staff will be released from their regular duties with pay to participate in focus groups and committee meetings during their regular work hours. Staff who come in for a meeting during their off-shift hours will be compensated at their regular rate of pay.

As we agreed, I will report directly to you and we will have at least monthly progress meetings. Responses from employees will not be identified by name in any of my reports, nor will this information be made available without the participant's consent.

Would you please sign this letter and return it to me to indicate your acceptance of this project and its terms as outlined. Thank you for the opportunity to be involved in this project.

Sincerely,

Jeanne Paulson

Jeanne Paulson, RNC, MSN

Accepted:

Name: _____

Title: _____

Date: _____

Figure 17-8   Sample Memo of Understanding for an Internal Nursing Consultation Engagement.
This memo identifies tasks, goals, and processes and requests acceptance of terms by the nurse-manager. The memo illustrates how contract components can be incorporated into an informal presentation format.

consultation situation, even if it is just a brief memo (Kurpius et al., 1993; Metzger, 1993). In all nursing consultation situations, it is essential that all signing parties (e.g., the nurse consultant and consultee or representative of the client system) keep a copy of any signed contract and/or letter of acceptance.

CHAPTER SUMMARY

As the services that nurse consultants can offer in today's health care environment gain recognition, more and more advanced practice nurses will opt to establish consultation practices. These nurse consultants will need to develop an additional knowledge base and take on a new set of skills—marketing, promotion, fees, and contracts—if they are to be successful. While nursing consultation has always been a part of advanced nursing practice, to a great extent, it remains an "emerging" role and profession. Nurses who wish to take advantage of the growing opportunities for nurse consultants need to develop "business savvy" and familiarity with business issues if they are to become recognized and valued as professional nurse consultants.

APPLYING CHAPTER CONTENT

1. Develop a consulting vita and capability statement that you could use for promoting nursing consultation services. Have a peer critique these for completeness and presentation.
2. Critique the contracts that appear in Figures 17-5, 17-6, 17-7, and 17-8. What changes would you make in each of these contracts?

References

Barron, A. (1989). The CNS as consultant. In A. Hamric & J. Spross (Eds.), *The clinical nurse specialist in theory and practice* (2nd ed.) (pp. 125–146). Philadelphia: Saunders.

Cosier, R., & Dalton, D. (1993). Management consulting: Planning, entry, performance. *Journal of Counseling and Development, 72,* 191–197.

Doughty, S., & Keller, J. (2000). Marketing and contracting considerations. In A. Hamric, J. Spross, & C. Hanson (Eds.), *Advanced nursing practice: An integrative approach* (2nd ed.). Philadelphia: Saunders.

Finnigan, S. (1996). Getting started in business: From fantasy to reality. *Advanced Practice Nursing Quarterly, 2*(1), 1–8.

Franck, J. (1995, January). Know the who, what, and when of consulting clients. *Hospital Infection Control,* 10.

Frings, C. (1991, October). What it takes to be a successful consultant. *Medical Laboratory Observer,* 47–50.

Kurpius, D., Fuqua, D., & Rozecki, T. (1993). The consulting process: A multidimensional approach. *Journal of Counseling and Development, 71,* 601–606.

Lachmann, V. (1996). Positioning your business in the marketplace. *Advanced Practice Nursing Quarterly, 2*(1), 27–32.

Lanza, M. (1996). Money: Personal issues affect professional practice. *Clinical Nurse Specialist, 10*(6), 310–317.

Lewin, M. (1995). *The overnight consultant.* New York: John Wiley & Sons.

Lippitt, G., & Lippitt, R. (1986). *The consulting process in action* (2nd ed.). San Diego: University Associates.

Longworth, J., & DiNardo, E. (1995). Marketing your services. In M. Snyder & M. Mirr (Eds.), *Advanced practice nursing: A guide to professional development* (pp. 241–251). New York: Springer.

Metzger, R. (1993). *Developing a consulting practice*. Newbury Park, CA: Sage.

Remley, T. (1993). Consultation contracts. *Journal of Counseling and Development, 72,* 157–158.

Schein, E. (1987). *Process consultation, volume II: Lessons for managers and consultants.* Reading, MA: Addison-Wesley.

Scott, L., & Beare, P. (1993). Nurse consultants and professional liability. *Clinical Nurse Specialist, 7*(6), 331–334.

Schulmeister, L. (1999). The challenges of a home-based nursing consultation business. *Clinical Nurse Specialist, 13*(2), 101–103.

Tepper, R. (1985). *Become a top consultant: How the experts do it.* New York: John Wiley & Sons.

18

....

Working with Consultants

The worst of all worlds is spending the money on consultants and not getting the benefit.
(Hammer & Stanton, 1995)

 KEY CONCEPTS:

consultation firms, standardized consultation services, consultative partnership

---

 KEY TERMS FOR YOUR SEARCH ENGINE:

consultation and (issue for which consultation is being sought)

INTRODUCTION

Knowing when and how to use consultation services is increasingly important for community leaders, nurses in leadership roles, and health care providers. In today's rapidly changing health care environment, consultants are needed for both their expertise and their ability to facilitate a community's timely response to changes that are forced on it by its external environments. Indeed, health care management consultants often are identified as the chief architects of restructuring plans (*California Nurse*, 1995). For individual health care providers and nurse leaders, knowing how to choose and work effectively with consultants is equally important. Nurse practitioners, for example, may find themselves needing consultation for patient care as well as practice management issues. Indeed, for all nurses, knowing when to seek consultation

and how to work effectively with consultants is a professional and ethical responsibility and can prevent malpractice problems related to practicing outside of one's scope of competency (Norwood, 1998b).

Some indication of the need for nurses to know how to work with consultants is indicated by the amount of business that consultants generate. In 1993, 80,000 consultants in all industries sold $17 billion in advice. This was up 10 percent from the previous year (*California Nurse*, 1995). In 1994, consultants working just on reengineering projects, including those in health care, generated an estimated $1.4 to $2.6 billion (Hammer & Stanton, 1995). These figures suggest not only that consultation is big business, they also suggest that the likelihood of working with a consultant is high.

325

Working with a consultant involves a commitment of time, energy, and resources on the part of both systems (e.g., communities) and individuals. Seeking consultation also entails a certain degree of personal and political risk. While seeking consultation implies personal or organizational "neediness," it also indicates the ability to recognize one's limitations. However, hiring a consultant when one is not needed, choosing the wrong consultant, or being unable to work effectively with a consultant can raise concerns about one's judgment as well as general competence. Satisfaction with the results of a consultation relationship is due to a combination of common sense and rigor in making decisions about when to hire a consultant, whom to hire, what the consultant is to do, how he is to do it, and how to help him do it (Frankenhuis, 1981).

It makes some sense to assume that if you know how to provide nursing consultation, you also should be able to be an effective buyer and user of consultation services. To some extent this is true, and the content presented thus far in this text should, at the very least, provide some insight into what it means to be on the receiving end of consultation. Being a savvy consumer or participant in consultation services, however, requires a different set of considerations and behaviors. This chapter is about these "consumer skills." More specifically, this chapter focuses on making the decision to seek consultation, choosing a consultant, and maximizing the benefits that can be derived from a consultation relationship. The content in this chapter should be equally useful to nurses who find themselves needing to seek and hire a consultant and those who find themselves having consultation imposed on them by organizational superiors. Some questions to think about as you read this chapter are:

- In your own nursing practice situation, for what specific reasons might you seek consultation? What would you look for in a consultant?
- What difficulties might you have working with a consultant? How could you address these?

DO I NEED A CONSULTANT?

The initial decision to seek consultation often is made on an emotional basis. That is, consultation is usually sought only after a crisis is reached or one feels at wit's end for solving a problem. The danger with this is that a consultant may be hired unnecessarily, may not be hired when needed, or may be hired for the wrong reason. Think, for example, of situations in which you may have been involved when considerable time and money was spent on having a consultant focus on team building or communication, when dealing with a personnel issue (such as a weak manager) was what was needed to solve a problem.

The decision to seek consultation deserves careful consideration because becoming involved in a consultation relationship involves a commitment of time, energy, and money. In general, nurses, health care organizations, and communities enlist the help of consultants for four reasons: to acquire human resources, to secure cost savings, to ensure objectivity, and to address political considerations in a problem situation.

Acquiring Human Resources

The most common reason for seeking consultation is to acquire the human resources that are needed to resolve a particular problem. The needed resources might be vision and motivation, knowledge and information, technical or managerial skill, or staff utilization (Norwood, 1998a). At the individual level, a nurse practitioner might seek consultation to supplement his or her own diagnostic and care management skills. Likewise, a nurse administrator might seek technical and process expertise in order to increase an organization's ability to handle a complex, widespread organizational change (such as restructuring) involving multiple simultaneous changes and competing priorities.

At other times, additional resources are needed not to fill gaps in skill or knowledge, but because community members who have the needed expertise and skill are too busy or are unwilling to be involved in problem-solving efforts (Distasio, 1988). For example, it makes good sense to hire a consultant when a community's members have the abilities and expertise needed to resolve a problem on their own but are resistant to the community's goals and objectives or deny that a problem exists. In this situation, a consultant often can provide the vision and enthusiasm that is needed to stimulate participation in problem solving. In other situations, there might be persons within a community or organization who are qualified to work on a problem, but these same individuals may already be overextended and unable or unwilling to respond within the desired time frame. In this situation, a consultant can provide the organizational skills needed to coordinate and implement a project.

Securing Cost Savings

Hiring a consultant sometimes is the most cost-effective way for a community to resolve a problem. For example, to develop a one-time project such as facility redesign, cross-training, or program evaluation, it may be more cost effective to hire a consultant than to hire a permanent employee with skills for which there is no ongoing need (Norwood, 1998a). A consultant can be hired as a temporary resource, thus, to work on a specific problem and provide specialty assistance that can be ended once the project is self-sustaining or completed (Shelley, 1994). For example, a consultant's expertise and assistance might be useful in the development and initiation phases of a school-based clinic project. However, once the clinic is operational, the consultant's expertise (e.g., in program development and facility design) may no longer be needed. The nature of a consultation contract precludes any need to worry about long-term employment and financial obligations. Hiring a consultant, however, will be cost effective only if a community avoids paying for more service than it needs and avoids hiring a consultant to provide services already available through existing (and accessible) resources (Bader & Stich, 1993). Thus, real needs and in-house resources need to be assessed to determine if hiring a consultant is the most cost-effective way to solve a specific problem.

Ensuring Objectivity

Another valid reason for hiring a consultant is to get an objective and broad view of a problem situation. Because consultants do not have a vested interest in a problem or a particular outcome, they often are able to present more options for consideration as problem solutions. Consultants also are more accustomed to taking risks than are members of a community (Windle & Boyd, 1989). Because of their independence, consultants often are able to propose more imaginative problem solutions than are members of the community (Frankenhuis, 1981).

The independent and objective view that a consultant brings to a problem situation often is perceived as more credible than the same view would be if it was offered by a member of the community. In other words, sometimes "hearing a prophet from another country" promote ideas facilitates their acceptance by members of a community. Likewise, changes that are recommended by an outsider who has "seen it all" and can tell war stories as well as success stories frequently will function as a wake-up call and be accepted when the same changes recommended by an insider would be resisted (Hansten, 1994).

The independence and objectivity of consultants also makes them useful as an "executive sounding board" or someone on whom to test ideas before they are shared with members of a community (Shelley, 1994). Finally, the independence of a consultant from the community can help facilitate access to internal and external resources that might not otherwise be available to help with both problem identification and solution generation.

Addressing Political Considerations

A final reason for seeking consultation can be the politics of a problem situation. Specifically, a consultant can help diffuse some of the personal and political risk involved in a change situation. Often, it is difficult for members of a community to identify problems because doing so can be perceived as an admission of failure of some sort. Likewise, proposing some problem solutions—especially those that entail personnel or process changes—can be interpreted as protecting self-interests or as "getting even" with a co-worker or superior.

Consultants also can be used as a focal point or "lightning rod" for the anxiety related to a problem solution. In this role, a consultant can serve as a shield against the emotional backlash that might be associated with a problem diagnosis or recommendation for change if it is advocated by someone from within the community (Shelley, 1994). Finally, seeking consultation makes political sense when having a community member respond to a problem could create even the appear-

ance of a dual relationship or be interpreted as jockeying for a more powerful position within the community. While these political considerations might appear to be less worthy reasons for hiring a consultant, they reflect realities of community and organizational life that may need to be addressed if a problem really is to be solved.

When *Not* to Seek Consultation

A consultation relationship is likely to be successful only if it is really needed and will be supported by the community. For this reason, it is important to recognize situations in which seeking consultation is inappropriate.

Consultation is likely to be unsuccessful when community members have already reached a definite conclusion about a problem's cause and the needed solution (Norwood, 1998a). This suggests a certain inflexibility and lack of openness that will likely undermine any consultation relationship. Even in a purchase-of-expertise interaction pattern, consultees need to be open to exploring other possible problem causes and solutions with a consultant. Consultation is equally likely to be unsuccessful when no one wants to make a decision about a problem's cause or possible solution. This can signal a lack of commitment or energy to deal with a problem or disagreement about whether a problem exists or is worth solving. Inflexibility, lack of openness, and lack of commitment are issues that should be resolved before consultation is sought (Bader & Stich, 1993). Finally, if the community lacks the resources (time, money, and human resources) to facilitate the consultation process or implement any type of problem solution, hiring a consultant may be an unnecessary drain on the community's already stretched resources (Collins, 1989). Box 18-1 summarizes factors to consider when deciding whether or not to seek consultation.

BOX 18-1   SHOULD I HIRE A CONSULTANT?

Consultation is likely to be helpful when:
- The consultee or community lacks the knowledge or skill to resolve a problem on its own.
- The consultee or community lacks the manpower to resolve a problem in a timely manner.
- Management or process expertise is needed to facilitate widespread change in the client system.
- Temporary assistance with a specific short-term project is needed.
- Hiring a consultant would be less expensive than hiring a permanent employee.
- An independent and broad view of a problem situation is needed.
- A consultant will be able to access resources that are not available to members of the community.
- Hearing an outsider will increase the credibility of an idea.
- A change situation is likely to create a political or emotional backlash and a "shield" is needed.

Consultation is *not* likely to be helpful when:
- The community and its members are closed to exploring problem explanations and possible solutions.
- No one in the community is willing to make decisions about the problem.
- There is disagreement about whether a problem exists or is worth solving.
- There is a lack of resources to complete the consultation process or implement any likely problem solution.

CHOOSING A CONSULTANT

Once the decision has been made to seek consultation, the process of choosing the right consultant for the problem situation begins. This process entails deciding whether to use an internal or external consultant, identifying where to find an external consultant, determining what to look for in the consultant, deciding whether to use standardized services and consultation firms, and screening potential consultants.

Internal or External Consultation?

The relative advantages of internal and external consultation were discussed in Chapter 1. Selecting an internal consultant can be advantageous if a problem solution will require long-term management and monitoring. A new computerized patient information system, for example, likely will require permanent on-site availability of expertise—an in-house consultant—for troubleshooting, staff training, and system revisions. Internal consultation also should be considered if it will foster growth and development and in-house availability of long-term problem-solving skills.

It is a mistake to think that assigning a current community member to function as an internal consultant will always be more cost effective than using an external consultant. Depending on the scope of a consultation project and the internal consultant's usual role within the community, assigning an individual to be an internal consultant can involve overtime pay as well as expenses for finding someone to assume the internal consultant's usual work responsibilities (Norwood, 1998b). For example, a nurse who is asked to provide consultation in terms of developing new educational programs for a home care agency will likely be working overtime unless her or his usual patient care and/or supervisory responsibilities are assumed by someone else.

An external consultant often is perceived as more objective and independent than an internal consultant. Outsider status also may carry with it increased credibility. An external consultant is likely to be more effective than an internal consultant if an issue is not well defined and process skills are needed to arrive at a problem definition. An external consultant should also be hired any time using an internal consultant would create a dual relationship (see Chapter 16) or other conflict of interest. Finally, it may be easier for consultees to "save face" if they work with an external rather than internal consultant. Seeking external consultation implies a gap in not only the problem-solving skills of the consultee (e.g., nurse administrator or a direct care provider), but in the abilities of the community as a whole.

There is a growing trend toward using both an internal and external consultant in a single problem situation (Bader & Stich, 1993; Shelley, 1994). Initially, this may be more expensive, but it enables a community to take advantage of both insider and outsider knowledge and expertise simultaneously. The internal consultant can facilitate the external consultant's ability to navigate a complex and unfamiliar community or organizational client system and, thus, expedite the problem identification phase of the consultation process. At the same time, an external consultant can help a internal consultant acquire the knowledge and skills needed for long-term management of a potentially recurring problem situation.

Finding a Consultant

Most consultants are hired as a result of word-of-mouth recommendations from colleagues. However, the right consultant for a colleague's situation may not necessarily be the best choice for one's own situation. Among possible sources for an external consultant are health care consulting firms, professional organizations and networks, and universities. Professional journals also can be valuable resources for finding a consultant. Journal articles also can help identify nurses and other individuals with specific areas of expertise. For technical consultation problems such as remodeling and facility design, equipment vendors can be helpful as a resource for identifying potential consultants. Finally, individuals or institutions or communities with similar characteristics that have faced a similar problem situation can help one develop a list of potential consultants.

What to Look for in a Consultant

Knowing what you want and why you want it (or what you don't want and why) is essential when choosing a consultant. The success of a consultation relationship is due, in large part, to the consultees' abilities to express *what* is needed and translate this into *who* is needed for a specific problem situation. The scope of the problem, the desired timeline for a problem solution, and the type of support available from the community should shape the selection criteria for a specific consultation project. The specific criteria that should be developed to identify an appropriate consultant are expertise, experience, and fit. The key to a successful consultation relationship is selecting a consultant who has the needed expertise and relevant experience, and who can relate effectively to the problem situation and members of community.

Expertise

Identifying the scope of a consultation project and the roles a consultant will need to fill helps to clarify the knowledge and skills that a consultant will need in order to be effective in a consultation situation. If a consultant is being sought to help address a community-wide health issue, for example, knowledge of communities and systems theory would likely be included on a list of necessary qualifications. On the other hand, if consultation is being sought to help with the management of a particular patient problem, expertise in that problem area is essential. The expertise that is needed also depends on the roles a consultant is expected to play in the consultant project. For example, if a consultant is expected to train staff as well as develop a new patient information system, needed expertise would include teaching and evaluation skills as well as expertise on the specific information system. Assessing existing limits and capabilities within one's own community also helps to more accurately identify the expertise a consultant needs to bring to a problem situation. For example, perhaps training staff to use a new patient information system could be carried out by an internal consultant. If so, the expertise sought in an external consultant would be redefined and narrower in scope. Consultation is most cost effective when services community members can provide are not duplicated by an external consultant. Knowing the set of skills a community needs to supplement its own prevents duplication and facilitates taking advantage of its own experts as well as involving members in problem solving; this, in turn, facilitates buy-in and the development of problem-solving skills for future use.

Experience

Experience is a crucial criterion in selecting a consultant (Cerne, 1993; Windle & Boyd, 1989). A consultant who is being asked to help resolve a health care problem needs experience working with health care systems and the specific specialty area involved. Community and health care settings generally have different philosophies, cultures, politics, and problems than other organizational systems. Because of this, for community consultation, a consultant with general business and management experience, but lacking in health care knowledge and community experiences, is unlikely to be the most effective consultant. Conversely, a consultant who has extensive clinical expertise, but lacks business experience, also may be unable to effectively help solve a management problem. Likewise, a consultant with work experience in only urban medical centers may have trouble helping to address problems in a rural community, and consultants who have worked only with hospitals may be unfamiliar with the problems faced by ambulatory or home health care settings.

Fit

In addition to expertise and experience, the success of a consultation relationship is determined by a consultant's "fit" with the community. To have a successful working relationship, a consultant's style and approach to problem solving needs to match that of both the community as a whole and the individuals who will be involved most directly in the consultation project. In other words, there must be a "personal chemistry" between the consultant and members of the community, particularly the consultees. Fit can be determined, in part, by a potential consultant's sensitivity to and respect for a community's culture. This can be reflected in dress, manner, tone of voice, sense of humor, and philosophy of consultation (Distasio, 1988).

Fit also means there is a congruence between the preferred problem-solving strategies of the consultant and consultees. For example, health care cost containment issues generally are resolved through one of three approaches: reengineering/work redesign, changes in compensation and wage structures, and information management (*California Nurse*, 1995). Each of these approaches make different assumptions about the causes of a health care system's cost containment problems and how they should be addressed. These assumptions must fit with the beliefs of the community if the consultation relationship is to be a success. Individual health care providers such as nurse practitioners who are seeking consultation for assistance with a specific patient management issue also need to screen potential consultants for fit in terms of philosophy of health care, preferred treatment strategies, and so forth.

Screening Consultant Candidates

Once qualifications for a consultant have been determined and potential candidates have been identified, the screening process begins. The screening process should culminate in a decision about who specifically to hire. The screening process also includes making decisions about the desirability of using standardized consultation interventions and about using an independent consultant versus the services of a consulting firm.

The screening process itself should begin with a review of prospective consultants' written proposals for the needed consultation services. Allowing consultant candidates to develop their own proposal rather than dictating the proposal's format provides an opportunity to evaluate a candidate's creativity, conciseness, clarity of presentation, and ability to translate general needs and goals into a specific and customized project (Distasio, 1988). The proposal also provides an opportunity to get some idea of a candidate's alignment with the mission, values, and strategic objectives of the community.

The second part of the screening process should be a face-to-face interview. For a community-wide consultation project, managers/

leaders of affected neighborhoods and agencies as well as at least some of the individuals who will be working most closely with the consultant should be involved in the interview process. This can be done through either a group interview or a series of individual interviews between the consultant candidate and key members of the community. Interviews provide an opportunity to gather further information about a candidate's expertise and experience (e.g. what does "participated in" mean and who was the "major health care organization" that the candidate has had experience with). An interview also provides an opportunity to assess communication style, comfort with the community's culture, attitudes, credibility, and personal chemistry with those who will be involved in the consultation process. Additional issues that can be explored during the interview process are identified in Box 18-2.

The third component of the screening process should be a check of references from communities with whom a consultant previously has worked. A candidate's willingness to identify previous consultees is an indication of trust in the potential ("hiring") client system's discretion as well as faith in the quality of previous work. Examples of questions that can be asked during a reference check are listed in Box 18-3.

Using Standardized Consultation Services

A consultation relationship will be effective only if there is a fit between what a community needs and what a prospective consultant can offer. Thus, consultees need to carefully examine any proposal to use a standardized approach to solving a community's problems. "Canned" interventions are particularly dangerous when they are proposed as the answer to a problem before the consultant conducts a thorough assessment and explores the range of possible problem solutions.

BOX 18-2   THE SCREENING PROCESS: INTERVIEW QUESTIONS FOR CONSULTANT CANDIDATES

In addition to verifying and clarifying experience and expertise and exploring a candidate's fit with the community, a face-to-face interview provides the opportunity to ask questions such as:

- Is the candidate more interested in doing the project or establishing a personal relationship with the community or some of its members? How does this fit with the needs of the community?
- How flexible does the candidate seem? How will they respond to examples of problem issues that might arise during the consultation process?
- How will the candidate go about understanding how the community functions?
- How will the candidate address issues such as disruption of the consultation process to the client system and education and training for those involved in the consultation process?
- What are the candidate's expectations for "in-house" support? Will there be a need for an internal liaison to coordinate the project, secretarial support, staff assistance with data collection, or a "demonstration unit" for the problem solution? (These would all add to the cost of the consultation process.)
- What is the candidate's proposed budget for the project—fees, travel, other expenses?
- How much on-site versus off-site time will the project involve? What specific components of the project will be carried out on- versus off-site?

BOX 18-3   THE SCREENING PROCESS: CHECKING REFERENCES

Questions that should be asked of consultees and communities/client systems with whom a consultant has worked include the following:

- Do you think you got a positive return on your investment with this consultant? What indicators are you using to come to this conclusion?
- What could this consultant have done better?
- How would you work differently with this consultant next time? Why?
- Did you implement this consultant's recommendations? If not, why not? If yes, did you receive adequate support and guidance? What adjustments did you need to make to the recommendations and why were they needed?
- Would you recommend this consultant or use this consultant again?

It is important to keep in mind that standardized consultation interventions are problem solutions that were originally developed and used to meet the needs of another community. Because of the intervention's previous success, and because it is quicker to implement a standardized problem solution than to develop a customized one, the intervention is offered for use repeatedly in different settings and situations. Work redesign and cross-training are two contemporary examples of standardized approaches to the current health care problem of cost containment. The appropriateness of standardized consultation interventions for a specific community's problems depends on how similar the present system and problem situation are to the conditions and setting for which the solution originally was developed. Effectiveness also depends on how much flexibility is built into the intervention and how willing a prospective consultant is to adapt it to the needs of a different setting and system.

Using a Consulting Firm

Screening a consulting firm to provide consultation services should involve screening both the firm itself and the individual(s) the firm will assign to actually do the work of a consultation project. As in screening individual consultant candidates, the process should involve review of the proposal, face-to-face interviews, and reference checks. It is particularly important to verify the expertise and experience of the individual(s) in the firm who will be working most directly with the members of the community. Again, vague phrases on resumes such as "participated in" or "assisted with" need to be clarified. Individuals who provide consultation services as a member of a consultation firm need to be held to the same expectations for experience and expertise as individual consultant candidates. If there are weak areas in their qualifications, there should be plans

for covering them with other consultants in the firm.

MAXIMIZING A CONSULTATION RELATIONSHIP

Seeking consultation for appropriate reasons and choosing the right consultant for a problem situation are just two thirds of what it takes to have an effective consultation relationship. Working with consultants to maximize their ability to resolve problems and create change involves approaching the consultation relationship as a partnership, preparing the community for the consultation process, orienting the consultant to the community, and monitoring the consultation process as it progresses. How a community works with a consultant is the single most important variable in maximizing a return on an investment in a consultation relationship (Shelley, 1994).

Creating a Partnership

Once a consultant has been hired, it often is tempting to want to relinquish all control of the problem situation to the consultant. This is particularly likely to occur when a purchase-of-expertise or doctor–patient interaction pattern is being used to guide the consultation process. Consultation, however, is more likely to be successful if it is treated as a partnership and a two-way process. This means an effort should be made to relate to the consultant as an "intellectual peer" and to create an atmosphere that encourages critique of each other's thinking (Shelley, 1994). Approaching consultation as a partnership also means sharing responsibility for any "tough decisions" (such as layoffs) that need to be made—even if consultation originally was sought to provide a shield against backlash from unpopular decisions.

Another dimension of approaching a consultation relationship as a partnership is openness. It is particularly important to be candid about any mixed emotions regarding the consultation. Often, when consultation is sought, help is needed and wanted—but there is still a desire to resolve a problem independently. It also is important to share concerns about exposure of gaps in competence ("loss of face") and loss of control.

Preparing the Community

Members of a community can react to news of an impending consultation with responses that range from a sigh of relief to suspiciousness. Whatever the initial response, all members of a community (or any other client system) who stand to be affected by the consultation process (stakeholders as well as consultees) need to be informed about the reasons for the consultation, its purpose, timelines, and expectations for participation. There also needs to be sensitivity to the feelings of those who actually will be working with the consultant, and an effort should be made to be empathetic to their concerns. Factual information should be given, rumors should be dispelled, and false reassurances should be avoided.

Orienting the Consultant

In organizational or community-wide consultation situations, orienting the consultant to the community will facilitate both physical and psychological entry into the community. Orientation is most effective when it is carried out by whomever is assigned to work with the consultant as a liaison or internal consultant on an ongoing basis. A consultant's orientation needs to address practical matters such as the logistics of phone use, copying, invoicing, and secretarial support. An orientation also should include a discussion of the community's culture and protocols as well as boundaries on access to information (Bader & Stich, 1993). A consultant should be advised about information sources, potential pitfalls, politics and interpersonal sensitivities, capabilities of the community, and champions and resistors to the consultation relationship.

BOX 18-4   MANAGING THE CONSULTATION RELATIONSHIP

- Be an active participant in the consultation relationship. Ask (and expect) to be educated and involved.
- Make an effort to understand each other's needs and objectives.
- Facilitate gaining entry—orient the community to the nature of the consultation relationship and orient the consultant to the community.
- Keep an open mind—be receptive to new ideas about problem causes and solutions.
- Agree on mechanisms for assessing progress, and carry these out.
- Uphold your end of the contract—keep promises about fees, time, and providing other resources.
- Keep lines of communication open.
- Know when to call it quits.

Monitoring Progress

A consultation relationship stands the best chance of being effective when its progress is monitored and reviewed on an ongoing basis. If formative evaluation activities (Chapter 13) are being carried out, progress can be monitored by reviewing evaluation findings. Progress also can be monitored by establishing key milestones and "deliverables"—and staying on top of them (Hammer & Stanton, 1995). Regularly scheduled progress report sessions are one strategy that can be used to ensure that the consultation process is progressing as desired. Progress report sessions should focus on a discussion of accomplishments of the consultation relationship to date as well as barriers encountered and additional help that is needed to facilitate the consultation. Progress report sessions also provide both the consultees (as well as the community as a whole) and consultant an opportunity to revise the nature of the consultation relationship (including termination) and the consultation contract as needed. Box 18-4 summarizes strategies for maximizing a consultation relationship.

CHAPTER SUMMARY

The current health care environment is characterized by an increased emphasis on a community perspective of health care, as well as by increasingly complex organizational issues. Health care administrators are being asked to respond to issues such as institutional cost containment and increased patient acuity. Communities are encountering health-related issues such as school violence, homelessness, air quality concerns, and the inability of citizens to access even basic health services. Likewise, individual health care providers such as nurse practitioners are faced with the challenge of needing to respond to complex and diverse health care delivery issues in their practices (Norwood, 1998b). Nurses in posi-

tions as direct care providers (e.g., as staff nurses, nurse practitioners, or clinical nurse specialists) are further challenged by individual patients with increasingly complex and diverse health care needs and by becoming the gatekeeper to a patient's access to specialty services. In all of these settings and situations, knowing and respecting one's limitations for dealing independently with these issues is a professional and ethical responsibility that can have legal ramifications.

Fortunately, at the same time that health care delivery and health care needs are becoming more complex, individuals (including nurses!) are developing the specialized knowledge and skills to respond to these issues and to provide consultation to others who need to address these issues. Developing skills in knowing when and how to access this expertise and work effectively with consultants has become an integral part of professional nursing practice for nurses in all roles and practice settings.

APPLYING CHAPTER CONTENT

1. Consider the following scenarios:
   A. You are a newly licensed nurse practitioner who is new to town. You are working in a practice with two physicians in a large multispecialty clinic. You have been working in this practice for only four months and, while you have a good working relationship with the physicians, you are still trying to establish your credibility. The office manager and support staff particularly need convincing that you "know your stuff."

   You have been seeing a patient for management of hypertension. The patient has been unresponsive to the "starter therapy" with which you are fairly comfortable. The patient has also been nonresponsive to suggestions regarding strategies for weight loss, exercise, stress reduction, and the like. You are feeling frustrated and lost.

Do you need a consultant? Why or why not?

How would you go about choosing a consultant for this problem?

Would you use an internal or external consultant? Why?

What would your selection criteria be for this consultant? How did you choose these criteria?

B. You are the director of a relatively small home health care agency. You have just received word that your agency will be merging with a competitor in the community. Rumors are flying about job losses; staff are angry and scared.

Do you need a consultant? Why or why not?

Would you seek internal or external consultation? Why?

How would you go about choosing a consultant?

What would your selection criteria be? Why?

C. You are the chairperson of the volunteer board of directors for a community health care agency that is having severe budget problems. One option the agency is considering in order to balance its budget is "downsizing" its services. You personally are resistant to this idea, as are agency staff, but the agency administrator seems to be in favor of it. The decision needs to be made within three months.

Do you need a consultant?

Would you seek internal or external consultation? Why?

How would you go about choosing a consultant?

What would your selection criteria be? Why?

2. Develop a list of consultation resources that are appropriate for problems you might encounter in your own nursing practice. Develop a list of screening criteria that would help you select a consultant for a typical problem in your practice role.

References

Bader, G., & Stich, T. (1993). Using external consultants wisely. *Seminars for Nurse Managers, 1*(1), 22–25.

California Nurse (1995, June). The unseen hand in cutting care—The healthcare consultant (pp. 16, 17).

Cerne, F. (1993, September). A call for consultants. *Hospital and Health Networks,* 33–35.

Collins, B. (1989). Do you need an external consultant? A model for decision making. *Clinical Nurse Specialist, 3*(2), 91–96.

Distasio, C. (1988). Consultative services: Guidelines for cost-effective utilization. *Healthcare Supervisor, 6*(4), 1–17.

Frankenhuis, J. (1981, November–December). How to get a good consultant. *Journal of Nursing Administration,* 56–60.

Hammer, M., & Stanton, S. (1995). *The reengineering revolution: A handbook.* New York: HarperBusiness.

Hansten, R. (1994). Consultants: Making your budget work. *Nursing Management, 25*(11), 10–11.

Norwood, S. (1998a). Making consultation work. *Journal of Nursing Administration, 28*(3), 44–47.

Norwood, S. (1998b). When the CNS needs a consultant. *Clinical Nurse Specialist, 12*(2), 53–58.

Shelley, S. (1994). Interactive consulting: Maximizing your consultant dollar. *Nursing Economics, 12*(5), 272–275.

19

The Future
and Nursing Consultation

Consultation is not a profession itself, but a way of practicing one. (Frings, 1991)

 KEY CONCEPTS:

entrepreneur, intrapreneur, trend, inductive reasoning, deductive reasoning

 KEY TERMS FOR YOUR SEARCH ENGINE:

entrepreneurism, intrapreneurism, health care and trends, futurists

INTRODUCTION

Nursing consultation is a way of practicing the profession of nursing: working with individuals and groups to help them solve actual or potential problems related to the health status of clients or health care delivery. Nurses' knowledge and competence as clinicians, managers, educators, and researchers provide them with both the content expertise and essential skills needed for success as nurse consultants (Hazelton, Boyum, & Frost, 1993). Clinical skills facilitate a nurse's ability to assess and identify nursing consultation problems. Management skills help a nurse manage time and resources during the nursing consultation process. Education skills are used when a nurse consultant interacts with consultees to help them learn problem-solving skills. Research skills facilitate a nurse's ability to interpret assessment data and evaluate the nursing consultation process. All nurses, thus, have the foundation needed to serve as consultants to anyone who seeks assistance with a problem or concern that is within the scope of their expertise.

So far, this text has presented a description of the nursing consultation process (Chapters 1 through 5 and 9 through 14) and a discussion of the contextual basis (Chapters 6 through 8) and professional issues (Chapters 15 through 18) associated with nursing consultation. In this final chapter, the focus is on envisioning how nursing consultation can become a part of one's personal practice of nursing. In a sense, the content in this chapter is a way of wrapping up, tying together, and moving into the future everything that has come before.

This chapter begins with an overview of strategies that can be used for envisioning opportunities in nursing consultation. Next, these strategies are applied to intrapreneurial and entrepreneurial practice patterns of nursing consultation. The final section of this chapter considers what is needed to turn a vision of consultation practice into a reality. As you read this chapter, think about the following questions:

- How are the trends identified in this chapter currently reflected in health care?
- What other trends can you identify? What are the implications of these trends for health care?
- What opportunities do these trends suggest for nursing consultation? What opportunities do they present for you personally as a nurse consultant?

THE ART OF FUTURETHINK FOR NURSE CONSULTANTS

You have to remember to stop and think. And think ahead. Or else you lose track of the future. (Popcorn, 1992)

Futurethink is the art of envisioning realistic opportunities. Futurethink means systematically identifying trends and speculating about alternate possible futures so that one's product or service will meet the likely needs and desires of its intended consumers. Services—such as nursing consultation—that are developed on the basis of futurethink have a greater chance of viability and longevity than do those based on hunches or meeting one's own personal needs.

Identifying Trends

Trends are pervasive ways of thinking and patterns of behavior that have a common underlying theme or meaning. Trends last an average of 10 years or more and appeal to the mainstream rather than just specific groups, although a trend may be stronger in some groups than in others (Popcorn, 1992). When considered together, trends provide a clear profile of the marketplace: what's starting to happen now and what will be happening in the immediate as well as more distant future (Popcorn & Marigold, 1996). Trends serve as predictors of what will be sought, what types of problems will need to be solved, and what types of problem solutions will be most desired. Trends also indicate where present need gaps are. In a very real sense, the ability to recognize trends is the ability to recognize the future (James, 1996).

Identifying trends means finding new patterns in everyday occurrences. It also means scanning the present culture for signs of the future. Cultural indicators of emerging trends can be found in children's literature, science fiction, television sitcoms, news magazines, symbols (clothes, jewelry, hair styles), new stores, and language (James, 1996). Often, "people messing with the rules" (Barker, 1992) can be an initial and early indicator of an evolving trend.

Identifying trends, then, involves applying inductive reasoning to specific observations to reach general conclusions about the observation's economic, social, political, and consumer significance (James, 1996). For nurse consultants, relevant trends are identified from observations of health care delivery practices as well as more general social and political patterns of behaving and thinking.

Becoming familiar with the thinking of current futurists is another way to get ideas about general trends as well as those that can be applied to health care and nursing consultation. It is important, however, to become familiar with the trends identified by a variety of futurists because every futurist tends to view the world differently and come to different conclusions about the future. Naisbitt and Aburdane (1990), for example, took a macroenvironmental approach and focused on global trends. The "mega-trends" they identified 10 years ago are listed in Box 19-1. In contrast, Popcorn (1992) and Popcorn and Marigold (1996) focused on social trends that are reflected in everyday behavior. The social trends that they have identified are highlighted in Box 19-2. As a third perspective on

trends, Schwartz (1996) identified "driving forces" (see Box 19-3) that can be used to speculate about needed goods, services, and modes of service delivery. Celente (1997) identified two trends that still have particular significance for health care providers: "Survival Strategies"—an emphasis on staying healthy and living longer, and "New Millennium Medicine"—recognition of the mind–body connection, acceptance of alternative treatment modalities, and an emphasis on nutrition, vitamins, and "clean food." All of these trends, which were identified as "emerging" 5 to 10 years ago, are facts of life today.

Other strategies that can be used for gathering information about emerging trends

BOX 19-1   GLOBAL TRENDS IN THE 1990S

In 1990, Naisbitt and Aburdane identified the following global trends. As you scan this list, ask yourself about (a) whether this trend materialized and is still present today, (b) the implications of the trend for health care, and (c) opportunities this trend could create for nurse consultants.

- *A booming global economy*—an increasing amount of disposable income
- *A renaissance in the arts*—a growing appreciation for the importance of the cultural side of life
- *Emergence of free market socialism*—the opening of new consumer markets in formerly socially and politically restrictive environments
- *Global lifestyles and cultural nationalism*—cultural blending and homogenization rather than isolated diversity
- *Privatization of the welfare state*—changes in funding sources for social welfare programs
- *Rise of the Pacific Rim*—growing importance of Asian markets as both consumers and producers
- *The decade of women in leadership*—increasing opportunities in the upper echelons of management for women
- *The age of biology*—increasing use of and advances in biotechnology
- *Religious revival*—increasing emphasis on the spiritual dimension of life
- *Triumph of the individual*—greater emphasis on and respect for individual rights

Source: Naisbitt, J., & Aburdane, J. (1990). *Megatrends 2000: Ten new directions for the 1990s.* New York: Avon Books.

BOX 19-2   SOCIAL TRENDS FOR THE 1990S AND BEYOND

Popcorn and Marigold (1996) identified the following 16 social trends. As you look at this list, consider how these trends are reflected in health care needs and health delivery issues. How are these trends reflected in the current health care system? What do these trends suggest in terms of health care delivery "wants" and potential problems? What ideas do these trends present for nursing consultation opportunities? What types of nursing consultation interventions do these trends suggest will be most successful?

1. *99 Lives*—the pressure to assume multiple roles
2. *Anchoring*—reaching back to what was comfortable in the past
3. *Being alive*—increasing awareness of the concept of wellness
4. *Cashing out*—questioning personal satisfaction and goals and opting for simpler living
5. *Clanning*—the inclination to "hang out" with groups of like kinds that can provide security and validation of one's own belief system
6. *Cocooning*—strategies to protect oneself from the harsh realities of the outside world
7. *Down-aging*—a nostalgia for childhood that is reflected in a lightness in adult lives
8. *Ego-nomics*—looking for ways to make a personal statement
9. *Fantasy adventure*—seeking excitement in risk-free adventures as a break from modern tension
10. *Femalethink*—an increasing emphasis on caring, sharing, and familial values
11. *Icon toppling*—active rejection of the monuments of government and business and the pillars of society
12. *Mancipation*—a new way of thinking for men that embraces the feeling of being an individual
13. *Pleasure revenge*—cutting loose and seeking "forbidden" pleasures
14. *Small indulgences*—rewarding oneself with small luxuries
15. *SOS (Save Our Society)*—a rediscovery of a social consciousness, including environmentalism
16. *Vigilante consumer*—an increased emphasis on consumerism: value, quality, safety

Source: Popcorn, F., & Marigold, L. (1996). *Clicking: 16 trends to fit your life, your work, and your business.* New York: HarperCollins.

include talking with "key players," reading widely both within one's discipline and in the popular literature, and travel (Popcorn & Marigold, 1996). Identifying trends and their implications also requires a certain type of mindset. Hamel and Prahalad (1994) describe this mindset as having the following characteristics:

- Curiosity
- Willingness to challenge assumptions
- Humility and willingness to engage in speculation
- A valuing of eclecticism
- A belief in the need to be "customer-led"
- Contrariness
- Empathy

BOX 19-3   DRIVING FORCES FOR THE NEXT TWO DECADES

"Driving forces" refer to the evolving realities of the business world. Driving forces occur in both the micro- and macroenvironment. Schwartz (1996) identified the following as the driving forces of the next two decades. Which of these forces do you recognize in today's health care delivery system? Which of these forces could keep the health care system going on as it is and which could influence it to change? What are the implications for these forces for nursing consultation services?

- Shuffling political alignments
- The technology explosion
- Global pragmatism ("whatever works") as a new political ideology
- Demographics—an increasing number of elders and teens; the number and proportion of teens will increase markedly in Asia, Africa, and South America
- Increasingly cautious energy consumption because of efficiency and perceived risk to the environment
- Public concern about the environment
- A global information economy—the possession of information will become the new measure of wealth

Source: Schwartz, P. (1996). *The art of the long view: Planning for the future in an uncertain world.* New York: Currency-Doubleday.

The implications of any identified trend for health care in general, and particularly for nursing consultation opportunities, can be speculated on by using deductive reasoning skills. That is, questions can be asked about how a specific trend is reflected in present patterns of health care delivery and how a trend might drive health care delivery to change. Nurses can use these observations and predictions about emerging patterns of changes in health care delivery to identify the types of problems and issues and consultation opportunities that might arise as a result of these changes. Trends can also give direction about how to package possible problem solutions. These possible problems and solutions can then be used to shape nursing consultation services. Serious futurists systematically keep a journal of their observations and thoughts about the implications of what they are observing.

Building Scenarios

Scenarios are myths about the future or stories about how the world might turn out (Schwartz, 1996). Scenarios can be thought of as alternate packages or combinations of trends. Scenarios help one recognize the reality to which one will need to adapt. Scenarios, thus, can function as tools for "taking the long view in a period of uncertainty" (Schwartz, 1996). For nurses, scenarios, like trends, can be used to identify what health care delivery might look like, what types of problems will most likely need solving, and, consequently, what types of nursing consultation services will be needed. Scenarios can help nurse consultants strategically position themselves and their services for the future.

Scenario building is most productive when a diverse group of people become involved in the envisioning process. Nurse consultants, for example, might want to consider the opinions of nurses, physicians, hospital administrators, patients, educators, legislators, insurance executives, health care consumers, and commuity activists in the development of scenarios. The first step in building a scenario is identifying forces in both the near and more remote environments that would support or hinder the success of a proposed service. These forces are then ranked in terms of their importance and their degree of certainty or uncertainty. The two or three most important driving forces are then put together in various combinations or themes to form a scenario. Themes around which scenarios tend to be built include:

- *Winners and losers*—a scenario of increasingly scarce resources and increasingly aggressive competition
- *Evolution*—a scenario of slow change that allows plenty of time for adaptation
- *Revolution*—a scenario of sudden and dramatic change
- *Challenge and response*—a scenario of serial unpredictable events, each calling for a different response
- *Infinite possibilities*—an optimistic scenario of increased resources
- *The "lone ranger"*—a scenario of the individual (or "little guy") versus the system (Schwartz, 1996)

NURSING CONSULTATION, INTRAPRENEURSHIP, AND ENTREPRENEURSHIP

[Insight is] the ability to look at the same landscape as someone else and see something original. (Popcorn & Marigold, 1996)

Intra- and Entrepreneurial Practice Patterns

Both intrapreneurship and entrepreneurship can provide opportunities for nurses who are risk takers in terms of offering an innovative service and responding to current or anticipated future need gaps in some sort of unique way. An intrapreneur is an "intracorporate entrepreneur" (Brandiet, 1995). That is, a nurse consultant who is an intrapreneur is employed by an organization such as a hospital or community health agency and offers consultation services to both internal and external client systems. Intrapreneurs have the freedom and flexibility to autonomously innovate while being able to take advantage of their employing organization's financial and resource supports and assuming little, if any, personal financial risk. In contrast, nurse consultants who are entrepreneurs are self-employed and assume full responsibility, accountability, and financial risk for the services they offer. An advantage, however, of being an entrepreneur is the opportunity to earn financial rewards that are commensurate with one's efforts and performance.

Nurse consultants who assume intra- and entrepreneurial practice patterns accelerate the evolution of the nursing profession by expanding its scope, territory, and visibility (Hazelton et al., 1993). Nurse consultants in entrepreneurial roles (consider, for example, nurse legal consultants) are often more visible than are nurse intrapreneurs. Intrapreneurial consultation practice, however, can be equally impressive. Malone's (1989) description of how clinical nurse specialists at one hospital established a consulting service is one example of an intrapreneurial practice pattern for nursing consultation. As consultants, the clinical nurse specialists secured internal and external consulting contracts with the hospital's nursing services department, private industries, community agencies, physicians, and a school of nursing. In just three years, the consulting income generated by the clinical nurse specialists reached $450,000. The ability of the clinical nurse specialists to become revenue generators saved their role by offsetting the cost of their salaries to nursing services and the hospital's overall budget.

Applying Trends

Trends can be used to identify and develop potential intra- and entrepreneurial nursing consultation (and other career) opportunities. For example, trends can be used to identify which services are likely to have the most profitable future. These trends can then be used to shape a consultation career. Trends can also be used to identify what visions and fantasies for an entrepreneurial nursing consultation practice are worth incubating as a "spare-time" business until the practice is strong enough to provide full-time income. Trends can be used to provide direction for how to reshape services already being offered so that they continue to be viable and profitable. Finally, nurse consultants can use trends to shape the problem solutions and advice they offer to consultees.

The exercise of "Clickscreen" or "trend discontinuity analysis" (Popcorn & Marigold, 1996) can be used to measure a proposed nursing consultation service against trends. The purpose of this analysis is to determine a proposed service's fit with trends and maximize its likelihood of success. Trend discontinuity analysis essentially serves as a screening device for "go" versus "no go" decisions and should be carried out before going on to the logistics of establishing a service.

One method for carrying out a trend discontinuity analysis is to list identified trends down the left-hand side of a page and then set up columns labeled "Yes," "No," "Maybe," and "Possible change." A proposed nursing consultation service or intervention is then evaluated against each trend. A service's likelihood of success is increased when it is driven by at least one trend and supported by at least three or four others (Popcorn & Marigold, 1996). If the proposed service or intervention is a poor fit with trends, consideration can be given as to how trend-supporting elements can be added (the process of "trend-bending"). In a similar way, existing nursing consultation services can be measured against trends and reshaped ("twisting the familiar") to make them more trend consistent and increase their longevity and success. Box 19-4 illustrates how trend discontinuity analysis (based on the trends identified in Box 19-2) could be used to help a nurse design a consultation practice.

Strategic Planning with Scenarios

Scenarios can also be used for strategically planning nursing consultation services. A proposed service or intervention is tested against a scenario to identify its strengths and vulnerabilities. Of additional interest is how many different scenarios a proposed service fits. Driving forces, inevitabilities, and uncertainties in each scenario are then identified and used to shape a proposed service so that it will be responsive to the widest possible variety of future situations. The process of using scenarios to plan a consulting service is illustrated in Box 19-5.

Making It Work

Trendworthiness and scenario viability are only two of the factors needed for a nursing consultation service to be successful. Careful planning, adequate support, and the right mindset are other factors that will influence the success of a nursing consultation venture. For planning purposes, the AFFIRM model (Rew, 1988) provides the following checklist of factors to consider when developing a consultation service:

BOX 19-4　TREND DISCONTINUITY ANALYSIS: DEVELOPING A CONSULTATION PRACTICE

Proposed Service: A nursing consultation service that specializes in research development, research facilitation, data analysis and interpretation, and packaging research findings for publication and presentation. The target market is health care providers.

Trend	Yes	No	Maybe
99 Lives	X		

Comment: This service could help busy health care providers respond to pressures to discover and disseminate new knowledge.

Anchoring		X	
Being Alive	X		

Comment: This service offers health care providers opportunities to increase understanding and teach others about wellness and health promotion.

Cashing Out		X	

Comment: Health care providers can simplify their lives by turning research responsibilities over to someone else.

Clanning		X	

Comment: Research may offer health care providers an opportunity to network with others who have similar interests.

Cocooning		X	
Down-Aging		X	
Ego-nomics	X		

Comment: Interpreting and presenting research findings is one way of making a personal statement. There is a certain amount of prestige associated with doing research.

Fantasy Adventure		X	

Comment: The adventure of learning new skills and making discoveries?

Femalethink		X	

Comment: Could doing research be one way to promote this agenda?

Icon-Toppling	X		

Comment: The opportunity to discover new knowledge that can "knock-down" old ways of practicing medicine.

Mancipation		X	

Comment: As is the case with Femalethink, research could offer opportunities to promote this agenda.

Pleasure Revenge		X	
Small Indulgences		X	

Comment: Doing "something different" (e.g., research) and having help with it might be perceived as a luxury.

Save Our Society	X		

Comment: Research is a social and professional responsibility.

Vigilante Consumer	X		

Comment: Research is a strategy for informing consumers about safety, values, and quality of health care.

Conclusion: This proposed consultation service stands a good chance of success since it is driven by six trends and supported by six others. "Trend-bending" can be used to further strengthen the service by developing promotion strategies that emphasize consistency of the service with trends that received only a "maybe" rating.

BOX 19-5 USING SCENARIOS TO PLAN A NURSING CONSULTATION SERVICE

Proposed Service

Consultation services that specialize in working with health care providers and health care delivery systems to resolve issues such as poor morale, staff burnout, and communication problems. The service will be based on a philosophy that emphasizes a process consultation interaction pattern.

Relevant Environmental Forces

- Local emphasis on cost containment and "belt-tightening"
- Needs for these services are currently met by out-of-town consultants
- A local hospital and home health care agency are talking about merging their administrative services and nursing staff
- The local nursing programs have experienced decreasing enrollments the past couple of years; this means that there is almost no back-up pool of new potential workers

Scenario 1—Winners and Losers

As competition becomes fiercer among local health care providers, morale problems and burnout are likely to increase. Since there is only a minimal pool of back-up workers, this scenario would support the consultation service.

Scenario 2—Evolution

With a slow, steady change in health care delivery practices, health care workers would have time to adjust to changes on their own. This scenario might not support the proposed consultation service.

Scenario 3—Revolution

In a scenario of sudden and dramatic upheaval, morale and communication problems are likely. However, there might not be enough time to resolve these problems with a process consultation interaction pattern. The proposed service might not be realistic for this scenario.

Scenario 4—Infinite Possibilities

In a scenario of increasing resources, there would be little or no need for the proposed services.

Conclusion

1. The environment needs to be monitored for indicators of each impending scenario.
2. The nurse consultant needs to consider redesigning the proposed services so that they would be responsive to more possible scenarios.

- *Availability:* Are the proposed services already available? If yes, how will these additional services be unique? If no, are the proposed services needed? Are the resources needed to offer the proposed service available? Institutional resources needed in order for an intrapreneurial consultation venture to be successful include strong administrative support for autonomous nursing practice and for generating new sources of revenue (Brandiet, 1995).
- *Formulation:* Exactly what will the proposed service look like? What will it cost? To whom will it be offered and under what circumstances? Where will it be offered?
- *Factual Information:* What information and skills are needed to develop and maintain the consultation service?
- *Referrals:* From whom will the consultation service receive referrals? To whom, in turn, will it refer? Realizing the limitations of one's services and forming strategic alliances and complementary collaborative relationships with others is key to a successful consultation practice.
- *Monitoring:* How will the success of the consultation service as a whole be determined?

Other issues such as setting fees and marketing that are part of planning either an intra- or entrepreneurial nursing consultation practice were discussed in Chapter 17. Nurses who want to establish intrapreneurial nursing consultation services also need to plan how their time will be divided between revenue-generating and non–revenue-generating activities so that nonbillable institutional needs such as providing consultation to nursing staff don't go unmet. As an example of addressing this issue, Malone (1989) described an arrangement in which clinical nurse specialists' time was allocated to nonbillable clinical services (50 percent), building and developing the structure and processes of hospital-based nursing consulta-

tion services (20 percent), external consultation and revenue-generating activities (20 percent), and professional development (10 percent).

Just as identifying trends and their implications takes a certain mindset, so too, does taking advantage of opportunities the future holds for nursing consultation. Skills and attributes needed for success as a nurse consultant were discussed in Chapter 5; however, they are worth repeating here. Nurses planning careers as nurse consultants need characteristics such as flexibility, ingenuity, fast footwork, and the ability to balance multiple agendas (James, 1996). They also need a strong sense of self-worth and a belief that their services are needed and valuable—and they must be able to communicate this sense of worth to others (Brandiet, 1995). Successful intrapreneurial and entrepreneurial nurse consultants have expertise in a prescribed area, excellent interpersonal skills, self-confidence, and the ability to prioritize and organize. They are risk takers who are resourceful and motivate, self-directed, perseverant, perceptive, innovative, and flexible (Schulmeister, 1999).

CLOSING THOUGHTS (SUMMARY)

Hard work, long hours, and perseverance are necessary prerequisites in this undertaking and will help prepare the determined professional to assume the challenge of success, achievement, and life balance. (Mackniesh, 1989)

Incorporating the consultation process into one's practice of nursing provides additional opportunities for responding to both current health care needs and emerging health care delivery issues. Opportunities for independent nurse consultants exist in many areas, including patient advocacy, corporate wellness, child care, elder care, ethics, chronic disease management, and pain management.

Nurses who want to incorporate consultation into their practice can find opportunities in such diverse community settings as schools, correctional facilities, law enforcement agencies, geriatric day care centers, retirement centers, hospices, businesses, and fitness clinics (Schulmeister, 1999). Futurethink—consideration of the implications of health care reform, global ("mega") trends, social trends, possible futures, and driving forces—can be used to identify opportunities for nursing consultation services and shape them to be successful. Careful planning, creativity, and motivation that is based on both a desire for challenge and a desire to fill a void will help to further ensure the success of one's practice of nursing consultation.

APPLYING CHAPTER CONTENT

Consider the following scenarios:

- *Scenario 1:* You are a nurse-manager who has been asked to work with two home health care agencies that are considering a merger. Use trend discontinuity analysis to speculate on the likely success of this merger. Based on this analysis, what advice would you share with these agencies about this proposed merger? Based on a consideration of trends, how would you suggest that they carry out this merger? What specific interventions and strategies would you propose to enhance the success of the merger?
- *Scenario 2:* You are consulting with a group of nurse practitioners who want to establish an independent nurse practitioner clinic. Besides considering the usual economic factors, you do a trend discontinuity analysis to predict the likely success of this clinic. What do you think your findings would show? How could you apply "trend-bending" to this situation? Are there any specific or addi-

tional services you would suggest that the nurse practitioners offer?
- *Scenario 3:* You are a nurse practitioner who is consulting with a family about how to support lifestyle changes needed by the father (age 48) who has just suffered a stroke. How could you use trend discontinuity analysis in this situation? How could "trend-bending" and "twisting the familiar" be used?
- *Scenario 4:* You are a nurse-educator who is providing consultation to a school of nursing that wants to revise their baccalaureate curriculum and develop a master's program. Based on a consideration of possible scenarios and emerging social trends as well as trends in health care, what types of curriculum revisions do you suggest they consider? What types of graduate programs do you recommend that they offer?

References

Barker, J. (1992). *Paradigms: The business of discovering the future.* New York: Harper-Business.

Brandiet, L. (1995). Entrepreneurial and intrapreneurial initiatives. In M. Snyder & M. Mirr (Eds.), *Advanced practice nursing: A guide to professional development* (pp. 271–285). New York: Springer.

Celente, G. (1997). *Trends 2000.* New York: Warner Books.

Frings, C. (1991, October). What it takes to be a successful consultant. *Medical Laboratory Observer*, 47–50.

Hamel, G., & Prahalad, C. (1994). *Competing for the future.* Boston: Harvard Business School Press.

Hazelton, J., Boyum, C., & Frost, M. (1993). Clinical nurse specialist subroles: Foundations for entrepreneurship. *Clinical Nurse Specialist*, 7(1), 40–45.

James, J. (1996). *Thinking in the future tense: Leadership skills for a new age.* New York: Simon & Schuster.

Mackniesh, J. (1989). Issues and concerns of a health promotion consultant. *Occupational Therapy in Health Care, 5*(4), 101–113.

Malone, B. (1989). The CNS in a consultation department. In A. Hamric & J. Spross (Eds.), *The clinical nurse specialist in theory and practice* (2nd ed.) (pp. 397–413). Philadelphia: Saunders.

Naisbitt, J., & Aburdane, J. (1990). *Megatrends 2000: Ten new directions for the 1990s.* New York: Avon Books.

Popcorn, F. (1992). *The Popcorn report.* New York: HarperBusiness.

Popcorn, F., & Marigold, L. (1996). *Clicking: 16 trends to fit your life, your work, and your business.* New York: HarperCollins.

Rew, L. (1988). AFFIRM the role of clinical nurse specialist in private practice. *Clinical Nurse Specialist, 2*(1), 39–43.

Schulmeister, L. (1999). Starting a nursing consultation practice. *Clinical Nurse Specialist, 13*(2), 94–100.

Schwartz, P. (1996). *The art of the long view: Planning for the future in an uncertain world.* New York: Currency-Doubleday.

Page numbers followed by f indicate figure or box. Page numbers followed by t indicate table.